T0204531

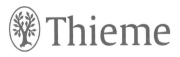

Handbook of Neuroscience Nursing

Care of the Adult Neurosurgical Patient

Denita Ryan, MN, ANP-C, CNRN
Neuroscience Nurse Practitioner
Barrow Neurological Institute
St. Joseph's Hospital and Medical Center
Phoenix, Arizona

Thieme
New York • Stuttgart • Delhi • Rio de Janeiro

Executive Editor: Timothy Y. Hiscock
Managing Editor: Elizabeth Palumbo
Director, Editorial Services: Mary Jo Casey
Editorial Assistant: Keith Palumbo
Production Editor: Sean Woznicki
International Production Director: Andreas Schabert
Editorial Director: Sue Hodgson
International Marketing Director: Fiona Henderson
International Sales Director: Louisa Turrell
Director of Institutional Sales: Adam Bernacki
Senior Vice President and Chief Operating Officer:
   Sarah Vanderbilt
President: Brian D. Scanlan

Library of Congress Cataloging-in-Publication Data
Names: Ryan, Denita, author.
Title: Handbook of neuroscience nursing : care of the
   adult neurosurgical patient / Denita Ryan, MN,
   ANP-C, CNRN, Barrow Neurological Institute,
   St. Joseph's Hospital and Medical Center, Phoenix,
   Arizona. Other titles: Neuroscience nursing
Description: New York : Thieme, [2017]
Identifiers: LCCN 2017006178| ISBN 9781626233782
   (print) | ISBN 9781626233799 (ebook)
Subjects: LCSH: Neurological nursing–Handbooks,
   manuals, etc.
Classification: LCC RC350.5 .R93 2017 | DDC 616.8/
   04231–dc23 LC record available at https://lccn.loc
   .gov/2017006178

© 2019 Thieme Medical Publishers, Inc.

Thieme Publishers New York
333 Seventh Avenue, New York, NY 10001 USA
+1 800 782 3488, customerservice@thieme.com

Thieme Publishers Stuttgart
Rüdigerstrasse 14, 70469 Stuttgart, Germany
+49 [0]711 8931 421, customerservice@thieme.de

Thieme Publishers Delhi
A-12, Second Floor, Sector-2, Noida-201301
Uttar Pradesh, India
+91 120 45 566 00, customerservice@thieme.in

Thieme Publishers Rio de Janeiro, Thieme Publica-
ções Ltda.
Edifício Rodolpho de Paoli, 25º andar
Av. Nilo Peçanha, 50 – Sala 2508
Rio de Janeiro 20020-906 Brasil
+55 21 3172-2297 / +55 21 3172-1896
www.thiemerevinter.com.br

Cover art by Michael Hickman and Cassandra Todd
Typesetting by Thomson Digital, India

Printed in the United States by
King Printing Co., Inc.   5 4 3 2

ISBN 978-1-62623-378-2

Also available as an e-book:
eISBN 978-1-62623-379-9

Important note: Medicine is an ever-changing science undergoing continual development. Research
and clinical experience are continually expanding
our knowledge, in particular our knowledge of proper
treatment and drug therapy. Insofar as this book
mentions any dosage or application, readers may rest
assured that the authors, editors, and publishers have
made every effort to ensure that such references are
in accordance with **the state of knowledge at the
time of production of the book.**

Nevertheless, this does not involve, imply, or
express any guarantee or responsibility on the part
of the publishers in respect to any dosage instructions and forms of applications stated in the book.
Every user is requested to examine carefully the
manufacturers' leaflets accompanying each drug and
to check, if necessary in consultation with a physician
or specialist, whether the dosage schedules men-
tioned therein or the contraindications stated by the
manufacturers differ from the statements made in
the present book. Such examination is particularly
important with drugs that are either rarely used or
have been newly released on the market. Every dosage schedule or every form of application used is
entirely at the user's own risk and responsibility. The
authors and publishers request every user to report
to the publishers any discrepancies or inaccuracies
noticed. If errors in this work are found after publi-
cation, errata will be posted at www.thieme.com on
the product description page.

Some of the product names, patents, and registered
designs referred to in this book are in fact registered
trademarks or proprietary names even though specific reference to this fact is not always made in the
text. Therefore, the appearance of a name without
designation as proprietary is not to be construed as a
representation by the publisher that it is in the public
domain.

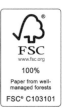

This book is dedicated to the nurses at Barrow Neurological Institute, both past and present, and to the patients we are privileged to serve.

In memory of Carol Johnson Chase, Jeanette Neubeck, and Marilyn Ricci. Friends, colleagues, mentors, and amazing nurses. You are missed.

Contents

Part III Disorders of the Central Nervous System

Part IV Diagnosis and Treatment of Central Nervous System Disorders

Part V Appendices

Video Contents

Foreword

I am honored to write the foreword for this handbook, which is long overdue in the nursing literature. It is an accessible, straightforward reference for nurses who work with patients with neurologic disorders—to carry in their pockets and consult during their busy days. Over the course of my 35-plus years as a neuroscience nurse, I have come to the realization that patients with neurologic disorders are treated not only in specialized neurologic units but also in emergency departments and on general medical floors and obstetrics units. Many of these nurses are called upon to think and act like neuroscience nurses, and I suspect that they will find this handbook to be of use in their daily practice.

To those nurses dedicated to caring for patients with neurologic disorders exclusively, this handbook is a must-have reference. The information in this volume was gleaned from many seasoned neuroscience nurses with decades of combined experience, and readers will learn much from the authors' expertise and insight into caring for this challenging subset of patients.

I am immeasurably proud that my colleague at Barrow Neurological Institute, which sets the bar for excellence in neuroscience nursing, should have produced this volume. Denita Ryan and I have worked together for more than 25 years. Over the course of our professional relationship, I have witnessed Denita's dedication to her ultimate goals: to provide the best possible care for neuroscience patients, and to mentor colleagues to help them achieve the same high level of expertise. Denita's years as a bedside nurse, followed by the past 15 years as a nurse practitioner within neurosurgery, make her uniquely suited to draft, compile, and edit this book.

In Section 1, Denita provides a painstaking overview of the anatomy of the central nervous system (CNS) and offers readers step-by-step instructions on performing a thorough assessment of a patient's neurologic status. Sections 2 and 3 outline common conditions and disorders that affect the CNS, covering everything from neoplasms to developmental disorders. Finally, Section 4 offers a practical description of how disorders of the CNS are diagnosed and describes the host of treatment options available to these patients. This handbook leaves no stone unturned, as its final chapter details a neurologic patient's oft-lengthy road to recovery. Each chapter in this handbook is enriched by a host of figures—diagnostic images, intraoperative photos, and illustrations—that bring concepts to life and offer a clear look at the structures described.

This handbook will undoubtedly set the standard for neuroscience nursing references for years to come. Although it was thoughtfully written for bedside nurses, it will be an indispensable resource in the library of every neuroscience intensive care unit, ward, and reference library for novice and expert nurses alike.

Virginia Prendergast, PhD, NP-C, FAAN, CNRN
Phoenix, AZ

Preface

The idea for this book emanates from my long history in neuroscience nursing. Forty-plus years ago, when I first discovered my love for patients with neurologic disorders, neuroscience nursing textbooks were rare. We had to learn as we went, meeting each new challenge with questions and searching far and wide for more information.

One of my most frustrating early experiences occurred when I was taking care of a patient with a brain tumor. The diagnosis itself did little to tell me what I wanted to know about my patient's condition and the proposed course of treatment. When I approached an oncologist with a request for information on types of brain tumors, treatment, and prognosis, I was given the name of a textbook—a very large oncology textbook. I managed to obtain a copy of that textbook, but I did not open it for months. What I really wanted was more concise information, presented succinctly, perhaps in a table, to make it easier to learn what I needed to know. I knew then that handy, easy-to-use reference materials, such as in a handbook like this one, would be most helpful to the bedside nurse.

The purpose of this book is not to teach the reader all there is to know about neuroscience nursing. Wonderful textbooks exist today to assist anyone wishing to learn more about this challenging field. Instead, the purpose of this book is to help the nurse, or the therapist, or clergy, or anyone else who is taking care of a patient with a neurosurgical disorder to take care of the patient more safely and confidently. The references at the end of each chapter will point the reader to additional resources for more thorough and comprehensive learning.

This handbook is divided into four sections. Section 1 covers anatomy and assessment of the central nervous system. The nurse is shown how to complete a neurologic assessment accurately and thoroughly, how to understand the clinical correlation of physical findings, and how to appropriately document those findings.

Section 2 is devoted to specific conditions associated with neurosurgical patients. These conditions include seizures, hydrocephalus, electrolyte disorders, and, most importantly, the principles of intracranial pressure. As these conditions may be seen in most, if not all, neurosurgical patients, much important information can be gleaned from these chapters.

Section 3 is concerned with neurologic disorders that frequently warrant neurosurgical intervention: tumors, cerebrovascular disorders, trauma, infection, and disorders of the spine and spinal cord. Each chapter discusses and outlines clinical manifestations of each disorder, as well as methods of diagnosis, treatment, and nursing management. Supplemental tables give added information on diagnostic tests, pharmacology, and multiple nursing interventions.

Finally, Section 4 deals with diagnostic tests and treatment of neurosurgical disorders. This section addresses neuroradiology, radiotherapy, surgical procedures such as craniotomy and spinal surgery, and rehabilitation.

The appendixes at the end of the book provide additional helpful information. They include tables of nursing management of multiple neurologic disorders, preoperative checklists, and discharge instructions.

This book is intended for anyone who takes care of adult patients with neurologic disorders that may require neurosurgical intervention. Nurses of all levels of experience will find much of use within its pages. It includes an abundance of helpful information for student nurses as well as for experienced neuroscience nurses. Other health care providers such as therapists, case managers, social workers, and clergy will also find it helpful. The handbook format makes it convenient to use by the provider taking care of the neurosurgical patient.

My sincere hope is that this book will give nurses and other health care providers who are taking care of neurosurgical patients more confidence and an increased ability to provide excellent care. May it also inspire them to continue learning throughout their careers.

Denita Ryan
Phoenix, Arizona

Acknowledgments

This book has come to fruition through the work of many people. Many of my advanced practice colleagues have contributed chapters to this book. They have devoted not only their considerable knowledge and expertise but also their unlimited support to this project. They include Virginia Prendergast, Bryan Lee, Charlotte S. Myers, Donna Wallace, Estelle Doris, Laurie Baker, Michele Grigaitis, Madona Plueger, Maeve Dargush, Manny Mejia, Nancy White, Simon Parkinson, Tammy Tyree, Sara Stephenson, and Risa Maruyama. It is an honor and a privilege to work with this wonderful group of professionals.

I must also thank my physician colleagues who helped with reviewing material and contributed imaging studies from their personal collections. They include Lynn Ashby, Cornelia Drees, Omar Gonzalez, U. Kumar Kakarla, Cameron G. McDougall, Peter Nakaji, Harold Rekate, Nicholas Theodore, Kris A. Smith, Volker K. H. Sonntag, Robert F. Spetzler, Marc Staman, David Treimann, Bill White, Eman Youssef, and Joseph M. Zabramski. I thank them for their patience and generosity with their time.

A special thank you to the great group in Neuroscience Publications at Barrow Neurological Institute for the comprehensive editing, marvelous illustrations, and meticulous coordination of this project. Clare Sonntag and Cassandra Todd deserve special recognition for spearheading the editorial and illustration aspects of this project, respectively. Thanks also to Jaime-Lynn Canales, Marie Clarkson, Mary Ann Clifft, Michael Hickman, Shelley Kick, Gena Lake, Kristen Larson Keil, Marco Marchionni, Joseph Mills, Dawn Mutchler, Lynda Orescanin, Mark Schornak, and Samantha Soto. You all have been more than generous with your time, patience, and expertise.

The many wonderful nurses and therapists at Barrow Neurological Institute inspired this work, and without them the project never would have become a reality. These pioneers in the care of neurologic patients have given much of their time helping review these chapters and making sure that we were on target about what bedside nurses really need and want to know. They include Jan Anderson, Terry Bachman, Cindi Bordson, Sarah Christopher, Jane Fitzgerald-Hines, Jessie Francisco, Amber Green, Tim Hilliard, Cindy Hoffman, Corrie Husack, Jenise Johnson, Kim Jones, Mary King, Rachael Nathan, Erin O'Brien, Lisa Ortiz, Flora Rich, Cindy Sullivan, Amanda Tessier, Heather Thomas, and Sarah Ward.

I would like to add a special thank you to Brandon Brown, who provided many beautiful preliminary illustrations in the initial stages of this project. His help is greatly appreciated.

Thank you to my children, Corry, Kelly, Brandon, and Angie, and to my grandchildren, Carter, Mackenzie, Madelyn, Kendall, and Morgan. Your patience and support for this project made it a little easier for me to spend so much time away from home.

Contributors

Laurie Baker, DNP, RN, ANP-BC
Nurse Practitioner
Barrow Brain and Spine
Barrow Neurological Institute
St. Joseph Hospital and Medical Center
Phoenix, Arizona

Maeve Dargush, MSN, ANP-C
Nurse Practitioner
Program in Women's Oncology
Women and Infants Hospital
Providence, Rhode Island

Estelle Doris, MSN, FNP-C, CNRN
Family Nurse Practitioner
Barrow Neurological Institute
St. Joseph's Hospital and Medical Center
Phoenix, Arizona

Michele Grigaitis, DNP, FNP-BC, CNRN
Advanced Nurse Practitioner
Banner Alzheimer's Institute
University of Arizona Medical Center
Phoenix, Arizona

Bryan Lee, MEd, PA-C
Physician Assistant
Department of Radiation Oncology
St. Joseph's Hospital and Medical Center
Phoenix, Arizona

Manuel F. Mejia, Jr., ACNP-C
Acute Care Nurse Practitioner
Neuroscience Nurse Practitioner Manager
Barrow Neurological Institute
St. Joseph's Hospital and Medical Center
Phoenix, Arizona

Risa Maruyama, PT, MPT, NCS
Acute Care Therapy Manager
St. Joseph's Hospital and Medical Center
Phoenix, Arizona

Charlotte S. Myers, MS, ANP-C, CNRN
Nurse Practitioner
Barrow Neurological Institute
St. Joseph's Hospital and Medical Center
Phoenix, Arizona

Simon Parkinson, MSN, FNP-C, CNRN
Nurse Practitioner
Brain and Spine Center
Chandler, Arizona

Madona Plueger ACNS-BC, APRN, CNRN
Adult Health Clinical Nurse Specialist
Neuroscience Nursing
Barrow Neurological Institute
St. Joseph's Hospital and Medical Center
Phoenix, Arizona

Denita Ryan, MN, ANP-C, CNRN
Neuroscience Nurse Practitioner
Barrow Neurological Institute
St. Joseph's Hospital and Medical Center
Phoenix, Arizona

Sara Stephenson, OTD, OTR/L, BCPR
Occupational Therapist
St. Joseph's Hospital and Medical Center
Phoenix, Arizona

Tammy Tyree, ACNP-C, CCRN, CNRN, RFNA
Neurosurgery Nurse Practitioner
Barrow Neurological Institute
St. Joseph's Hospital and Medical Center
Phoenix, Arizona

Donna Wallace, RN, MS, PNP-C
Nurse Practitioner
Barrow Neurological Institute
St. Joseph's Hospital and Medical Center
Phoenix, Arizona

Nancy White, NP-C, CRNFA, CNOR, CNRN
Nurse Practitioner
Barrow Neurological Institute
St. Joseph's Hospital and Medical Center
Phoenix, Arizona

Joseph M. Zabramski, MD
Professor
Neurological Surgery
Barrow Neurological Institute
St. Joseph's Hospital and Medical Center
Phoenix, Arizona

Abbreviations

3D-CRT:	three-dimensional conformal radiotherapy	GCSE:	generalized convulsive status epilepticus
AANN:	American Association of Neuro-science Nurses	GTR:	gross total resection
		Gy:	gray
ABG:	arterial blood gas	ICH:	intracerebral hemorrhage
ADH:	antidiuretic hormone	ICP:	intracranial pressure
ADLs:	activities of daily living	ICU:	intensive care unit
AED:	antiepileptic drug	IMRT:	intensity-modulated radiotherapy
ANS:	autonomic nervous system		
AVF:	arteriovenous fistula	INR:	international normalized ratio
AVM:	arteriovenous malformation	IPH:	intraparenchymal hematoma
CBC:	compete blood count	IV:	intravenous
CBF:	cerebral blood flow	LOC:	level of consciousness
CJD:	Creutzfeldt-Jakob disease	LP:	lumbar puncture
CN:	cranial nerve	LPS:	lumboperitoneal shunt
CNS:	central nervous system	LSO:	lumbosacral orthosis
CPP:	cerebral perfusion pressure	MRA:	magnetic resonance angiography
CRP:	C-reactive protein		
CSF:	cerebrospinal fluid	MRI:	magnetic resonance imaging
CSI:	craniospinal irradiation	NCSE:	nonconvulsive status epilepticus
CT:	computed tomography	NF1:	neurofibromatosis 1
CTA:	computed tomography angiography	NPH:	normal pressure hydrocephalus
		NPO:	nil per os
DAVF:	dural arteriovenous fistula	NSAID:	nonsteroidal anti-inflammatory drug
DDD:	degenerative disk disease		
DI:	diabetes insipidus	OT:	occupational therapy
DSA:	digital subtraction angiography	PACU:	postanesthesia care unit
DVT:	deep vein thrombosis	PNS:	peripheral nervous system
EBRT:	external beam radiotherapy	POD:	postoperative day
ECG:	electrocardiogram	PT:	prothrombin time
EDH:	epidural hematoma	PTC:	pseudotumor cerebri
EEG:	electroencephalogram	PTT:	partial thromboplastin time
EMU:	epilepsy monitoring unit	QOL:	quality of life
EOMs:	extraocular movements	RA:	rheumatoid arthritis
ESR:	erythrocyte sedimentation rate	ROM:	range of motion
ETV:	endoscopic third ventriculostomy	SAH:	subarachnoid hemorrhage
		SCI:	spinal cord injury
EVD:	external ventricular drain	SDH:	subdural hematoma
FDA:	U.S. Food and Drug Administration	SIADH:	syndrome of inappropriate antidiuretic hormone
GBM:	glioblastoma multiforme	SLP:	speech and language pathology
GCS:	Glasgow Coma Scale	SRS:	stereotactic radiosurgery

STA-MCA:	superficial temporal artery–middle cerebral artery	TLSO:	thoracic lumbosacral orthosis
		tPA:	tissue plasminogen activator
SUDEP:	sudden unexpected death in epilepsy	UTI:	urinary tract infection
		VAS:	ventriculoatrial shunt
TBI:	traumatic brain injury	VPS:	ventriculoperitoneal shunt
TCD:	transcranial Doppler	WBI:	whole brain irradiation
TIA:	transient ischemic attack	WHO:	World Health Organization

Part I

Anatomy and Assessment of the Nervous System

I

1 Anatomy

Denita Ryan

Abstract

Knowledge of the anatomy of the nervous system is crucial for nurses caring for patients with neurologic diseases or disorders because they must thoroughly understand the normal neuroanatomy to make meaningful correlations between anatomical and clinical findings. The nervous system consists of the central nervous system and the peripheral nervous system. This overview of the normal neuroanatomy includes basic surface structure, the ventricular system, and the vasculature of both the brain and the spine.

Keywords: autonomic nervous system, brain, cranial nerves, peripheral nervous system, spinal cord, vertebrae

1.1 Nervous System

The nervous system, widely thought to be the most complicated system in the human body, is divided into two parts: the central nervous system (CNS) and the peripheral nervous system (PNS) (Box 1.1 Components of the Nervous System). Nurses caring for patients with neurologic diseases or disorders must possess a thorough knowledge of normal neuroanatomy, including the cranial nerves (CN), so that they can recognize anatomical abnormalities. This knowledge will allow nurses to make meaningful correlations between anatomical and clinical findings.

Box 1.1 Components of the Nervous System

- Central nervous system
  - Brain
  - Spinal cord
- Peripheral nervous system
  - Spinal nerves
  - Cranial nerves
  - Autonomic nervous system
    - Sympathetic nervous system
    - Parasympathetic nervous system

1.1.1 Cellular Anatomy

The nervous system comprises two fundamental cell types: neurons
(▶ Fig. 1.1) and neuroglial cells (▶ Fig. 1.2).

Neurons

- Fundamental building blocks
- Highly specialized
- Conduct and receive nerve impulses, as well as release chemical
  transmitters
  - Soma: Cell body of the neuron
  - Dendrites: Receive impulses
  - Axons: Carry impulses away from the cell

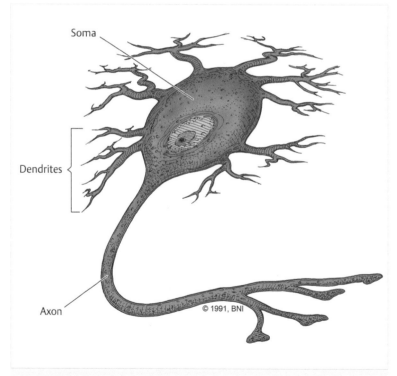

Fig. 1.1 Neuron.

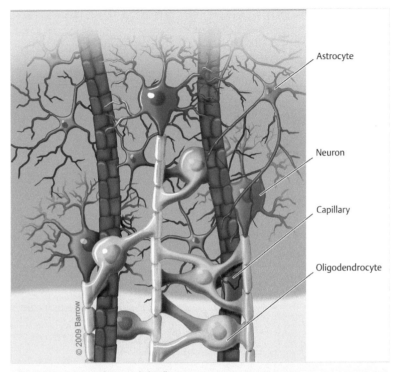

Fig. 1.2 Neurons and neuroglial cells.

- Myelin sheath (Box 1.2 Clinical Correlation: Demyelinating Disease)
  - Formed by Schwann's cells
  - Composed of a lipid substance
  - Provides insulation for nerve impulses
- Synapse
  - The junction between neurons, in which impulses are transmitted
- Neurotransmitters
  - Chemical substances that promote, inhibit, or alter cellular response
  - Over 100 neurotransmitters have been identified, including
    - Amines (e.g., acetylcholine and serotonin)
    - Catecholamines (e.g., dopamine and norepinephrine)

Box 1.2 Clinical Correlation: Demyelinating Disease

- Multiple sclerosis is an example of a demyelinating disease
- In demyelination, the protective Schwann's cells lose their myelin sheaths, making them less effective in shielding the nerves

Neuroglial Cells

- Specialized support cells. They include
  - Astrocytes: Supply nutrients to the brain
  - Ependymal cells: Line the ventricles and help produce cerebrospinal fluid (CSF)
  - Oligodendrocytes: Form protective myelin sheath around the axons
  - Microglial cells: Scavengers; associated with immune response
  - Schwann's cells: Form the myelin sheath around the peripheral nerves

1.2 Central Nervous System

The CNS includes the brain and spinal cord (Video 1.1). Of all the systems in the body, the CNS has the largest number of axons and synapses. The brain alone consists of approximately 100 billion cells. The brain is encased and protected by the skull. In turn, the skull is covered and cushioned by the scalp, which consists of multiple layers. Both the scalp and the skull protect the brain.

1.2.1 Scalp

The scalp consists of several layers that cover the skull.
- Skin (dermal) layer
  - Protects the skull
  - Contains hair
- Subcutaneous layer
  - Vascular; may bleed profusely
- Galea
  - Tough innermost layer
  - Subgaleal space: Potential location for blood to collect, commonly called a *goose egg*
- Periosteum
  - Thin layer of connective tissue that covers the skull

1.2.2 Skull

The skull (▶ Fig. 1.3) is composed of eight fused bone plates.

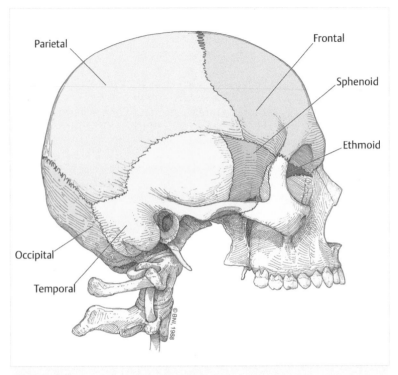

Fig. 1.3 Skull.

Cranial Bones (*n* = 8)

- Frontal
- Temporal (*n* = 2); thinnest portion of bone
- Parietal (*n* = 2)
- Occipital
- Sphenoid
- Ethmoid

Fourteen facial bones form the anterior portion of the skull.

Other Important Bone Segments

- Clivus: The thin bone that rests against the brainstem
- Sella turcica: Houses the pituitary gland, which is not considered part of the brain

1.2.3 Brain

The brain (Box 1.3 Just the Facts: The Brain), largely recognized as the most complex organ in the human body, has a complicated anatomy. Sulci (singular, sulcus) are small separations between brain tissue. Gyri (singular, gyrus) are folds (i.e., wrinkles) on the surface of the brain. The purpose of the sulci and gyri is to increase the surface area of the brain.

Fissures are deep separations between the cerebral hemispheres (or lobes) of the brain, commonly used as geographical markers. The best-known fissures are as follows:
- Great longitudinal fissure
- Lateral fissure of Sylvius
- Central fissure of Rolando
- Parieto-occipital fissure

Box 1.3 Just the Facts: The Brain

- The adult brain weighs about 3 lb
- Brain tissue is also called parenchyma
- The brain is composed of 78% water, 10% fat, 8% protein, and 4% organic and inorganic substances
- The brain makes up only about 2% of the body's total weight, but it uses about 20% of its oxygen supply and 20% of its blood flow
- The brain consists of 40% gray matter and 60% white matter
- The adult brain has the consistency of thickened JELL-O

Meninges

The meninges (▶ Fig. 1.4) are the three layers of thick connective tissue that cover the entire brain and spinal cord.
- Pia mater
  - Delicate innermost layer
  - Adheres to the brain
- Arachnoid mater
  - Situated above the pia mater
  - Space below the arachnoid is called the *subarachnoid space* (Box 1.4 Clinical Correlation: Subarachnoid Hemorrhage)
  - Contains CSF
- Dura mater
  - Latin for "tough mother"
  - Tough, fibrous layer between the arachnoid mater and the skull bone

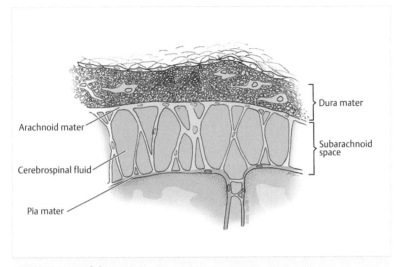

Fig. 1.4 Layers of the meninges.

- Spaces above (epidural) and below (subdural) the dura are typical locations for dural hematomas, a common type of brain injury (Box 1.5 Clinical Correlation: Dural Hematomas)
  - The tentorium, a tent-like fold of dura that separates the cerebrum and cerebellum, serves as an important anatomical marker

Box 1.4 Clinical Correlation: Subarachnoid Hemorrhage

- Defined as bleeding into the space below the arachnoid layer
- Common causes of subarachnoid hemorrhage are trauma and aneurysmal rupture

Box 1.5 Clinical Correlation: Epidural and Subdural Hematomas

- The main cause of cerebral and spinal hematomas is trauma
- This common traumatic brain injury involves bleeding into the space above or below the dura
  - Epidural hematoma: Bleeding above the dura
  - Subdural hematoma: Bleeding below the dura
- May result from surgery or rapid decompression of ventricles

Ventricular System

The ventricular system produces and circulates CSF (Box 1.6 Cerebrospinal Fluid). It includes four cavities (i.e., ventricles) that contain CSF and the transport system that circulates CSF throughout the brain and spinal cord (Box 1.7 Clinical Correlation: Disorders of the Ventricular System). The components of the ventricular system are

- Ventricles
  - Situated in the center of the brain
  - The four ventricles include the right and left lateral ventricles, the third ventricle, and the fourth ventricle (▶ Fig. 1.5. and ▶ Fig. 1.6)
  - Communicate with other ventricles
  - Composed of ependymal cells
- Choroid plexus
  - Refers to the group of blood vessels in each ventricle
  - Produces CSF (approximately 22 mL/h)

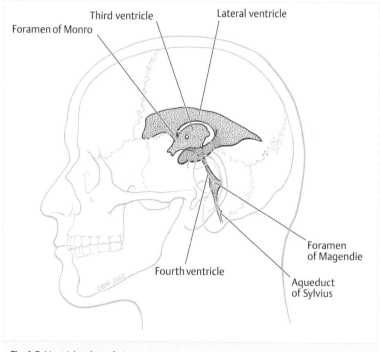

Fig. 1.5 Ventricles, lateral view.

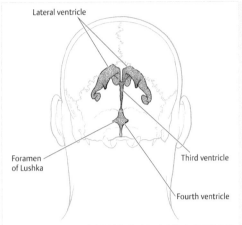

Fig. 1.6 Ventricles, posterior view.

- Cisterns
  - CSF reservoirs
- Foramina of Monro
  - Connect the lateral ventricles with the third ventricle
  - Also called the interventricular foramina
- Cerebral aqueduct of Sylvius
  - Passageway from the third to fourth ventricle
  - Also called the sylvian aqueduct
- Foramen of Magendie and foramen of Luschka
  - Openings from the fourth ventricle into the subarachnoid space
- Arachnoid villi
  - Reabsorb CSF into blood
  - Transport CSF to dural sinus

Box 1.6 Cerebrospinal Fluid

- Produced by the choroid plexus
- Circulates through the ventricular system and in the subarachnoid space
- Cushions the brain and spinal cord
- Produced at a rate of 500 mL/day
- The body contains about 150 mL of CSF at any one time
- Absorbed by the arachnoid granules
- Intracranial pressure is commonly measured in the ventricular CSF

Cerebrum

The cerebrum consists of two cerebral hemispheres, right and left.
• Separated by the great longitudinal fissure
• Surface of the brain is covered by gray matter, which is composed of millions of neurons
• Deeper brain tissue contains white matter, which is composed of millions of highly specialized neuroglial cells
• Pathways carrying information to the cerebral hemispheres cross over from one hemisphere to the other (Box 1.8 Clinical Concern)

The hemispheres are further divided into two parts.
• Supratentorial (above the tentorium)
• Infratentorial (below the tentorium)

Supratentorial Region

The supratentorial area of the brain consists of the frontal, parietal, temporal, and occipital lobes (▶ Fig. 1.7) and the corpus callosum.
• The frontal lobe controls
  ○ Emotions and behavior
  ○ Attention
  ○ Motivation
  ○ Judgment
  ○ Broca's area: Motor aspect of speech (i.e., expressive speech)
  ○ Initiation of motor integration

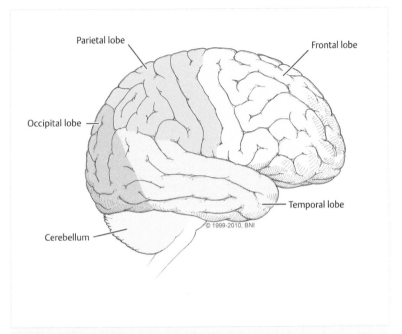

Fig. 1.7 Lobes of the brain.

- ○ Problem-solving
- ○ Bowel and bladder function
- The parietal lobe controls
  - ○ Interpretation of characteristics of sensory input (e.g., pain, temperature, and touch)
  - ○ Processing of visual–spatial information (nondominant hemisphere)
  - ○ Praxis (dominant hemisphere)
- The temporal lobe controls
  - ○ Hearing
  - ○ Wernicke's area: Interpretation of language (i.e., receptive speech)
  - ○ Memory
  - ○ Musical awareness
  - ○ Sequencing
- The occipital lobe controls
  - ○ Visual perception
  - ○ Interpretation of the written word
- The corpus callosum is a thick band of nerve fibers running longitudinally that connects the hemispheres

Diencephalon

Located in the posterior portion of the forebrain, the diencephalon (▶ Fig. 1.8) contains several important structures, primarily the thalamus and the hypothalamus that form the floor of the third ventricle.

Thalamus

- Sensory relay system
- Integrative center that connects various areas of the brain
- Pain awareness

Hypothalamus

- Deep structure forming the wall of the third ventricle
- Regulates basic instincts such as hunger, thirst, sex drive, anger, and aggression (part of limbic system)
- Controls secretion of pituitary hormones
- Autonomic nervous system (ANS) center (sympathetic), which regulates
  ○ Body temperature
  ○ Water metabolism (antidiuretic hormone)
  ○ Sleep cycles; see also section on ANS in this chapter

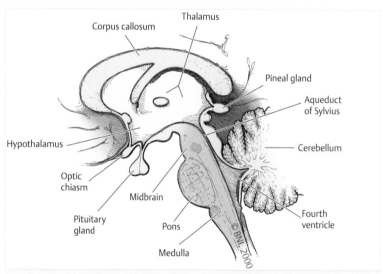

Fig. 1.8 Diencephalon (consisting primarily of the thalamus and hypothalamus), brainstem (consisting of medulla, pons, and midbrain), and cerebellum.

Internal Capsule

The internal capsule is a large bundle of nerve fibers, both motor and sensory, that connect the various areas of the brain and spinal cord.

- Composed of white matter
- Anatomically critical; controls major motor and sensory functions
- Occupies a very small area of the brain

Pituitary Gland (Hypophysis)

- Endocrine gland (▶ Table 1.1) located in the sella turcica, at the base of the brain
- Connected to the hypothalamus

Basal Ganglia

The basal ganglia (▶ Fig. 1.9) are located deep within the cerebrum (Box 1.9 Clinical Correlation: Disorders of the Basal Ganglia). They control fine motor function, particularly in the hands and arms. The basal ganglia consist of several subcortical nuclei.

Table 1.1 Pituitary gland function

Lobe of pituitary gland	Hormone secreted	Implications of hormone deficiency
Anterior	Adrenocorticotropic hormone	Cushing's syndrome
		Adrenal hyperplasia
	Growth hormone	Acromegaly
	Thyrotropin	Thyrotoxicosis (rare)
	Prolactin	Galactorrhea
		Amenorrhea
		Infertility
	Follicle-stimulating hormone	Usually does not produce clinical symptoms
	Luteinizing hormone	Usually does not produce clinical symptoms
Posterior	Vasopressin or antidiuretic hormone	Controls rate of water secretion into urine
		Implicated in diabetes insipidus and SIADH
	Oxytocin	Uterine contraction

Abbreviation: SIADH, syndrome of inappropriate antidiuretic hormone.

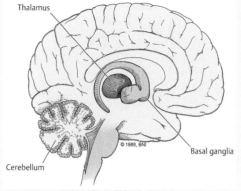

Thalamus

Cerebellum

Basal ganglia

© 1988, BNI

Fig. 1.9 Thalamus and basal ganglia.

- Lenticular nuclei
  - Globus pallidus (regulates voluntary movement)
  - Substantia nigra (stores dopamine)
  - Putamen (affects learning and helps regulate voluntary movement)
- Caudate nucleus
- Amygdala

Box 1.9 Clinical Correlation: Disorders of the Basal Ganglia

- Parkinson's disease
- Athetosis
- Hemiballismus
- Huntington's chorea

Infratentorial Region

Brainstem

The brainstem is a very small area of the brain that contains extremely eloquent brain tissue. The brainstem is composed of

- Midbrain
  - Origin of oculomotor and trochlear nerves (cranial nerve [CN] III and CN IV)
- Pons
  - Origin of trigeminal, abducens, facial, and vestibulocochlear nerves (CNs V-VIII)
  - Located between the midbrain and medulla

- Medulla
  - Located below the pons and above the spinal cord
  - Origin of CN glossopharyngeal, vagus, spinal accessory, and hypoglossal nerves (CNs IX-XII)
  - Includes the cardiac and respiratory centers, as well as the ANS, which regulate
    - Heart rate
    - Blood pressure
    - Respiration

Cerebellum

The cerebellum, located in the posterior fossa and attached to the brainstem, influences the following:
- Coordination and fine motor movement
- Balance and equilibrium
- Tone and posture
- Eye movement (ocular disorders such as nystagmus may result from damage to the cerebellum) (Box 1.10 Clinical Correlation: Disorders of the Cerebellum)

Box 1.10 Clinical Correlation: Disorders of the Cerebellum

- Ataxia
- Nystagmus
- Tremors (intention)

Specific Systems in the Brain

Reticular Activating System

- Diffuse system within the deep structures of the brain
- Extends from the cerebral cortex to the brainstem
- Controls sleep–wake cycles
- Regulates consciousness

Limbic System

- Complex system that includes
  - Hypothalamus
  - Hippocampus
  - Amygdala

- Regulates primitive emotions and instincts
  - Behavior and emotions (e.g., fear and anger)
  - Sex drive
  - Short-term memory
  - Self-preservation (e.g., hunger and sleep)

Vasculature of the Brain

Arterial System

Circle of Willis

- Located at the base of the brain (▶ Fig. 1.10)
- Consists of anterior (carotid) and posterior (vertebrobasilar) components
- Connects the anterior and posterior circulations
  - Anterior component
    - Middle cerebral arteries ($n = 2$)
    - Anterior cerebral arteries ($n = 2$)
    - Anterior communicating artery
  - Posterior component
    - Posterior communicating arteries ($n = 2$)
    - Posterior cerebral arteries ($n = 2$)

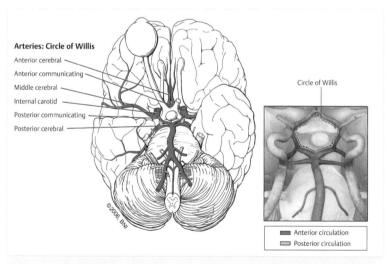

Fig. 1.10 Circle of Willis.

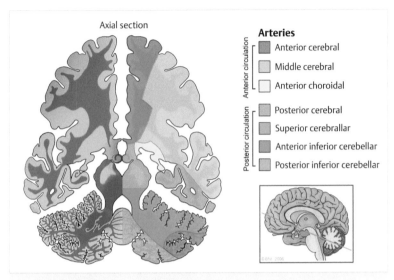

Fig. 1.11 Blood supply to cerebrum and cerebellum.

Anterior Circulation

The anterior circulation supplies the cerebrum anterior to the posterior edge of the temporal lobe (▶ Fig. 1.11). It includes arteries originating from the carotid arteries.

- Internal carotid arteries
- Middle cerebral arteries
- Anterior communicating artery
- Anterior cerebral arteries
- Posterior communicating artery

Posterior Circulation

The posterior arterial circulation supplies the inferior portion of the temporal lobe, the brainstem, the cerebellum, and the spinal cord (Box 1.11 Clinical Correlation: Disorders of the Cerebrovascular System). It consists of arteries arising from the subclavian artery.

- Vertebral arteries
- Basilar artery
- Posterior cerebral arteries
- Superior cerebellar arteries
- Anterior inferior cerebellar arteries
- Posterior inferior cerebellar arteries

> ## Box 1.11 Clinical Correlation: Disorders of the Cerebrovascular System
>
> - Aneurysms
> - Arteriovenous malformations
> - Atherosclerosis
> - Arteritis
> - Hemorrhagic stroke
> - Ischemic stroke
> - Moyamoya disease
> - Stenosis

Venous System

The venous circulation courses primarily through the dural sinuses.
- Cavernous sinus
  - Includes oculomotor, trochlear, trigeminal, and abducens nerves (CN III–VI)
  - Internal carotid arteries pass through the cavernous sinus
  - Collects blood from the inferior surface of the brain, including orbits
- Superior sagittal sinus
  - Collects blood from the cortical veins on the convexity of the brain
  - Drains CSF
- Bridging veins
  - Connect the brain and the dural sinuses
  - Common location of subdural hemorrhage

1.2.4 Spine

- Consists of multiple bony structures called *vertebrae* (▶ Fig. 1.12)
- Vertebrae are stacked on top of each other, providing support for the head and the body
- The 33 vertebrae make up the 5 areas of the spine
  - Cervical ($n = 7$)
  - Thoracic ($n = 12$)
  - Lumbar ($n = 5$)
  - Sacrum ($n = 5$, fused into 1 segment)
  - Coccyx ($n = 4$, fused into 1 segment)

Anatomy and Sections of Individual Vertebra

Body

- Anterior portion of the vertebra
- Largest portion of the vertebra

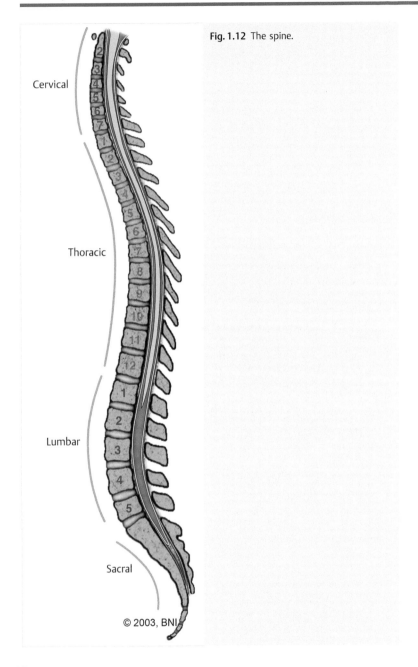

Fig. 1.12 The spine.

© 2003, BNI

Arch

- Posterior portion of the vertebra
- Each arch consists of
  - Pedicles
  - Lamina
  - Spinous and transverse processes
  - Articulating surfaces or facets

Articulation

- Vertical alignment of the vertebral bodies, with the disk in between and the facets on either side

Cervical Vertebrae

- Topmost vertebrae ($n = 7$) (▶ Fig. 1.13)
- Smallest vertebrae
- The first cervical vertebra (C1) is called the atlas
- The second cervical vertebra (C2) is called the axis
  - C2 contains the odontoid process, on which the atlas rests

Thoracic Vertebrae

- Trunk-level vertebrae ($n = 12$) (▶ Fig. 1.14)
- Slender part of the spinal cord

Lumbar Vertebrae

- Low-back vertebrae ($n = 5$) (▶ Fig. 1.15)
- Largest vertebrae
- End at conus medullaris (i.e., the cone-shaped end of the spinal cord)

Sacral Vertebrae and Coccyx

- Bottommost vertebrae ($n = 5$)
- Include the conus medullaris

Supportive and Protective Structures

Ligaments

- Control spine movements
- Best-known spinal ligaments
  - Anterior longitudinal ligament
  - Posterior longitudinal ligament
  - Ligamenta flava

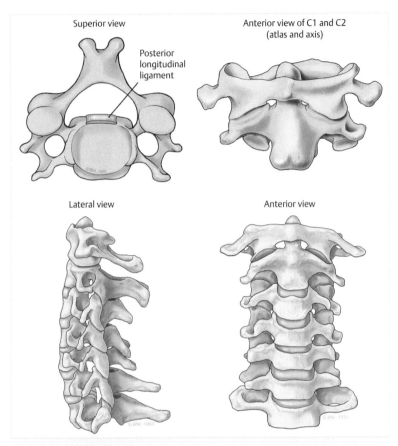

Fig. 1.13 Cervical vertebrae.

Meninges

- Membranes that cover the spinal cord and the brain

Intervertebral Disks

- Cartilaginous cushions between vertebrae; center of disk is nucleus pulposus (Box 1.12 Clinical Correlation: Herniated Disk)
- Differ in size and shape, depending on the size of vertebrae
- Serve to cushion and absorb movement and stress

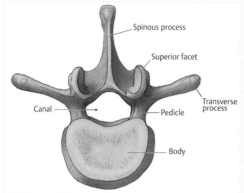

Fig. 1.14 Thoracic vertebrae.

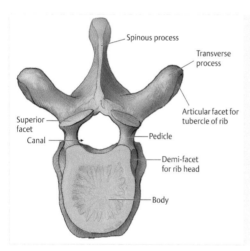

Fig. 1.15 Lumbar vertebrae.

Box 1.12 Clinical Correlation: Herniated Disk

- The nucleus pulposus loses moisture and becomes dry (i.e., desiccates) with age or trauma
- Herniated nucleus pulposus is a common spine disorder; see also Chapter 11, Spine Disorders

Spinal Cord

- Elongated mass of nerve tissue
- Extends from C1 to L1 or L2 in adults
- Terminates at the conus medullaris, around L1
- Serves as the primary pathway between the peripheral (nonvisceral) areas of the body and the brain
- Segmented by region and groups of nerves, and numbered by level of vertebral column
- Covered by meninges and cushioned by CSF, which fills the central canal of the spinal cord and the space between the spinal cord and the meninges
- A cross-section of the spinal cord reveals a butterfly- or **H**-shaped central area of gray matter (dorsal and ventral horns) surrounded by white matter (myelinated axons)
- Protected by the vertebrae

Spinal Nerves

- Part of the PNS; see also section on PNS in this chapter
- Exit the spinal cord in bilateral pairs

Sensory Pathways

- Afferent (i.e., ascending) pathways carry sensory information from specific areas of the body (i.e., dermatomes) to the sensory cortex in the brain
- These sensations travel along one of the two major pathways
  - The dorsal column: Pain and temperature sensations travel via the dorsal column to the medulla, where they cross to the opposite side and enter the thalamus (▶ Fig. 1.16)
  - The ganglia: Touch, pressure, and vibration sensations travel via the ganglia to the medulla, where they cross to the opposite side and enter the thalamus
- The thalamus is the relay station that transmits all impulses to the sensory cortex for interpretation

Motor Pathways

- Ventral, efferent, and descending motor pathways transmit motor impulses from the brain to specific muscles
- These pathways originate in the motor cortex of the frontal lobe of the brain
- Voluntary motor activity is regulated by the interaction between the pyramidal and extrapyramidal systems
  - Pyramidal: Responsible for fine motor movement (▶ Fig. 1.17)
  - Extrapyramidal: Responsible for gross motor movement
- Motor impulses cross at the medulla to the opposite side and progress along descending pathways, affecting contralateral motor function

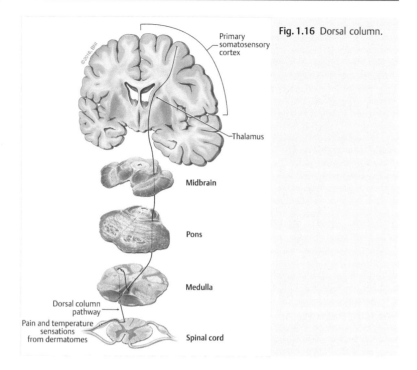

Primary somatosensory cortex

Thalamus

Midbrain

Pons

Medulla

Dorsal column pathway

Pain and temperature sensations from dermatomes

Spinal cord

Fig. 1.16 Dorsal column.

Vasculature of the Spine

Arterial System

The vertebral arteries first supply the upper cervical spinal cord and then supply the anterior ($n = 1$) and posterior ($n = 2$) spinal arteries. All three arteries run along the length of the spinal cord.

- The radicular and radiculospinal arteries also contribute blood to various nerve roots
- The artery of Adamkiewicz, which originates from the aorta, supplies about one-third of the superior portion of the spinal cord

Venous System

- Intradural system: Consistent with arterial pathways
- Extradural system: Empties into the vena cava

1.3 Peripheral Nervous System

The PNS connects the CNS with the motor and sensory structures.

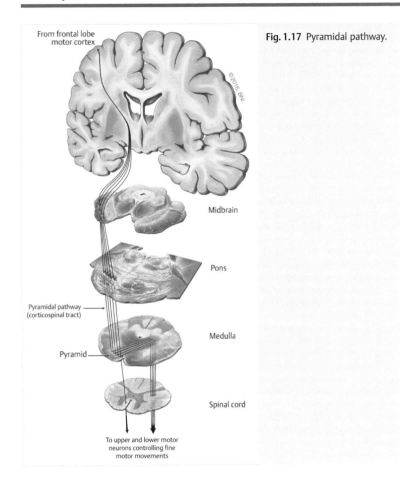

Fig. 1.17 Pyramidal pathway.

From frontal lobe motor cortex

©2016 BNI

Midbrain

Pons

Pyramidal pathway (corticospinal tract)

Medulla

Pyramid

Spinal cord

To upper and lower motor neurons controlling fine motor movements

1.3.1 Spinal Nerves

- Bilateral pairs ($n = 31$)
  - Cervical ($n = 8$)
  - Thoracic ($n = 12$)
  - Lumbar ($n = 5$)
  - Sacral ($n = 5$)
  - Coccygeal ($n = 1$)
- Transmit sensory stimuli from receptors in skin, muscles, viscera, and sensory organs to the dorsal column of the spinal cord

Cauda Equina

- Means "horse's tail" in Latin
- Collective term for nerve root cluster at inferior edge of spinal cord

1.3.2 Cranial Nerves

- Exist in pairs ($n = 12$) (▶ Table 1.2)
- Transmit the motor and sensory impulses
- Originate in the brainstem, except for the olfactory (CN I) and optic (CN II) nerves (▶ Fig. 1.18)

Table 1.2 Origin and function of cranial nerves

Cranial nerve	Origin	Function
Olfactory (CN I)	Olfactory tract	Smell
Optic (CN II)	Retina	Vision
Oculomotor (CN III)	Midbrain	Eye movement (medial, superior, and inferior)
		Pupil constriction
		Elevation of eyelids
Trochlear (CN IV)	Midbrain	Eye movement (downward and inward)
Trigeminal (CN V)	Pons	Corneal reflex
		Facial sensation
		Chewing
Abducens (CN VI)	Pons	Eye movement (lateral)
Facial (CN VII)	Pons	Elevation of forehead (wrinkling forehead and raising eyebrows)
		Eye closure
		Taste
Vestibulocochlear (CN VIII)	Pons	Hearing
Glossopharyngeal (CN IX)	Medulla	Swallowing
		Taste
Vagus (CN X)	Medulla	Swallowing
		Gag reflex
		Visceral sensations (peristalsis and heart rate)
Spinal accessory (CN XI)	Medulla	Shoulder shrug
Hypoglossal (CN XII)	Medulla	Tongue protrusion

Abbreviation: CN, cranial nerve.

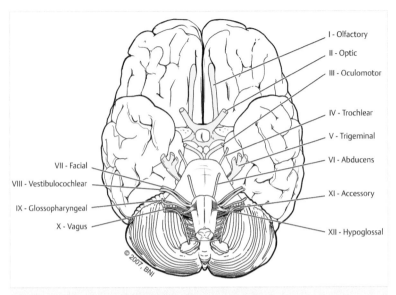

Fig. 1.18 Origin of cranial nerves.

I - Olfactory
II - Optic
III - Oculomotor
IV - Trochlear
V - Trigeminal
VI - Abducens
XI - Accessory
XII - Hypoglossal
VII - Facial
VIII - Vestibulocochlear
IX - Glossopharyngeal
X - Vagus
© 2007, BNI

1.3.3 Autonomic Nervous System

The ANS contains neurons that can detect changes in, and maintain control of, the viscera (i.e., internal organs). Its purpose is to provide a stable internal environment within the body. The ANS is further divided into the sympathetic and parasympathetic nervous systems. Awareness of the ANS and its role is essential when caring for patients with spinal cord injuries.

Sympathetic Nervous System

• Acts globally to activate body responses in fight-or-flight situations

Parasympathetic Nervous System

• Acts focally to activate basic instincts, such as hunger and sex drive
 (► Table 1.3)

1.4 Anatomy of the Nervous System

An in-depth understanding of neuroanatomy is critical for nurses who care for patients with neurologic disorders. In fact, the rest of the information in this

Table 1.3 Sympathetic and parasympathetic responses to stimulus

Structure	Sympathetic response	Parasympathetic response
Eyes	Pupil dilation	Pupil constriction
Heart	Increased heart rate	Decreased heart rate
Lungs	Bronchodilation	Bronchoconstriction
Digestive tract	Decreased peristalsis	Increased peristalsis
Salivary glands	Decreased secretion	Increased secretion
Urinary system	Decreased urine production	Contracted bladder
		Increased urine production

handbook builds on the information provided in this chapter. Although the basics of neuroanatomical structures and components have been briefly described here, this chapter is intended to serve as a handy, basic reference for the bedside care of patients with neurologic disorders. The references below may offer additional information, and the reader is encouraged to refer to them to learn more about this challenging, awe-inspiring topic.

Video

Video 1.1 The brain and spinal cord.

Suggested Readings

[1] Goldberg S, Ouellette H. Clinical Anatomy Made Ridiculously Simple. Miami, FL: MedMaster; 2016

[2] Grigaitis M. Nursing assessment of patients with neurological disorders. In: Osborn KS, Wraa CE, Watson A, eds. Medical Surgical Nursing: Preparation for Practice. 2nd ed. Boston, MA: Pearson; 2013

[3] Hansen JT. Netter's Clinical Anatomy. 3rd ed. Philadelphia, PA: Elsevier Saunders; 2014

[4] Hickey J. Clinical Practice of Neurological and Neurosurgical Nursing. 7th ed. Philadelphia, PA: Wolters Kluwer Health; 2013

[5] Iannotti JP, Parker R. The Netter Collection of Medical Illustrations: Musculoskeletal System, Volume 6, Part II—Spine and Lower Limb. 2nd ed. Philadelphia, PA: Elsevier Saunders; 2013

[6] McIlwain H, Bachelard HS. Biochemistry and the Central Nervous System. 5th ed. Edinburgh: Churchill Livingstone; 1985

[7] Netter FH. The CIBA Collection of Medical Illustrations. Summit, NJ: CIBA-Geigy Corp.; 1991

[8] Wilson-Pauwels L, Akesson EJ, Stewart PA, Spacey SD. Cranial Nerves in Health and Disease. 3rd ed. Shelton, CT: People's Medical Publishing House—USA; 2010

[9] Inner Body. http://www.innerbody.com. Accessed June 9, 2017

[10] University of British Columbia. Anatomy of the brain. http://www.neuroanatomy.ca. Accessed June 9, 2017

2 Assessment

Denita Ryan

Abstract

Assessment by the nurse is a critical component of caring for conscious and unconscious patients with neurologic disorders. A comprehensive assessment includes medical history, mental status examination, review of speech patterns, motor and sensory examination, and evaluation of cerebellar function.

Keywords: cerebellar assessment, cranial nerves, Glasgow Coma Scale, intracranial pressure, level of consciousness, motor assessment, reflexes, sensory assessment

2.1 History

The nurse is the single most valuable asset for assessing patients in the health care setting. Therefore, all nurses must master good assessment skills. Many diverse components contribute to an adequate assessment of patients with neurologic disorders (Box 2.1 Components of a Neurologic Assessment).

Before a physical examination is performed, a thorough history should be obtained from the chart, the patient, and the family. Nurses should strive to gather as much information as possible when interviewing the patient or family. The following topics should be covered: current complaint, health history, family history, social history, and current medications.

Box 2.1 Components of a Neurologic Assessment

- Patient history
- Vital signs
- Mental status
- Level of consciousness
- Speech
- Cranial nerve testing
- Motor assessment
- Sensory assessment
- Reflex assessment
- Cerebellar function

2.1.1 Current Complaint

- Chief complaint or problem
- Symptoms and their duration
- What causes aggravation or relief of symptoms

2.1.2 Health History

- Other recent or past illnesses or diseases (e.g., diabetes mellitus, hypertension, and infectious diseases)
- Any childhood diseases (e.g., measles, mumps, and chickenpox)
- Detailed report of the patient's surgical history

2.1.3 Family History

- Medical history of the patient's parents, siblings, and children
- Age and health status of each family member (noting cause of death for any deceased immediate family members)

2.1.4 Social History

- Occupation
- Marital and family status
- Ethnicity
- Social habits (e.g., tobacco, alcohol, and drug use); indicate type, amount, and frequency of consumption, if appropriate
- Recent international travel

2.1.5 Current Medications

- Include a list of over-the-counter medications and herbal supplements
- Inquire about history of allergic reactions to any medications

2.2 Vital Signs

Routine assessment of vital signs (e.g., temperature, heart rate, respiration, and blood pressure) is an appropriate way to begin the physical examination, as vital signs may reveal important information about patients with known or suspected neurologic impairment.

2.3 Mental Status

In *Taber's Cyclopedic Medical Dictionary*, the term *mental status* is defined as "The functional state of the mind as judged by the individual's behavior, appearance, responsiveness to stimuli of all kinds, speech, memory, and judgment."

Assessment of mental status begins in the first meeting with the patient. The patient's demeanor, attentiveness, and ability to answer both simple and complex questions should be closely observed. The mental status examination offers insights on the patient's thinking, reasoning, and other functions.

- Attention
- Memory
- Appearance
- Behavior
- Orientation
- Affect
- Abstraction

If there is any uncertainty or concern about a patient's mental status, other screening tests may offer a more detailed and advanced evaluation (Box 2.2 Mental Status Screening Test Options). Any patient with a neurologic disorder should be screened for cognitive impairment.

Box 2.2 Mental Status Screening Test Options

- Mini-Mental State Examination
- Rankin Scale
- Karnofsky Performance Status Scale
- Barthel Index of Activities of Daily Living
- National Institutes of Health Stroke Scale

2.4 Level of Alertness

The most basic level of assessment is the level of alertness, which can be divided into two categories: cognition and consciousness.

2.4.1 Cognition

Cognition refers to the intellect and to the ability to gather and process information. It includes the capacity for various mental processes.

- Attention
- Organization
- Planning
- Perception
- Judgment
- Learning
- Memory
- Safety awareness

Cognitive deficits are commonly associated with cases of neurologic impairment. These deficits can be obvious (e.g., short-term memory loss), or they can be subtle (e.g., impaired safety awareness). In all patients with neurologic impairment, cognitive deficits must be identified to ensure that the patient receives appropriate care and is well-versed in safety at the time of discharge.

Altered States of Cognition

Dementia

Dementia refers to the deterioration of cognitive function with a clear sensorium. It is associated with a variety of pathologic processes that progressively damage and destroy brain cells. According to the Alzheimer's Association, a patient must meet specific criteria to receive a diagnosis of dementia.

- Decline is noted in at least two of the following cognitive functions: memory; ability to speak and understand spoken language; capacity to plan, make judgments, and carry out plans; and ability to process and interpret visual information
- Decline is severe enough to interfere with daily life

Most forms of dementia are progressive and irreversible. However, dementia may be reversible with prompt treatment when it is associated with a pathologic process.

- Drug intoxication
- Depression
- Certain vitamin deficiencies
- Normal pressure hydrocephalus

Delirium

Delirium is a transient condition characterized by disorientation and fluctuation in levels of awareness and consciousness throughout the day. Patients with delirium may exhibit various symptoms.

- Restlessness
- Agitation
- Emotional lability
- Paranoid or delusional thoughts
- Decreased cognition
- Inability to focus and maintain attention
- Hallucinations (visual, auditory, or tactile)
- Altered sleep-wake cycles
- "Sundowning" (i.e., increased levels of confusion as the day progresses)

Delirium is usually transient (lasting anywhere from several hours to many days) and is caused by an underlying condition. Possible underlying conditions may include the following:

- Infection, especially urinary tract infection (UTI), pneumonia, or viral illness (Box 2.3 Age Awareness: Urinary Tract Infection and Delirium)
- Drug or alcohol withdrawal
- Cerebral hypoxia
- Structural causes (e.g., vascular blockage, subdural hematoma, and brain tumors)
- Metabolic encephalopathy
- Certain medical conditions (e.g., hypothyroidism, hyperthyroidism, hypokalemia, anoxia, and hyponatremia)
- Prolonged intensive care unit (ICU) stay ("ICU psychosis")
- Change of environment, especially in elderly patients
- Overmedication, especially in elderly patients
- Chemical poisoning (e.g., carbon monoxide, lead, or mercury)
- Vitamin deficiency (e.g., thiamine and vitamin B1)
- Adverse reaction to a common medication (e.g., antiepileptic drugs, digoxin, cimetidine, aspirin, corticosteroids [dexamethasone], narcotics, tricyclic antidepressants, or medications used to treat Parkinson's disease)

Box 2.3 Age Awareness: Urinary Tract Infection and Delirium

- Work-up for unexplained delirium in elderly patients should always include testing for a UTI

Dementia and delirium are not the same (▶ Table 2.1).

Table 2.1 Comparison of dementia and delirium

Variable	Dementia	Delirium
Onset	Insidious and gradual	Acute and fluctuating
Level of consciousness	May be unchanged	Decreased
Medical condition	Alzheimer's disease, neurologic injury (e.g., stroke and trauma)	May include infection, drug toxicity, and hypoxia
Mood	Flat affect	Labile, irritable, and confused

2.4.2 Consciousness

Consciousness refers to one's state of awareness to self and to the environment. Alterations in consciousness may be multifactorial. They may occur slowly, over the course of several months, or they may occur rapidly, over the span of several minutes (Box 2.4 Terms to Describe Decreased Level of Consciousness).

A decline in neurologic status often starts with a decrease in the level of consciousness (LOC). Neurologic decline is frequently preceded by increased lethargy, but it can sometimes commence with restlessness, confusion, or agitation. These changes are warning signs, especially if they are new and different for the patient. Decreased LOC can have many causes, and not all causes are neurologic (Box 2.5 Common Nonneurologic Causes of Altered Level of Consciousness).

Box 2.4 Terms to Describe Decreased Level of Consciousness

- Drowsy
- Sleepy
- Lethargic
- Obtunded
- Stuporous
- Coma

Box 2.5 Common Nonneurologic Causes of Altered Level of Consciousness

- Infection
- Medication
- Fever
- Metabolic factors
- Hypoxia

Glasgow Coma Scale

The Glasgow Coma Scale (GCS) is a standardized scale often used to describe LOC in patients with neurologic disorders. It was developed in Scotland in 1974 to allow clinicians everywhere to report LOC in a uniform way. The GCS evaluates patients' responses in three areas.

- Eye opening (E)
- Verbal response (V)
- Motor response (M)

Table 2.2 Glasgow Coma Scale

Points	Eye opening (E)	Verbal response (V)	Motor response (M)
6			Obeys commands
5		Oriented	Moves purposefully
4	Eyes open spontaneously	Confused	Withdraws to pain
3	Eyes open to voice	Inappropriate speech	Decorticate positioning
2	Eyes open to pain	Incomprehensible speech	Decerebrate positioning
1	No eye opening	No verbal output	No response to pain

Note: Patients are scored on four eye responses, five verbal responses, and six motor responses. Glasgow Coma Scale (GCS) values will total 3–15, with 3 being the worst and 15 being the best. A GCS score of 8 or less indicates a severe injury, 9–12 indicates a moderate injury, and 13 or higher indicates a mild brain injury.

The patient receives points in each category based on best response. The GCS score is the sum of these points (▶ Table 2.2).

The GCS is a useful reporting tool for the assessment of neurologic function, but it is not appropriate for all patients. For example, it will not be useful for reporting neurologic function for patients with spinal cord injuries. It is most useful for patients with actual or suspected brain trauma or disease.

Altered States of Consciousness

Persistent Vegetative State

The term *vegetative state* refers to a condition that follows a period of depressed consciousness. Plum and Posner describe a vegetative state as being the return of alertness but without awareness or cognition. Patients in this state may have spontaneous eye opening and complete sleep–wake cycles but do not communicate, follow commands, or exhibit purposeful movements. Brainstem functions such as breathing remain intact. The term *persistent vegetative state* refers to a permanent vegetative state. Patients in a persistent vegetative state who receive outstanding nursing and medical care may live for many years.

Locked-In Syndrome

Locked-in syndrome is characterized by paralysis of all four extremities, resulting in the inability to move one's limbs. Affected patients are often mistakenly deemed unresponsive, because it is exceedingly difficult for those in this condition to communicate. Locked-in patients may only be able to move their eyes. Neither consciousness nor cognitive function is affected. This syndrome results from a lesion or a neurologic event (e.g., stroke) in the pontine region of the brainstem. See Chapter 1: Anatomy.

Brain Death

Brain death is defined as the permanent and irreversible absence of all brain functions, including brainstem functions, which results in apnea and coma. Brain death is a clinical diagnosis made by a physician following a strict protocol, which may vary slightly among institutions. When brain death is suspected or imminent, the nurse should contact the appropriate donor procurement organization, provided that organ donation is in accordance with the patient's advance directive (Box 2.6 Ethical Considerations: Brain Death).

Box 2.6 Ethical Considerations: Brain Death

- Brain death is determined by a physician and is based on the following criteria
  - Absence of brainstem reflexes
    - Fixed pupils
    - Absent corneal reflexes
    - Absent vestibuloocular reflexes (cold calorics)
    - Absent oculocephalic reflex (doll's eyes)
    - Absent gag reflex
    - No spontaneous respirations upon apnea challenge testing[*]
    - No response to deep central pain
- Determination of brain death is inappropriate in patients who may be intoxicated from alcohol or drug abuse
- It is critical to distinguish between brain death and conditions that can mimic brain death (e.g., alcohol intoxication, barbiturate overdose, sedative overdose, and hypothermia)
- Organ donation should be considered for patients in whom brain death is an imminent possibility

[*]Diagnostic criteria for apnea testing may differ by institutional policy and guidelines.

2.5 Speech

An important component of the neurologic assessment is determining the patient's ability to communicate. Language is a basic tool of communication, and it is often one of the first areas affected by neurologic deficits. The patient must demonstrate the ability to express thoughts and ideas, in both speech

Table 2.3 Testing speech

Speech characteristic	Testing mechanism
Fluency	Listen to the patient's flow of speech.
Repetition	Ask the patient to repeat words or phrases (e.g., "No ifs, ands, or buts").
Naming	Ask the patient to name several common objects (e.g., watch, pen, clock, and ring).
Word comprehension	Ask the patient to follow simple commands. Start with a one-step command, such as "Stick out your tongue." Progress to a two-step command, such as "Pick up the paper and set it on the floor."
Reading comprehension	Have the patient read an instruction written by the examiner or a sentence taken from a newspaper and then ask the patient to follow the instruction or explain the meaning of the sentence.

and writing (▶ Table 2.3). It is also necessary for the patient to understand both the spoken and the written word. Speech deficits are categorized according to the disorders listed below.

2.5.1 Aphasia

- Reduction or loss of language skills resulting from brain injury (▶ Table 2.4)
  - Nonfluent (expressive)
    - A type of aphasia in which the person can understand speech but has difficulty formulating words
    - Grammar may become simplified, with expressions limited to one or two words
  - Fluent (receptive)
    - A type of aphasia in which verbal expression (i.e., talking speed, grammar, and intonation) remains normal
    - Comprehension is markedly reduced, but patients with aphasia may be unaware of their language deficits

2.5.2 Apraxia

- Not a language deficit; rather, a motor planning disruption
- Involves the loss of ability to properly sequence or process the voluntary muscle movements that produce speech

Table 2.4 Types of aphasia

Diagnosis	Primary characteristics	Location of associated lesion
Broca's aphasia	Impaired verbal expression Writing ability same as speech	Broca's area of the left frontal lobe
Wernicke's aphasia	Impaired auditory comprehension Fluent speech Poor error awareness Writing ability mirrors speech ability	Wernicke's area of the temporal lobe
Global aphasia	Severely impaired spontaneous speech, auditory comprehension, naming, writing, and reading	Left middle cerebral artery territory lesions involving Broca's and Wernicke's areas

2.5.3 Dysarthria

- Not a language deficit; rather, a deficit of motor control of speech
- Refers to a group of speech disorders that result in disruption of muscle control of the speech mechanism
- Patients with dysarthria are unable to perform motor functions of speech, which can affect speed, strength, range, and coordination of speech
- Dysarthria may also affect breathing, resonation, and rhythm of speech

2.5.4 Mutism

- Inability to speak
- Results from a deficit in speech production

2.5.5 Dysphonia

- Characterized by a reduction in vocal quality
- May be caused by surgical trauma; see Chapter 1: Anatomy

2.6 Cranial Nerve Assessment

Cranial nerve assessment is an integral part of the neurologic examination, because it provides revelatory information about the functioning of various areas of the brain. This assessment is especially useful in determining whether there is damage to the brainstem, the region where most of the cranial nerves originate (▶ Table 2.5 and ▶ Table 2.6).

- There are 12 cranial nerves
- They come in pairs, a left and a right

Table 2.5 Cranial nerve function

Cranial nerve	Motor function	Sensory function
Olfactory (CN I)	None	Smell
Optic (CN II)	None	Vision
Oculomotor (CN III)	Medial, inferior, and superior rectus	None
	Inferior oblique (all extraocular muscles, except superior oblique and lateral rectus)	
	Pupillary constriction	
	Levator palpebrae (controls eyelid elevation)	
Trochlear (CN IV)	Superior oblique extraocular muscle	None
Trigeminal (CN V)	Muscles of mastication	Its three branches supply sensation to face, scalp, nasal and oral cavities, and the anterior two-thirds of the tongue
Abducens (CN VI)	Lateral rectus	None
Facial (CN VII)	Facial expression, eyelid closure, and eyebrows	Taste from anterior two-thirds of tongue
Vestibulocochlear (CN VIII)	None	Balance and hearing
Glossopharyngeal (CN IX)	Swallow	Taste from posterior one-third of tongue
Vagus (CN X)	Swallow	Sensory for pharynx and larynx (involved with swallowing)
Spinal accessory (CN XI)	Shoulder shrugs	None
Hypoglossal (CN XII)	Intrinsic and extrinsic muscles of tongue	None

Abbreviation: CN, cranial nerve.

- Some cranial nerves serve purely motor functions, some purely sensory, and some both
- They are denoted with Roman numerals (i.e., CN I–CN XII)
- The function of each cranial nerve should be tested separately, but some can be examined together
- They are always tested bilaterally

Table 2.6 Documentation and chart annotation for cranial nerve assessment

Testing method	Documentation of normal findings	Documentation of abnormal findings
CN I		
Identification of specific odors	Sense of smell present bilaterally	Unable to identify odors (indicate whether this inability is present in the left or right nostril, or bilaterally)
CN II		
Visual acuity	Visual acuity grossly intact	Document decreased visual acuity in left eye, right eye, or both eyes
Snellen chart	Document visual acuity (e.g., 20/20)	Document test score for each eye
Visual field	Visual fields full to confrontation	Document presence of visual field deficit (may use drawings)
CN III, CN IV, and CN VI		
Bilateral pupil response to light	Pupils equal and reactive to light (PERL) May document size of pupil, before and after response to light	Document size and response of each pupil to light if pupils are unequal
Extraocular movements	Extraocular movements intact (EOMI) bilaterally	Document deficit in movement of each eye, indicating direction
CN V		
Facial sensation in all three branch distributions (V1, V2, and V3)	Light touch intact in V1, V2, and V3 bilaterally	Document deficit in light touch sensation by area (V1, V2, and V3) bilaterally
Corneal reflex	Corneal reflex present bilaterally	Corneal reflex absent (right or left)
CN VII		
Facial symmetry	Face symmetric	Presence of facial weakness (indicate side) (may use House-Brackmann scale)
CN VIII		
Hearing	Hearing intact bilaterally	Decreased hearing (right or left)
CN IX and CN X		
Swallow	Swallow present bilaterally; palate raises bilaterally	Decreased swallow noted (right or left)

Table 2.6 (*continued*)

Testing method	Documentation of normal findings	Documentation of abnormal findings
CN XI		
Shoulder shrugs	Shoulder shrugs intact bilaterally	Shoulder shrugs decreased (right or left)
CN XII		
Tongue protrusion	Tongue midline	Tongue deviation (to right or left)

Abbreviation: CN, cranial nerve.

2.6.1 Examination of Cranial Nerves

In this section, we present the cranial nerves not in numerical order but rather in groups according to which nerves they should be tested with. For example, CN VI is presented directly after CN III and CN IV, with CN V presented later.

CN I: Olfactory Nerve

Often overlooked, the olfactory nerve (CN I) provides the sense of smell, the loss of which is called *anosmia* (Box 2.7 Clinical Correlation: Potential Causes of CN I Dysfunction). To test CN I

- Present nonirritating scents such as peppermint, vanilla, citrus, and coffee for the patient to identify; occlude the patient's nostrils one at a time to test both sides
- Do not test CN I with agents such as ammonia because they can irritate the sensitive nasal mucosa

---

Box 2.7 Clinical Correlation: Potential Causes of CN I Dysfunction

- Tumors such as olfactory groove meningioma
- Skull fracture causing rhinorrhea
- Aneurysm of anterior circulation

CN II: Optic Nerve

The optic nerve (CN II) is responsible for the sense of vision (Box 2.8 Clinical Correlation: Potential Causes of CN II Dysfunction). To test CN II

- Test visual acuity using a Snellen chart
  - Test each eye separately
    - Patients should wear their corrective glasses or contacts, if available and if appropriate

- Test visual fields
  - May be done grossly at the bedside
  - Compare the patient's visual fields with those of the examiner
    - Vision should be tested in quadrants. The examiner should sit directly across from the patient. The patient closes one eye, and the examiner closes the opposite eye. The examiner brings a finger into the patient's visual field, asking the patient to confirm when it is visible. Patients who do not see the finger when the examiner sees it are considered to have a field cut (deficit) (Box 2.9 Therapy Thought: Visual Field Deficits).
  - Formal visual field testing should be done by an ophthalmologist in an office with more sophisticated equipment
- Test pupillary constriction by shining a light into each eye, noting
  - Constriction of pupil (direct reflex)
  - Constriction of opposite pupil (consensual reflex)
  - These reactions are referred to as the *pupillary light reflex*
- Visualize the fundus by using an ophthalmoscope
  - Usually performed by a physician, but can be done by any member of the health care team who is trained to use an ophthalmoscope
  - The fundus may appear abnormal when there is increased intracranial pressure (ICP)

Box 2.8 Clinical Correlation: Potential Causes of CN II Dysfunction

- Optic neuritis
- Cerebral aneurysms in the anterior circulation
- Lesion (e.g., brain tumor) on or compressing the optic nerve
- Demyelinating diseases (e.g., multiple sclerosis)
- Trauma
- Stroke
- Increased ICP (e.g., from hydrocephalus or from pseudotumor cerebri)

Box 2.9 Therapy Thought: Visual Field Deficits

- Patients with visual field deficits may benefit from a consultation with an occupational therapist, who can
  - Evaluate visual deficits and functional impairments
  - Determine safety risks
  - Provide adaptive training such as visual scanning

CN III: Oculomotor Nerve

The oculomotor nerve (CN III) is responsible for several different types of eye movement. It controls medial and up-and-down extraocular movements (EOMs), and it is also responsible for pupillary constriction and raising of the eyelid (Box 2.10 Clinical Correlation: Potential Causes of CN III Dysfunction). CN III is usually tested in conjunction with the trochlear nerve (CN IV) and the abducens nerve (CN VI). To test CN III

- Test EOMs, specifically noting medial movement, as well as upward and downward movements (▶ Fig. 2.1 and ▶ Fig. 2.2)
- Observe raising of the eyelid
  ○ Inability to raise the eyelid is called *ptosis* (▶ Fig. 2.3)
- Check for pupillary restriction by shining a light into the patient's eye and observing the pupillary reaction

Box 2.10 Clinical Correlation: Potential Causes of CN III Dysfunction

- Cerebral aneurysms or arteriovenous malformations
- Brain tumors
- Demyelinating diseases (e.g., multiple sclerosis)
- Trauma
- Diabetes mellitus
- Stroke
- Infections
- Increased ICP

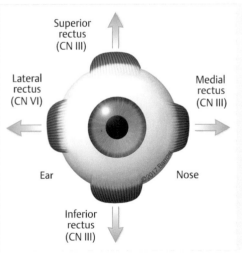

Fig. 2.1 Extraocular movement.

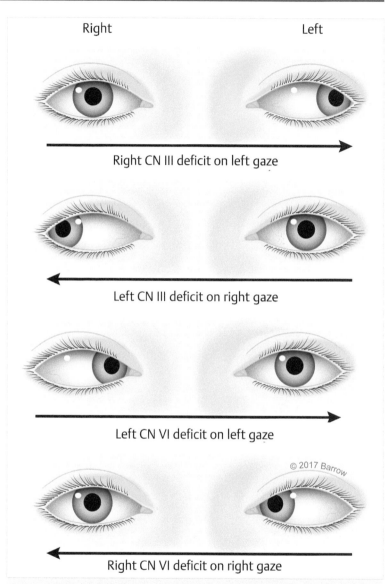

Fig. 2.2 Testing of extraocular movements.

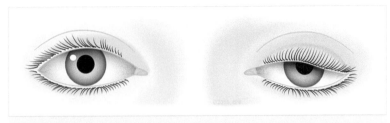

Fig. 2.3 Ptosis.

CN IV: Trochlear Nerve

The trochlear nerve controls downward and inward eye movements. CN IV is usually tested with CN III and CN VI, and deficiency of CN IV is rarely found alone. To test CN IV

• Test EOMs (in conjunction with CN III and CN VI)

If possible, observe the patient performing tasks that require downward and inward eye movements, such as reading and descending a staircase.

CN VI: Abducens Nerve

The abducens nerve, which is responsible for lateral eye movement, is tested with CN III and CN IV (Box 2.11 Clinical Correlation: Potential Causes of CN VI Dysfunction). To test CN VI

• Test EOMs (in conjunction with CN III and CN IV)

Box 2.11 Clinical Correlation: Potential Causes of CN VI Dysfunction

• Cavernous sinus lesion (e.g., tumor, aneurysm, and infection)
• Stroke
• Demyelinating diseases (e.g., multiple sclerosis)
• Lesions in upper brainstem
• Tumor
• Anterior circulation aneurysm
• Infection
• Diabetes mellitus

Conjugate Gaze

The term *conjugate gaze* refers to horizontal eye movement, which is controlled by the medial and lateral rectus muscles. Eyes must move in a coordinated (i.e., conjugate) fashion (in same direction and at same speed) to provide coordinated movement.

- Weakness in either muscle results in dysconjugate gaze and double vision (i.e., diplopia)
  - Conjugate gaze is controlled by the brainstem
    - Lateral gaze is controlled by the paramedian pontine reticular formation
    - Vertical gaze is controlled by the medial longitudinal fasciculus

Abnormal Findings for CN II, CN III, CN IV, and CN VI Tests

Anisocoria

Anisocoria refers to unequal pupil size (▶ Fig. 2.4).

- Physiologic anisocoria, or pupils that are unequal by 1 mm or less, occurs in approximately 20% of the population
- Pharmacologic anisocoria is a sudden change in pupil size due to exposure to certain drugs or medications, such as mydriatics (e.g., atropine and scopolamine) and miotics (e.g., pilocarpine)
- A new diagnosis of anisocoria may be meaningful when it occurs in conjunction with other neurologic deficits
- Pupils should be evaluated for size, shape, and rate of constriction (▶ Table 2.7)
- An enlarged pupil with a slower rate of constriction may indicate oculomotor nerve (CN III) compression and possible imminent neurologic decline

Afferent Pupillary Defect

Afferent pupillary defect occurs when light is shone in the affected pupil without eliciting either a direct response in the affected pupil or a consensual response in the opposite pupil.

- Caused by a lesion on the ipsilateral CN II
- Also referred to as *Marcus Gunn pupil*

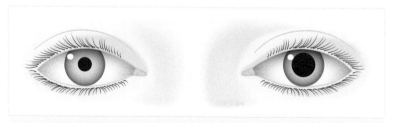

Fig. 2.4 Anisocoria.

Table 2.7 Pupillary size and characteristics

Pupil characteristic	Indication
Anisocoria (i.e., unequal pupil size)	May be physiologic
	May indicate increased ICP if new or increasing in asymmetry
	Further neurologic assessment is warranted
Dilated nonreactive pupil (one)	Increased ICP
	Possible brainstem compression
	May be precursor to herniation
Dilated nonreactive pupils (both)	Midbrain damage
	Ominous sign
	Precursor to death
Midposition nonreactive pupils	Midbrain involvement
	Further neurologic assessment is warranted, especially if nonreaction is new
Pinpoint nonreactive pupils	Pontine involvement
	Morphine reaction
Unilateral sluggishly reactive pupil	May be an early sign of increasing ICP

Abbreviation: ICP, intracranial pressure.

Parinaud's Syndrome

• Characterized by bilateral upward gaze palsy (CN III deficit)
• Bilateral lid retraction may also be present
• Bilateral upward gaze palsy and bilateral lid retraction seen together are referred to as the *setting sun* sign (▶ Fig. 2.5)
• Parinaud's syndrome may be observed in patients with pineal tumors or hydrocephalus

Horner's Syndrome

• Caused by an interruption of the sympathetic fibers of the face and eyes
• Results in ptosis, one smaller pupil, and the inability to sweat on one side of the face (▶ Fig. 2.6)
• May occur in patients who have undergone neck surgery (Box 2.12 Horner's Syndrome)

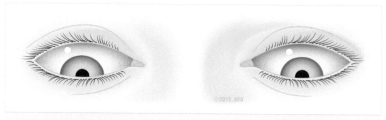

Fig. 2.5 Parinaud's syndrome.

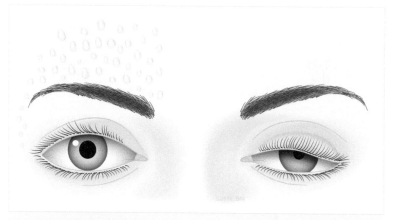

Fig. 2.6 Horner's syndrome.

Internuclear Ophthalmoplegia

- Caused by a lesion in the medial longitudinal fasciculus (the brainstem)
- Characterized by paresis in medial movement (adduction) in the affected eye (ipsilateral to the lesion) and by weakness and nystagmus in the opposite eye on abduction
- Convergence is not affected (▶ Table 2.8)

Table 2.8 Types of eye movements

Movement	Definition
Smooth pursuit	Smooth movements that keep object fixed when object or head moves
Saccades	Rapid eye movements when looking toward new object
Nystagmus	Alternating smooth pursuit movements with saccadic movements
	Can be normal or abnormal
	Nystagmus may be horizontal, vertical, or rotary
Conjugate	Eyes move together in same direction and at same speed
Dysconjugate (convergent or divergent)	Eyes move in different directions or at different speeds

CN V: Trigeminal Nerve

The trigeminal nerve (CN V) has three main branches: the ophthalmic (V1), maxillary (V2), and mandibular (V3) nerves (▶ Fig. 2.7). The trigeminal nerve is the major sensory nerve of the face, and it controls the muscles of mastication (Box 2.13 Clinical Correlation: Potential Causes of CN V Dysfunction). Each branch should be tested when CN V deficit is suspected. To test CN V:

- Lightly touch the V1, V2, and V3 distributions of the face, asking the patient to report whether sensation is felt with each touch (▶ Fig. 2.8)
- Ask the patient to clamp the jaw tightly to gauge the effectiveness of mastication muscles (masseter and temporalis muscles)
- Lightly touch the cornea with a wisp of cotton to elicit the blink reflex (Box 2.14 Blink Reflex: Nursing Implications)

Box 2.13 Clinical Correlation: Potential Causes of CN V Dysfunction

- Trigeminal neuralgia
- Tumors
- Aneurysms
- Viral infections (e.g., herpes)
- Head trauma

Box 2.14 Blink Reflex: Nursing Implications

- The blink reflex refers to the response to stimuli, either tactical or sensory. It is useful because it can help the nurse assess the brainstem response in an unconscious patient.
- When the blink reflex is absent, artificial tears or ointment can be used to protect the cornea from dryness.

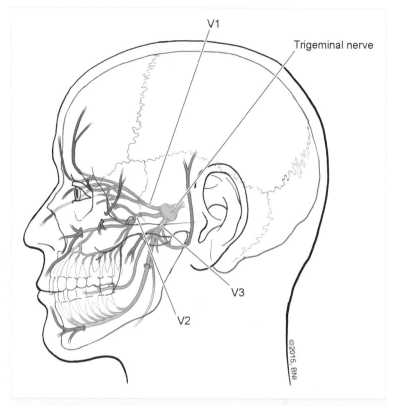

Fig. 2.7 Trigeminal nerve branches.

CN VII: Facial Nerve

The facial nerve (CN VII) controls the facial muscles (Box 2.15 Clinical Correlation: Potential Causes of CN VII Dysfunction). This nerve is also responsible for eye closure and the sense of taste on the anterior two-thirds of the tongue. To test CN VII

- Ask the patient to smile or show teeth and to raise eyebrows
- Assess eye closure by asking the patient to close both eyes tightly
- Facial weakness or the inability to close the eye is abnormal. Facial weakness is called *droop* (▶ Table 2.9; Box 2.16 Facial Weakness: Nursing Implications)

Table 2.9 House-Brackmann Grading Scale

Grade	Function	Description
1	Normal	Normal facial function
2	Mild dysfunction	Slight facial weakness
3	Moderate dysfunction	Obvious but no facial disfigurement
4	Moderate–severe dysfunction	Obvious/disfiguring facial asymmetry and incomplete eye closure
5	Severe dysfunction	Barely perceptible facial movement
6	Total paralysis	No facial movement

Box 2.15 Clinical Correlation: Potential Causes of CN VII Dysfunction

- Acoustic or vestibular lesion (e.g., acoustic neuroma)
- Skull fracture
- Infection
- Stroke
- Tumor
- Bell's palsy

Box 2.16 Facial Weakness: Nursing Implications

If a patient does not have adequate eye closure, the following tools can be helpful:
- Artificial tears during the day, as needed, and ophthalmic eye ointment at night
- Plastic bubble
- Protection of the eye and avoidance of corneal abrasion are the primary concerns
- Avoid use of eye patch

Consider evaluating the patient's swallowing if facial weakness causes pocketing of food.

Abnormal Findings for CN V and CN VII Tests

Trigeminal Neuralgia

- Also known as *tic douloureux* (French for "painful spasm")
- Painful condition in which the patient experiences a sharp, lancinating pain on the face in one or more regions related to branches of the trigeminal nerve

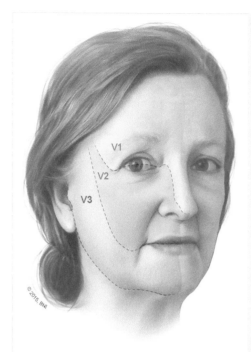

Fig. 2.8 Sensory abnormality regions: V1 to V3 in trigeminal neuralgia.

- Chewing, talking, smiling, or feeling a cold breeze may trigger neuralgia, but it can also occur spontaneously
- Painful attacks may last only a few seconds, but they can occur many times an hour, with no pain between attacks
- Pain may occur in one or more of the three main branches of the trigeminal nerve, affecting the ophthalmic (V1), maxillary (V2), or mandibular (V3) regions (▶ Fig. 2.8)

Facial Nerve Palsy

Peripheral
- Facial asymmetry; involves incomplete eye closure, weakness of forehead muscles, and facial droop on the ipsilateral side

Central
- Facial asymmetry on the lower portion of the face, on the contralateral side

Bell's Palsy

- Idiopathic facial nerve palsy (peripheral)
- Cause is unknown, but viral etiology is suspected

CN VIII: Acoustic Nerve (or Vestibulocochlear Nerve)

The acoustic nerve (CN VIII), also called the vestibulocochlear nerve, has two components. The cochlear portion controls hearing and the vestibular portion controls balance (Box 2.17 Clinical Correlation: Potential Causes of CN VIII Dysfunction). To test the cochlear portion of CN VIII:

- Assess hearing in each ear
  - After covering one of the patient's ears, the examiner should rub his or her fingers together next to the patient's other ear. The examiner can also perform further testing by snapping the fingers next to each ear and recording the patient's ability to hear those sounds.
  - An audiogram (hearing examination by an audiologist) may be needed to test the patient's hearing ability more thoroughly

To test the vestibular portion of CN VIII:

- Observe the patient's eye movements for signs of nystagmus (i.e., involuntary, rapid, and rhythmic eye movement)

Although only one component of CN VIII may be affected, both the vestibular and cochlear portions of CN VIII should be tested. Other cranial nerves, such as the facial (CN VII) and the abducens (CN VI) nerves, are nearby so other deficits resulting from those cranial nerves may also be present.

> ### Box 2.17 Clinical Correlation: Potential Causes of CN VIII Dysfunction
>
> - Tumor (e.g., acoustic neuroma)
> - Stroke
> - Trauma
> - Demyelinating diseases (e.g., multiple sclerosis)

CN IX: Glossopharyngeal Nerve

Along with the vagus nerve (CN X) and the hypoglossal nerve (CN XII), the glossopharyngeal nerve (CN IX) is involved with the mechanism of swallowing (Box 2.18 Clinical Correlation: Potential Causes of CN IX Dysfunction). It also senses taste on the posterior one-third of the tongue and processes sensation from the pharynx, controlling the gag reflex. CN IX is usually tested along with CN X and CN XII. To test CN IX

- Elicit the gag reflex by touching the back of the patient's throat lightly with a tongue depressor or a similar instrument; elevation of the pharynx indicates a positive gag reflex

Box 2.18 Clinical Correlation: Potential Causes of CN IX Dysfunction

- Brainstem lesions (e.g., stroke, tumor, and vascular lesion)
- Glomus jugulare tumor
- Glossopharyngeal neuralgia
- Infection

CN X: Vagus Nerve

The vagus nerve, along with CN IX and CN XII, controls the gag and swallow reflexes (Box 2.19 Clinical Correlation: Potential Causes of CN X Dysfunction). The vagus nerve elevates the soft palate and processes sensations from the larynx and pharynx. CN X is usually tested along with CN IX and CN XII. To test CN X:
- Elicit the gag reflex by touching the back of the patient's throat lightly with a tongue depressor or a similar instrument
  - Check for elevation of the palate; CN IX or CN X impairment causes diminished elevation

Box 2.19 Clinical Correlation: Potential Causes of CN X Dysfunction

- Brainstem lesion
- Glomus jugulare tumor

CN XII: Hypoglossal Nerve

The hypoglossal nerve innervates the tongue muscles (Box 2.20 Clinical Correlation: Potential Causes of CN XII Dysfunction). To test CN XII:
- Assess tongue protrusion by asking the patient to stick out the tongue
- Midline protrusion of the tongue is normal
- Tongue deviates to weak side if nerve deficit is present

Box 2.20 Clinical Correlation: Potential Causes of CN XII Dysfunction

- Aneurysm
- Stroke
- Tumor

Abnormal Findings for CN IX, CN X, and CN XII Tests

Dysphagia

Dysphagia is the impaired ability to swallow. It can be caused by several factors, including the following:

- Weakness of CN IX, CN X, or CN XII
- Decrease in LOC, rendering the patient too sleepy to protect the airway and swallow safely
- Cognitive impairment that causes swallowing difficulty, even when the patient is awake and alert
- The surgical approach and esophageal manipulation that may occur during anterior cervical diskectomy with fusion and plating

Perform bedside dysphagia screening for any patient who does not appear to be swallowing safely or who is at risk for unsafe swallowing. Enlist the help of a speech pathologist to conduct more sophisticated testing.

CN XI: Spinal Accessory Nerve

The spinal accessory nerve (CN XI) innervates the sternocleidomastoid muscle. It is responsible for our ability to shrug our shoulders (Box 2.21 Clinical Correlation: Potential Causes of CN XI Dysfunction). To test CN XI

- Place hands on the patient's shoulders and ask the patient to shrug

---

Box 2.21 Clinical Correlation: Potential Causes of CN XI Dysfunction

- Surgical procedures involving the neck
- Trauma

2.7 Motor Assessment

Motor strength assessment is an important part of any neurologic examination. A basic assessment should address various aspects of muscle strength.

- Muscle strength and symmetry
- Muscle tone
- Abnormal movement

2.7.1 Muscle Strength and Symmetry

Generalized testing of the strength of both the upper and lower extremities is warranted for patients with actual or suspected brain pathology. It is important to test the motor strength on each side of the body to check for symmetry

Table 2.10 Muscle Strength Grading Scale

Grade	Strength
0	No muscle contraction
1	Flicker or trace contraction
2	Active movement with gravity removed (severe weakness)
3	Active movement against gravity (anti-gravity)
4	Active movement against resistance (mild weakness)
5	Normal

(► Table 2.10). Motor weakness may be evident in patients with spinal compression or in patients with space-occupying lesions of the brain or spinal cord, including

- Tumors
- Aneurysms
- Hemorrhages
- Stroke
- Contusions
- Edema
- Intervertebral disks

Patients who have recently undergone spine surgery or who have had an actual or a suspected spinal cord injury should undergo a more thorough motor assessment. Testing should include the following:

- Each muscle group should be tested for strength on both sides of the body
- Specific muscle groups are classified according to their spinal nerve root. The spinal nerve roots should also be tested and results documented according to the scale shown in ► Table 2.11.
- Weakness on one side of the body may indicate a lesion in the contralateral side of the brain
- Weakness in a specific muscle group on one or both sides of the body may indicate a lesion in the spinal cord on the ipsilateral (same) side
- New findings of abnormalities in motor strength should be reported

2.7.2 Tone

The term *tone* refers to muscular resistance against passive movement (i.e., stretching).

- There should be slight resistance to passive range of motion
- Increased tone, which is also referred to as *hypertonicity* or *spasticity*, may
  - Be painful
  - Be severe, with possible joint dislocation

Table 2.11 Spinal nerve root motor assessment

Spinal level	Motor/muscle involvement	Muscle test
C4	Diaphragm	Respiratory inspiration
C5	Deltoid	Abduct arm
	Biceps	Elbow flexion
C6	Extensor carpi radialis	Wrist extension
C7	Triceps	Elbow extension
	Extensor digitorum	Finger extension
C8	Flexor digitorum profundus	Hand grip
	Hand intrinsics	Abduct little finger
L2	Iliopsoas	Hip flexion
L3	Quadriceps	Knee extension
L4	Hamstrings–medial Tibialis anterior	Ankle dorsiflexion
L5	Hamstrings–lateral	Knee flexion
	Posterior tibialis	Foot inversion
	Extensor hallucis longus	Extension of big toe
S1	Gastrocnemius	Ankle plantar flexion
S2	Bladder Anal sphincter	Rectal tone

○ Make it difficult to assess the patient's muscle strength
• Decreased tone is referred to as *hypotonicity* or *flaccidity*
• Degree of tone is categorized and documented as normal, increased, or decreased

2.7.3 Abnormal Movements

Observed movements, such as gait and posture, should be documented as part of the motor assessment.

Abnormal Gait Patterns

Ataxic

• Uncoordinated movement
• Wide-based stride
• Associated with cerebellar dysfunction

Parkinsonian

- Shuffling steps
- Head bowed and shoulders stooped
- Loss of arm swing
- Associated with Parkinson's disease

Hemiparetic

- Affected leg swings outward
- Possible foot drop

Spastic

- Stiff legs
- Shuffling steps
- Feet never leave ground

Other Abnormal Movements

Dystonia or Dyskinesia

A patient with dystonia or dyskinesia will have abnormal twisting or writhing movements of parts of the body, including the face.
- May be caused by degenerative neurologic disease
- May be caused by certain medications (e.g., antipsychotics)

Tremors

Tremors are involuntary trembling movements of the body or limbs (Video 2.1). There are many possible causes, including the following:
- Essential
  - Occur when muscles are required to perform a task, such as providing support and initiating movement
  - Absent at rest
- Resting
  - Occur only when the body is at rest
- Intention
  - Are triggered by or intensified with increased muscle activity
- Parkinsonian
  - Regular, rhythmic tremors
  - May be seen at rest
  - Associated with increased tone

2.8 Sensory Assessment

A comprehensive neurologic examination should also include a sensory assessment that tests the various senses.

- Sensitivity to light touch
- Assessment for presence of pain
- Testing for sensitivity to vibration
- Assessment for perception of temperature
- Testing for presence of proprioception (position sense)

When testing each above-mentioned component, each section of the dermatome diagram should be tested bilaterally, moving from head to toe. Findings should be documented using the dermatome diagram, with deficiencies indicated on the left and right sides of the body (▶ Fig. 2.9).

Knowledge of key anatomical landmarks may help determine a "rough estimate" of sensory level. However, these landmarks are not as accurate as the dermatome diagram (▶ Table 2.12). In most cases, light touch is a sufficient test; however, more advanced testing is occasionally required, such as when testing for sensitivity to pain, vibration, or temperature.

2.8.1 Light Touch

- Patient is lightly stroked with fingertips or a wispy piece of cotton

2.8.2 Pain

- Patient is lightly pricked with a sterile testing pin or other sharp object, such as a pinwheel
- The patient must describe the pinprick as "sharp"

2.8.3 Vibration

- A vibrating tuning fork is placed on various bony prominences, beginning with the fingers, moving up the arm, and then moving down the body
- Any loss of vibratory sensation should be documented; sensation should also be absent below the level where it is initially lost
- This portion of the sensory assessment can provide specific information about demyelinating disease and diabetic neuropathies

2.8.4 Temperature

- Test sensitivity to temperature only when the patient's perception of pain is impaired, because pain and temperature pathways are congruent

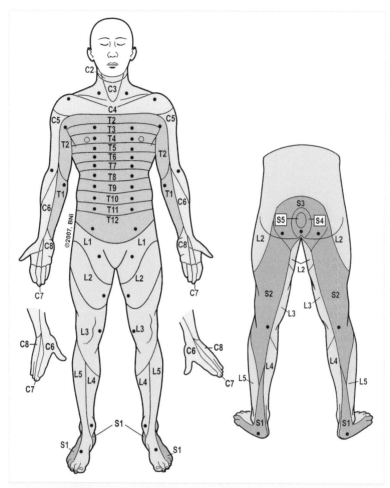

Fig. 2.9 Dermatomes.

- Use two test tubes filled with hot water and cold water, and ask the patient to describe the temperature of the water as the sides of the tubes are alternately touched to the patient's skin (beginning with the fingers, up the arm, and then down the body); randomly alternate the application of the hot and the cold tubes

Table 2.12 Sensory landmarks

Spinal level	Anatomical landmark
C4	Shoulders
C6	Thumb
C7	Middle finger
C8	Little finger
T4	Nipple line
T6	Xiphoid process
T10	Umbilicus
L3	Slightly above patella
L4	Medial malleolus
L5	Big toe
S1	Lateral malleolus
S4	Perianal

2.8.5 Proprioception

- The examiner should grasp the sides of the patient's toe or thumb and flex it up or down
- With eyes closed, the patient reports whether the toe is in a neutral position or is being moved up or down
- This portion of the sensory examination assesses the sensory pathways from the extremities through the spinal cord to the parietal lobe of the brain

2.9 Reflex Assessment

Reflex assessment is an important tool that can be used for all neuroscience patients, whether they are alert or unconscious. Types of reflexes include
- Muscle stretch reflexes
- Superficial reflexes
- Pathologic reflexes

2.9.1 Muscle Stretch Reflexes

Muscle stretch reflexes, also known as *deep tendon reflexes*, are reactions to sudden stimuli. For example, a reflex hammer striking a tendon should cause a sudden muscle stretch reflex. The reflex is the sudden movement of a limb that is innervated by muscle. Many muscles, tendons, and ligaments can be tested for reflexes, but only a few are commonly tested.

- Biceps
- Triceps
- Brachioradialis
- Patellar tendon
- Achilles tendon
- Plantar

The reflex is categorized on a 5-point scale from 0 to 4 (▶ Fig. 2.10).
- Absent (i.e., areflexive) (0)
- Diminished (1+)
- Normal (2+)
- Brisk (i.e., hyperreflexive) (3+)

Clonus, an abnormal response to muscle stretching, is indicated by a sudden jerking movement of the muscle in response to the stretching stimulus. It indicates damage to the nerve fibers that carry impulses from the brain to specific muscles.

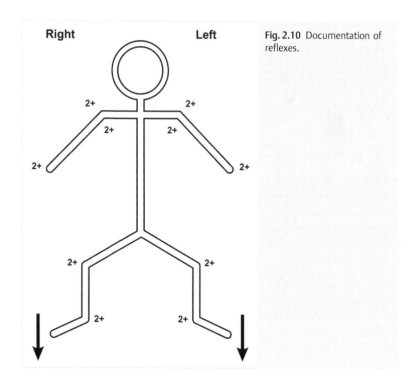

Fig. 2.10 Documentation of reflexes.

2.9.2 Superficial Reflexes

Superficial reflexes are elicited by cutaneous stimulation (e.g., touching and stroking). Document these reflexes simply as being either present or absent. Examples of superficial reflexes include
- Corneal (CN V)
- Gag (CN IX and CN X)
- Swallow (CN IX and CN X)
- Abdominal (evoked by abdominal stimulation next to the umbilicus)

2.9.3 Pathologic Reflexes

Pathologic reflexes are sometimes referred to as *primitive reflexes*, because they occur naturally in the early stages of human development and then disappear. These reflexes may also occur in neurologically impaired adults.
- Triple flex
  - Flexion of the hip, knee, and ankle all together, causing the patient to withdraw the entire leg
- Babinski reflex
  - The most common plantar reflex tested
    - Stimulation of the bottom lateral portion of the foot from heel to toe with a blunt object such as the end of a reflex hammer. Positive response is dorsiflexion of the foot, with fanning of the toes (especially the big toe and the toe next to it).
    - Downward motion of the toe or an absent response is normal, but a positive response is considered a pathologic reflex

2.10 Cerebellar Assessment

2.10.1 Nystagmus

Nystagmus is an involuntary rhythmic movement of the eyes. It is characterized by a slow drift in one direction, followed by fast corrective movements. It is described in terms of the direction (e.g., horizontal, vertical, and rotary) of the fast movements.
- Horizontal nystagmus is the most common and may indicate
  - Cerebellar dysfunction
  - Use of medications (e.g., sedatives and antiepileptics)
  - Alcohol intoxication
  - A normal finding in extreme lateral gaze (i.e., physiologic nystagmus)
- Vertical nystagmus is always pathologic and indicates posterior fossa dysfunction

2.10.2 Dysmetria

- Dysmetria is the inability to assess distance accurately from one point to another (e.g., overreaching for an object). Assess by asking the patient to touch his or her nose and then the examiner's finger.
- Dysdiadochokinesia is the inability to perform rapid, alternating tasks (e.g., turning the palm up or down)

2.10.3 Ataxia

Ataxia is the dyscoordination that is commonly noted as instability in gait or movements (Box 2.22 Clinical Alert: Ataxia). Ataxia is assessed by considering numerous components.

- Gait (ability to walk in a straight line)
- Romberg's test
  - The examiner stands behind the patient to steady the patient if balance is lost
  - The patient is asked to stand with heels together and eyes closed
  - Swaying or loss of balance with eyes closed indicates proprioceptive deficits
  - Loss of balance with eyes open indicates cerebellar ataxia

Box 2.22 Clinical Alert: Ataxia

- Public safety officers can be seen testing for ataxia (lack of muscular coordination) in roadside checks for alcohol intoxication. Persons with suspected intoxication are often asked to walk in a straight line or to touch their nose and then the officer's finger. Alcohol consumption affects cerebellar function and often results in ataxia.

2.11 Examination of an Unconscious Patient

Examining an unconscious patient involves many of the same components of the general neurologic examination. However, lack of the patient's involvement and cooperation will likely necessitate modifications.

2.11.1 Vital Signs

Vital signs, especially respiratory status, are crucial elements of the neurologic examination of an unconscious patient. Likewise, changes in blood pressure or heart rate are critical to note, because they may be late signs of increased ICP.

Table 2.13 Respiratory patterns associated with patients with decreased level of consciousness

Type	Description	Indication
Cheyne–Stokes	Period of increased respiratory rate, alternating with period of apnea	Increased ICP
Apneustic	Irregular breathing pattern characterized by gasping inspiration, with a pause on full inspiration, followed by expiration and then another pause before inspiration	Severe brainstem injury
Biot's sign	Irregular and unpredictable rate of respiration	Late sign indicating brainstem compression
Central neurogenic hyperventilation	Rapid rate over prolonged period	Damage to midbrain and upper pons
Cluster	Irregular rate, with periods of apnea	Damage to lower pons and upper medulla
Ataxic	Irregular, unpredictable pattern of respirations of various depths, alternating with periods of apnea	Damage to medulla

Abbreviation: ICP, intracranial pressure.

Respiration

- Although it is not usually an *early* indication of neurologic change, any variation in respiratory pattern may indicate changed neurologic status
- Respiratory centers are located in the pons and medulla in the brainstem
- Changes in respiratory rate or pattern of respiration may indicate pending neurologic decline (▶ Table 2.13)

2.11.2 Glasgow Coma Scale

- The first step in a thorough neurologic examination is to establish a patient's LOC by using the GCS
- Obtaining an accurate GCS score does not require the patient's cooperation
- The initial GCS score is used as the baseline for future examinations, so it is an important factor when communicating with other health care providers

2.11.3 Abnormal Posturing

A patient with severely decreased LOC may exhibit abnormal (i.e., decorticate and decerebrate) posturing when confronted with pain or noxious stimuli (▶ Fig. 2.11).

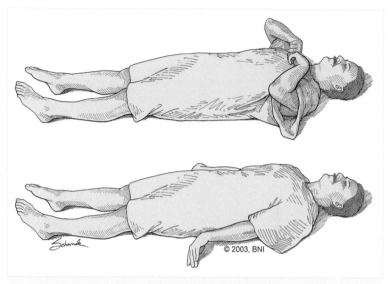

Fig. 2.11 Decorticate (*top*) and decerebrate (*bottom*) posturing.

Decorticate Posturing

Decorticate posturing, also referred to as *flexion*, is characterized by bending of the upper extremities and extension of the lower extremities.
• Seen in patients with dysfunction (i.e., lesion) above the upper brainstem
• Mandates a GCS motor score of 3

Decerebrate Posturing

Decerebrate posturing, also referred to as *extensor posturing*, is characterized by upper and lower extremity extension.
• Seen in patients with dysfunction in the lower brainstem
• Connotes a poor prognosis
• Mandates a GCS motor score of 2

2.11.4 Cranial Nerves

Pupillary Examination

• Should include examination of the pupils to assess the function of CN II and CN III; see also sections on pupil examination in Section 2.6.1 Examination of

Cranial Nerves in this chapter, specifically the subsections CN II: Optic Nerve and CN III: Oculomotor Nerve
- A change in pupils may be extremely significant, especially when combined with a low GCS score (Box 2.23 Anisocoria: Nursing Implications)

> **Box 2.23 Anisocoria: Nursing Implications**
>
> - Newly discovered pupil asymmetry (anisocoria) may be significant, especially when it occurs in conjunction with other neurologic deficits. It should be reported immediately. Anisocoria, or any change in pupillary reaction, can be an early sign of neurologic decline.

Extraocular Movements

EOMs may be assessed in various ways.
- If the patient is conscious but not cooperative, EOMs may be assessed by watching the patient's eye movement as the patient looks at his or her surroundings. This method is not ideal and should be used only when a voluntary examination cannot be elicited. Results should be documented as "tracking left" and "tracking right."
- If the patient is unconscious, the examiner may move the patient's head from side to side (**if neck injury has been ruled out**)
  - Both eyes should look completely in both directions at the same speed (conjugate gaze)
  - If eye movements are not completely coordinated, the movements are dysconjugate
  - Ideally, rotation of the head in each direction should produce eye movements in the opposite direction. This reaction, referred to as the *oculocephalic reflex* (or "doll's eye sign") is normal. Loss of this reflex is an ominous sign, because it indicates brainstem pathology.

2.12 Other Neurologic Assessment Signs

2.12.1 Kernig's Sign

- A positive response is an early sign of meningeal irritation
- The examiner attempts to extend the patient's leg at the knee, with the hip and knee flexed about 90 degrees
- A positive Kernig's sign is resistance with hamstring discomfort when leg extension is attempted

2.12.2 Brudzinski's Sign

• Also an indicator of meningeal irritation
• A positive Brudzinski's sign is flexion of the hips and knees when the neck is passively flexed while the patient is supine

Both Brudzinski's and Kernig's signs indicate meningeal irritation due to stretching and subsequent irritation of nerve roots of the neck and lower back (Box 2.24 Meningeal Signs: Nursing Implications).

Box 2.24 Meningeal Signs: Nursing Implications

• The presence of Kernig's sign or Brudzinski's sign indicates meningeal irritation, and further clinical correlation is required
• In the presence of recent neurologic surgery or trauma, nuchal rigidity or fever may alert the practitioner to the presence of meningitis

---

2.12.3 Battle's Sign

• The presence of bruising over the mastoid bone (▶ Fig. 2.12)
• Indicates basal skull fracture.

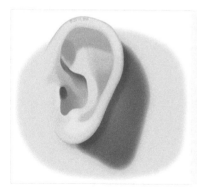

Fig. 2.12 Battle's sign.

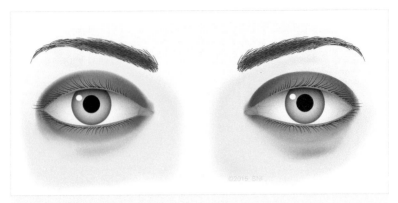

Fig. 2.13 Raccoon eyes.

2.12.4 Raccoon eyes

- Characterized by periorbital ecchymosis (bruising) (▶ Fig. 2.13)
- Indicates basal skull fracture
- May be seen in conjunction with Battle's sign; see Chapter 9: Traumatic Brain Injury.

2.13 Assessment of the Nervous System

Mastering the technical skills of a neurologic examination is important; however, knowledge of a standard examination is essential for the neuroscience nurse to effectively assess a patient who has an actual or suspected neurologic disorder. Proper identification and documentation of abnormal clinical findings should help the nurse understand the implications of these findings, thereby increasing confidence and enhancing one's ability to care for this challenging subset of patients (▶ Fig. 2.14).

This chapter is intended to be a basic reference for bedside care of patients with neurologic disorders. The references included at the end of this chapter may serve as additional helpful resources, and the reader is encouraged to consult them to learn more about specific areas of interest.

Video

Video 2.1 Brain signaling to muscles: tremor.

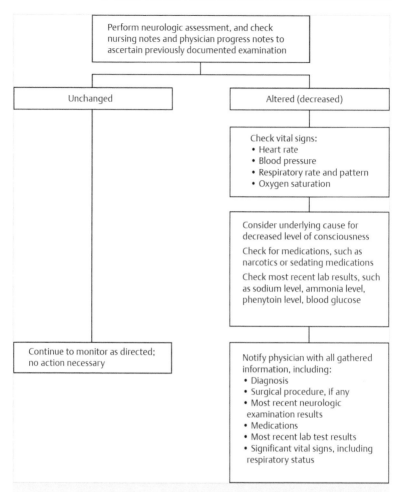

Fig. 2.14 Decision-making tree: suspected decreased level of consciousness.

Suggested Reading

[1] Alzheimer's Association. 2017 Alzheimer's disease facts and figures. 2017; http://www.alz.org/facts. Accessed July 10, 2017

[2] Booth JH. Delirium. Encyclopedia of Mental Disorders. 2017; http://www.minddisorders.com/Br-Del/Delirium.html. Accessed July 10, 2017

[3] Bowers B. Recognising metastatic spinal cord compression. Br J Community Nurs. 2015; 20(4): 162–165

[4] Braun-Janzen C, Baker S. Speech, language, swallowing and hearing disorders: what you need to know. Can Nurse. 2015; 111(4):14–15

[5] Goldberg S, Ouellette H. Clinical Anatomy Made Ridiculously Simple. 4th ed. Miami, FL: MedMaster; 2016

[6] Greenberg MS. Handbook of Neurosurgery. 8th ed. New York, NY: Thieme Medical Publishers; 2016

[7] Hickey J. Clinical Practice of Neurological & Neurosurgical Nursing. 7th ed. Philadelphia, PA: Wolters Kluwer Health; 2014

[8] Hobdell F, Stewart-Amidei C, McNair N, et al. Assessment. In: Bader MK, Littlejohns LR, eds. AANN Core Curriculum for Neuroscience Nursing. 4th ed. St. Louis, MO: Saunders; 2004

[9] Posner JB, Saper CB, Schiff ND, Plum F. Plum and Posner's Diagnosis of Stupor and Coma. 4th ed. New York, NY: Oxford University Press; 2007

[10] Venes D, ed. Taber's Cyclopedic Medical Dictionary. 23rd ed. Philadelphia, PA: F.A. Davis; 2017

[11] Voyer P. Communicating with people with dementia: Avoiding mistakes. Can Nurse. 2015; 111 (5):10

[12] Wilson-Pauwels L, Akesson EJ, Stewart PA, Spacey SD. Cranial Nerves in Health and Disease. 2nd ed. Hamilton, Ontario, Canada: B C Decker; 2002

[13] Yetzer E, Blake K, Goetsch N, Shook M, St Paul M. SAFE medication management for patients with physical impairments of stroke, part one. Rehabil Nurs. 2015; 40(4):260–266

Part II

Specific Conditions Associated with Neurologic Disorders

3 Principles of Intracranial Pressure

Denita Ryan

Abstract

The principles of intracranial pressure, including pathology, variations, and treatment, form the foundation to understanding neurologic function. Increased intracranial pressure may be a symptom or a side effect of a variety of neurologic diseases and injuries. Understanding these principles is essential for nurses caring for any patient with an actual or potential neurologic disorder.

Keywords: cerebral blood flow, cerebral perfusion pressure, cerebrospinal fluid, external ventricular drain, Glasgow Coma Scale, Monro–Kellie doctrine

3.1 Intracranial Pressure

Knowledge of the principles of intracranial pressure (ICP) and its variations is the foundation for understanding neurologic function. Increased pressure in the head has been known for centuries as a predictor of poor outcome—nearly 2,500 years ago, Hippocrates wrote that alleviating pressure in the head helped relieve "dropsy of the brain." This belief may have been the basis for the ancient practice of trepanation, that is, drilling holes in the skull to relieve pressure. Increased ICP can occur in many neurologic disorders and portends a poor neurologic outcome (Box 3.1 Conditions Associated with Increased Intracranial Pressure).

Intracranial pressure refers to the pressure exerted on the brain and its contents. Normal ICP is between 0 mm Hg and 15 mm Hg. Increased ICP, also referred to as intracranial hypertension, occurs when the pressure within the brain is increased to more than 15 mm Hg, as first described in the Monro–Kellie doctrine in 1783.

Box 3.1 Conditions Associated with Increased Intracranial Pressure

- Conditions that increase brain volume
  - A space-occupying lesion, such as intracranial tumor, hematoma, hemorrhagic stroke, abscess, aneurysm, vascular malformation, and cerebral edema
- Conditions that increase blood volume
  - Hyperemia
  - Increased intrathoracic or intra-abdominal pressure (Valsalva maneuver)
  - Venous outflow obstruction
- Conditions that increase cerebrospinal fluid (CSF) volume
  - Hydrocephalus due to obstruction, poor CSF resorption, tumor, increased production of CSF

3.1.1 Basic Principles of the Monro–Kellie Doctrine

- Intracranial contents include brain parenchyma, cerebrospinal fluid (CSF), and blood
- Intracranial contents are contained in a fixed vault (the skull); therefore, their total volume must remain constant
- A change in volume of any one component mandates a change in the other components

3.1.2 Compensatory Mechanisms

Compensatory mechanisms are a necessary part of the brain's ability to alter the volume of one of its components to regulate the volume of the others, thereby maintaining normal ICP. These mechanisms may include

- Alterations in blood volume
- Alterations in CSF volume
- Compression of brain tissue

Deterioration of these compensatory mechanisms results in neurologic decline.

Compliance

Compliance is described as a
- Measure of brain "stiffness"
- Measure of the brain's ability to maintain equilibrium in the presence of internal and external challenges
- Mechanism that allows the brain to accommodate slow-growing, space-occupying lesions (e.g., tumors)

Cerebral Blood Flow

Cerebral blood flow (CBF) refers to the amount of blood that passes through 100 g of brain tissue in 1 minute.
- Normal value is approximately 50 mL/min
- The brain uses approximately 20% of the body's oxygen

Cerebral Perfusion Pressure

Cerebral perfusion pressure (CPP) is the net pressure gradient driving the CBF that delivers oxygen and metabolites. It is defined as
- The difference between mean arterial pressure (MAP) and ICP
- Normal CPP is 70 to 100 mm Hg (Box 3.2 Calculation of Cerebral Perfusion Pressure)

Cerebral perfusion pressure serves as the stimulus for autoregulation to provide adequate CBF.

Box 3.2 Calculation of Cerebral Perfusion Pressure

- Cerebral perfusion pressure is the difference between mean arterial pressure (MAP) and intracranial pressure (ICP):
  CPP = MAP – ICP
- MAP can be calculated using systolic blood pressure (SBP) and diastolic blood pressure (DBP), using the formula
  MAP = DBP + 1/3 (SBP – DBP)
- Normal CPP = 70–100 mm Hg; Normal ICP = 0–15 mm Hg

Autoregulation

- Process in which the brain alters its own vasculature to accommodate changes in ICP
- Failure of the brain to autoregulate results in neurologic decline

Cerebral Edema

- Refers to an increase of water in the brain parenchyma
- Cytotoxic edema
  - Accumulation of intracellular water
  - Results from a hypoxic event
  - May or may not be reversible
- Vasogenic edema (▶ Fig. 3.1)
  - Alteration in vascular permeability, with disruption of the blood-brain barrier
  - Increased extracellular space
  - Frequently seen in neoplastic diseases
  - Treated with osmotic agents
  - May coexist with cytotoxic edema
  - May be irreversibly damaging

3.1.3 Herniation Syndromes

Herniation of the brain can occur when the intracranial contents are shifted away from their usual location in the skull (▶ Fig. 3.2). This shifting can be caused by numerous factors, such as abscess, hemorrhage, hydrocephalus, stroke, and radiotherapy.

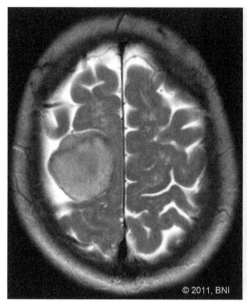

Fig. 3.1 Vasogenic edema.

Cingulate Herniation

- Also referred to as *subfalcine herniation*
- Caused by an expanding lesion in one hemisphere that causes it to shift toward the opposite hemisphere
- Causes compression, which restricts local blood flow
- May cause cerebral edema, local tissue ischemia, and increased ICP
- Resulting deficits depend on the specific location and extent of herniation

Transtentorial Herniation

- Also referred to as *central herniation*
- Caused by a lesion that displaces the brain downward through the tentorial notch
- May cause cerebral edema, local tissue ischemia, and hemorrhage
- May result in decreased level of consciousness (LOC), respiratory depression, and contralateral motor weakness
- Resulting deficits depend on the specific location and the extent of herniation

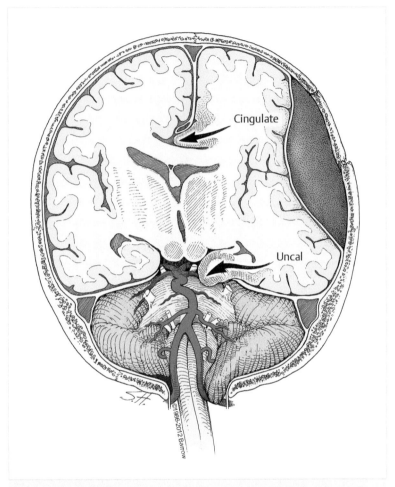

Fig. 3.2 Herniation syndromes.

Uncal Herniation

- Most common type of brain herniation
- Caused by an expanding lesion, often in the temporal lobe (Box 3.3 Conditions at Risk for Uncal Herniation)
- Pressure is exerted across the midline, pushing the uncus into the edge of the tentorium

- Sluggish ipsilateral pupil is a common early sign
- Contralateral hemiparesis, decreased LOC, and altered respiratory patterns are common late signs
- Brainstem compression may result
- A dilated nonreactive pupil is a very late sign of uncal herniation (Box 3.4 Herniation Syndromes: Nursing Implications)

Box 3.3 Conditions at Risk for Uncal Herniation

- Any supratentorial space-occupying lesion (especially in the temporal lobe), including
  - Tumor
  - Cerebral contusion
  - Intracranial hemorrhage
  - Subdural or epidural hemorrhage
  - Gunshot wound
  - Abscess

Box 3.4 Herniation Syndromes: Nursing Implications

- Herniation syndromes are a neurologic emergency and must be reported immediately
- Nursing intervention is aimed at early recognition and reporting of neurologic decline

---

3.1.4 Clinical Manifestations of Increased Intracranial Pressure

Clinical manifestations of increased ICP depend on the location within the brain where pressure is exerted and the rate and extent of increased ICP. Some areas of the brain called *eloquent areas*, which are directly involved in speech, motor function, sensory reception, and cranial nerve function, are less tolerant of increased ICP than others. The brainstem is particularly sensitive to ICP. It is the origin of many cranial nerves, and it is a small area with little room for edema. It is also the location of the brain's respiratory center. Clinical manifestations of ICP affecting the brainstem may include

- Decreased LOC
- Cranial nerve deficits
- Motor and/or sensory changes
  - Decorticate or decerebrate posturing

- Headache
- Nausea and vomiting
- Changes in vital signs (usually seen with increasing progression of brainstem compression); see also Chapter 2, Assessment

3.1.5 Diagnosis of Increased Intracranial Pressure

- Clinical assessment (Box 3.5 Clinical Alert: Early Diagnosis of Increased Intracranial Pressure)
- ICP monitoring
- Imaging studies, such as magnetic resonance imaging (MRI) and computed tomography (CT) (▶ Table 3.1)

Table 3.1 Diagnostic tests associated with intracranial pressure monitoring

Diagnostic tests	Expected findings	Nursing implications
CT and MRI	Can confirm presence of cerebral edema, hydrocephalus, and space-occupying lesion	Ask if the patient has allergy to contrast agents; notify physician if an allergy is present If the patient is undergoing an MRI, perform metal screening. In addition, determine whether the patient is claustrophobic; if so, notify physician for sedation orders NPO status for MRI with sedation
Lumbar puncture	Measures opening and closing pressure indications of ICP	Contraindicated in the presence of a space-occupying lesion (or suspicion of lesion) Informed consent required
TCD ultrasonography	Measures velocity of arterial and venous flows, indicative of ICP	Important to note TCD trends Elevated TCD may indicate vasospasm, which could lead to increased ICP
Cerebral angiography (performed if cerebrovascular abnormality is suspected)	Indicates vasospasm	Patient must be NPO before angiography Patient must lie flat for predetermined period (usually 4–6 hours) Close observation of puncture site (usually right or left femoral artery) is required to detect groin hematomas

Abbreviations: CT, computed tomography; ICP, intracranial pressure; MRI, magnetic resonance imaging; NPO, nil per os (nothing by mouth); TCD, transcranial Doppler.

Box 3.5 Clinical Alert: Early Diagnosis of Increased Intracranial Pressure

- The importance of early and accurate nursing assessment cannot be overstated
- Identification and reporting of early signs of increasing ICP can be the difference between recovery and neurologic devastation

3.1.6 Treatment of Increased Intracranial Pressure

Medical Treatment

- Hyperosmolar therapy
- Nursing interventions to decrease ICP (Box 3.6 Hospital Activities that May Exacerbate Increased Intracranial Pressure)
- Respiratory support
- Sedation (▶ Table 3.2)
- Barbiturate coma (Box 3.7 Barbiturate Coma)

Box 3.6 Hospital Activities that May Exacerbate Increased Intracranial Pressure

- Improper positioning of head and neck
- Straining (e.g., during a bowel movement)
- Coughing
- Suctioning
- Valsalva maneuver
- Emotional stress
- Excessive environmental stimuli (television, radio, and conversation)
- Nursing activities (assessment, positioning, administration of medications, and bathing)

Table 3.2 Pharmacology for management of patients with increased intracranial pressure

Drug	Category	Indication	Nursing implications
Dopamine (Intropin) Phenylephrine (Neo-Synephrine) Norepinephrine (Levophed) Epinephrine (Adrenalin)	Vasopressor	Increase blood pressure Support adequate CPP	Monitor for hypotension with arterial line
Mannitol (Osmitrol)	Hyperosmotic agent	Reduce vasogenic edema	Monitor for serum sodium and osmolality levels
Acetaminophen (Tylenol)	Antipyretic	Control fever	Use caution to avoid exceeding daily limits Monitor for liver toxicity
Propofol (Diprivan)	Sedative	Sedate Reduce anxiety Decrease CBF and oxygen demands	Masks neurologic examination Effects are short-lived; dosage may be suspended temporarily to allow for accurate neurologic examination
Pentobarbital (Nembutal)	Barbiturate	Trigger barbiturate-induced coma for refractory increased ICP Decrease metabolic demands	Impedes nurse's ability to perform neurologic assessment Closely monitor ICP, hemodynamic functions, and respiratory status

Abbreviations: CBF, cerebral blood flow; CPP, cerebral perfusion pressure; ICP, intracranial pressure; IV, intravenous.

Box 3.7 Barbiturate Coma

- Sometimes induced in patients with refractory increased ICP
- Intended to decrease metabolic demands
- Patients are given loading dose and then maintenance doses
- Neurologic examination is completely suspended
- Respiratory support is required
- Intensive nursing care (usually 1:1) is required; nurses should
  - Monitor ICP and immediately report increased ICP
  - Monitor hemodynamics and report arrhythmia and hypotension
  - Monitor barbiturate levels, as ordered
  - Monitor skin integrity
  - Educate family, if applicable

Surgical Treatment

- Placement of an ICP-monitoring device (Box 3.8 Intracranial Pressure Monitoring)
- Craniectomy

Box 3.8 Intracranial Pressure Monitoring

- The purposes of intracranial pressure monitoring are to
  - Obtain objective data to maintain adequate cerebral perfusion pressure
  - Monitor trends in neurologic status
  - Evaluate response to treatment

Intracranial Pressure Monitoring

Intracranial pressure–monitoring devices are used mainly to measure ICP (Box 3.9 Guidelines of the American Association of Neuroscience Nurses (AANN) for Insertion of Intracranial Pressure–Monitoring Devices). These devices may also lower ICP by draining excessive CSF. The goal of the monitoring is to gain information about ICP to ensure adequate CPP.

Box 3.9 Guidelines of the American Association of Neuroscience Nurses (AANN) for Insertion of Intracranial Pressure–Monitoring Devices

Patient Preparation
- Obtain informed consent for procedure per hospital policy
- Obtain most recent laboratory results, including coagulation profile
- Obtain and record most recent neurologic assessment findings
- Medicate or sedate the patient, if necessary
- If restraints are necessary, explain their purpose to the patient and the family, and observe hospital policies regarding restraints and proper documentation

Placement of Intracranial Pressure–Monitoring Device
- Procedure must be sterile, including a sterile field and the use of masks, gowns, and gloves
- The patient should be supine, with the head of the bed elevated at least 30 degrees
- The ICP-monitoring system should be calibrated and prepared according to the manufacturer's directions
- Surgical site should be shaved, prepared, and draped according to the physician's preference (site is usually anterior to the coronal suture and at the level of the right mid-pupil line)

• The ICP-monitoring device should be placed by a neurosurgeon or an accredited practitioner

Nursing Activities
• Attach the device to the previously prepared and calibrated system
• Apply the dressing according to hospital policy
• Record the initial ICP reading and waveform
• Document the date, time, site, and type of monitoring device, as well as the practitioner's name
• Maintain strict aseptic technique when working with the drain
• Recalibrate and rebalance the ICP device according to hospital policy
• Perform hourly neurologic assessments, including measurements of ICP and CPP
• Notify the physician immediately of any changes in ICP or neurologic assessment or of any breaks in the integrity of the ICP-monitoring system

*A brief, highlighted version of the AANN guidelines is presented in this handbook. The reader is strongly encouraged to refer to the AANN guidelines found in the AANN reference presented in the reference list of this chapter.

Indications

• Glasgow Coma Scale (GCS) score < 9
• Abnormal CT scan of the head, showing
  ○ Cerebral edema or cerebral ischemia, or both
  ○ Intracerebral hematoma
  ○ Subarachnoid hemorrhage
  ○ Brain tumor
  ○ Hydrocephalus
• Normal CT scan, with other predisposing factors, such as
  ○ Intracerebral pathology (e.g., stroke and tumor)
  ○ Poor neurologic examination
• Any patient thought to be at the risk of acute neurologic decompensation after the neurosurgeon reviews the patient's individual circumstances

Contraindications

• Coagulopathy
  ○ Abnormal results in tests such as prothrombin time (PT), partial thromboplastin time (PTT), and international normalized ratio (INR)
  ○ Low platelet count
• Immunosuppression

Potential Complications

- Hemorrhage
- Incorrect position of ICP-monitoring device
  - Catheter position (confirmed by CT scan)
  - Drain leveled at appropriate landmark
  - Analysis of ICP waveform
- Incorrect patient positioning after placement of monitoring device (Box 3.10 Intracranial Pressure Monitoring and Patient Transportation)
- Infection, most commonly resulting from one or more of the following
  - Extended duration of invasive monitoring (longer than 5 days)
  - CSF leakage (open system)
  - Concurrent systemic infection
  - Craniotomy

Box 3.10 Intracranial Pressure Monitoring and Patient Transportation

- The ICP-monitoring device should be turned to the "off" position when the patient is being transported (unless ICP is unstable), to prevent unintended CSF drainage
- Always confirm the advisability of stopping CSF drainage before changing device settings

---

Intracranial Pressure Monitoring Devices

There are several different categories of the ICP-monitoring devices (▶ Table 3.3).
- External ventricular drain (EVD) (▶ Fig. 3.3)
  - Most common device used
  - Usually placed on the right side of the head
  - Inserted into the ventricle (usually a lateral ventricle)
  - Attached to a continuous drainage system via an external transducer
  - Capable of adjusting the volume of CSF drained by the position of drain for therapeutic drainage
  - Capable of collecting fluid for testing
  - Most common risks associated with EVD are hemorrhage and infection
  - Capable of monitoring ICP
- Subarachnoid screw or bolt
  - Inserted into the subarachnoid space through a burr hole and attached to an external transducer
  - Cannot drain CSF
  - Capable of monitoring ICP

Table 3.3 Types of intracranial pressure–monitoring devices

Device type	Advantages	Disadvantages	Nursing considerations
EVD	Most common Most accurate Excellent ICP waveform Ability to drain CSF Allows for monitoring of CSF characteristics (e.g., quantity, color, and clarity) Allows access for administration of medicine	More difficult to insert Risk of infection Risk of hemorrhage Requires constant nursing monitoring	Patient requires ICU stay Must recalibrate EVD when patient's position changes Monitor EVD for signs of CSF leak and/or infection Requires informed consent and patient or family education Requires recent blood work (especially coagulation profile) May require sedation Nurse may assist with surgical procedure Insertion site must be kept clean and sterile at all times
Intraparenchymal catheter	Quick and easy to insert Offers accurate measurement of brain tissue pressure Useful when ventricular access is not an option	Does not measure ventricular pressure Does not monitor CSF characteristics (e.g., quantity, color, and clarity) Reflects only regional pressure	Patient requires ICU stay No recalibration required Requires informed consent and patient or family education May require sedation Requires recent blood work (especially coagulation profile) Nurse may assist with surgical procedure Insertion site must be kept clean and sterile at all times
Subarachnoid screw or bolt	Quick insertion Useful when ventricular access is not an option Decreased risk of infection and parenchymal damage	Easily occluded Does not drain CSF or monitor its characteristics Not advised for long-term use	Patient requires ICU stay Requires informed consent and patient or family education Requires recent blood work (especially coagulation profile) May require sedation Nurse may assist with surgical procedure Insertion site must be kept clean and sterile at all times

Table 3.3 (*continued*)

Device type	Advantages	Disadvantages	Nursing considerations
Epidural or subdural monitor	Quick and relatively easy to place Low risk of infection or hemorrhage	Placement is not as accurate as some of the other device types	Patient requires ICU stay Requires informed consent and patient or family education Requires recent blood work (especially coagulation profile) May require sedation Nurse may assist with surgical procedure Insertion site must be kept clean and sterile at all times
Multifunction monitoring device	Monitors ICP, brain tissue oxygenation, and brain temperature	Expensive Limited availability Reflects only regional measurements (e.g., ICP, oxygenation, and temperature)	Patient requires ICU stay Requires informed consent and patient or family education Requires recent blood work (especially coagulation profile) May require sedation Nurse may assist with surgical procedure Insertion site must be kept clean and sterile at all times

Abbreviations: CSF, cerebrospinal fluid; EVD, external ventricular drain; ICP, intracranial pressure; ICU, intensive care unit.

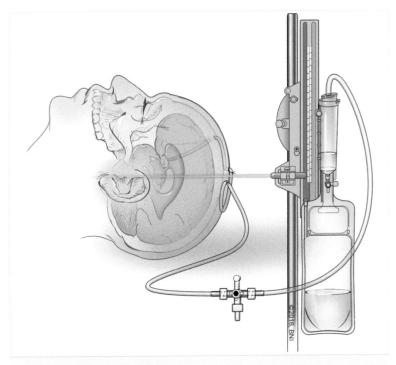

Fig. 3.3 External ventricular drain.

- Intraparenchymal catheter
  - Inserted into the brain parenchyma
  - Insertion is quick and accurate
  - Cannot drain CSF

Intracranial Pressure Waveform

ICP waveforms (▶ Fig. 3.4) normally correlate with arterial waveforms. They have three characteristic peaks of decreasing height.
- Percussion wave (P1)
  - Arterial in origin
  - Sharp peak
  - Fairly consistent height
- Tidal wave (P2)
  - Arterial in origin
  - Ends on dicrotic notch
  - Elevation usually indicates impaired autoregulation

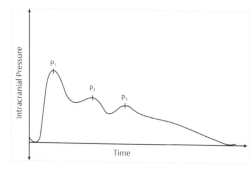

Fig. 3.4 Intracranial pressure waveforms (P1, percussion; P2, tidal; P3, dicrotic).

- Dicrotic wave (P3)
  - Venous in origin
  - Follows dicrotic notch

When a patient has increased ICP, the ICP waveform amplitude increases. The tidal wave increases more drastically than the percussion wave.

3.1.7 Special Conditions Associated with Increased Intracranial Pressure

Pseudotumor Cerebri

Pseudotumor cerebri (PTC), also called *idiopathic intracranial hypertension*, is a syndrome in which ICP is elevated. It is associated neither with hydrocephalus nor with an intracranial lesion (e.g., tumor).

Hydrocephalus

Hydrocephalus is a congenital condition found in neonates. It is also associated with most types of brain disorders, including stroke, trauma, tumors, and infections. It may be accompanied by increased ICP.

Because hydrocephalus is a condition commonly associated with most brain disorders, an entire chapter has been devoted to it. Both PTC and hydrocephalus are discussed in Chapter 4: Hydrocephalus.

3.2 Nursing Management of Patients with Increased Intracranial Pressure

Nursing management of patients with increased ICP is complex and multifaceted. Increased ICP may lead to dysfunction in many body systems. Thus, all body systems must be assessed (▶ Table 3.2 and ▶ Table 3.4). The importance

Table 3.4 Increased intracranial pressure

Complication	Indication	Nursing actions	Rationale
Decreased LOC	Increased ICP	Perform complete neurologic assessment frequently Check for other causes of decreased LOC, such as hypoxia, decreased hemoglobin, decreased ventilatory drive, infection, medications, and metabolic causes	Decreased LOC may be early indication of increasing ICP; however, there are many non-neurologic causes that must be ruled out

Hypoxia	Decreased oxygenation	Remember that the cause of hypoxia may be non-neurologic or neurologic. Determine the cause of hypoxia by using the following guidelines.
		Neurologic cause:
		  Decreased LOC
		  Decreased respiratory drive
		Respiratory cause:
		  Lack of oxygen
		  Decreased respiratory drive
		  Decreased ventilation
		  Pneumonia or atelectasis
		  Pulmonary embolus
		  Trauma to chest
		Cardiovascular cause:
		  Decreased hemoglobin
		  Hypotension
		  Arrhythmia
		  Heart failure
			Hypoxia leads to cerebral edema and is a strong indicator of poor outcome

Hyponatremia	SIADH	Report and take corrective measures, as directed	Hyponatremia may facilitate cerebral edema and result in increased ICP
Hyperglycemia	Increased blood glucose levels	Report and take corrective measures, as directed	Hyperglycemia may increase cerebral metabolic demand

Abbreviations: ICP, intracranial pressure; LOC, level of consciousness; SIADH, syndrome of inappropriate antidiuretic hormone.

of a thorough, accurate assessment cannot be overemphasized, and any change in condition between assessments and any abnormal findings should be reported (see also Chapter 2: Assessment). A comprehensive assessment should include the components described below (**Appendix A1: Nursing Management of Patients with Increased Intracranial Pressure**).

This chapter is meant to be a basic reference for nurses caring for patients with neurologic disorders who have increased ICP (or who have the potential to develop increased ICP). The reader is encouraged to consult the references found at the end of this chapter to learn more about specific subjects of interest.

3.2.1 Neurologic Assessment

- Evaluate LOC; see also Chapter 2: Assessment (Box 3.11 Clinical Alert: Level of Consciousness)
- Test motor function
- Monitor sensory function
- Assess cranial nerve function

Box 3.11 Clinical Alert: Level of Consciousness

- Sometimes, the first indication of decreased LOC is restlessness and/or agitation, rather than lethargy

3.2.2 Respiratory Assessment

- Monitor the patient's ability to protect the airway
- Observe respiratory rate and rhythm, perform visual inspection, and auscultate the lungs
- Monitor arterial blood gases, avoid hypercapnia (goal is normal $PaCO_2$: 35–45 mm Hg)
- Using O_2 saturation monitor, supplement O_2, as indicated
- Prepare for intubation and mechanical ventilation, if warranted

3.2.3 Cardiovascular Assessment

- Perform hemodynamic monitoring, if appropriate, via central line or arterial line
- Monitor electrocardiogram (ECG) for cardiac arrhythmias
- Monitor blood pressure closely to avoid hypotension
  - Administer vasopressors, if indicated
- Monitor complete blood count for hemoglobin/hematocrit

3.2.4 Fluid and Electrolyte Assessment

- Monitor serum sodium level; watch for hyponatremia
- Administer salt supplements or hyperosmolar solutions, as indicated

- Restrict fluids, if indicated
- Monitor strict intake and output
- Monitor glucose levels; administer insulin, as directed; see also Chapter 5: Electrolyte Disturbances

3.2.5 Fever Management

- Monitor vital signs for increased temperature
- Maintain normothermia; use cooling blankets, as indicated
- Administer antipyretics, as ordered

3.2.6 Pain Management

- Assess the patient frequently for possible pain
- Administer narcotics or sedation, as needed

3.2.7 Patient and Family Teaching

- Teach the patient and the family about the importance of minimizing stimulation
- Teach the patient and the family about ICP-monitoring devices and the contraindications to changing the patient's position without notifying nursing staff. The patient's head must be kept in a neutral, central position— not turned to either side
- Provide emotional support, as needed, for the patient and the family

3.2.8 Collaborative Management

Many different specialties may be called into action in the case of a patient with increased ICP. These specialties include

- Nursing
- Neurosurgery for surgical intervention (including insertion of ICP-monitoring devices)
- Critical care intensivists and internal medicine physicians for pulmonary and respiratory management and cardiovascular management
- Neurology service for the management of associated disorders (e.g., seizures)
- Clergy, chaplain, or other spiritual support
- Occupational, physical, and speech therapies are usually placed on hold when a patient has increased ICP
- Social work or case management
- Palliative care, if appropriate

Suggested Reading

[1] American Association of Neuroscience Nurses. Care of the Patient Undergoing Intracranial Pressure Monitoring/External Ventricular Drainage or Lumbar Drainage. Glenview, IL: American Association of Neuroscience Nurses; 2011

[2] American Association of Neuroscience Nurses. Guide to the Care of the Patient with Intracranial Pressure Monitoring. Glenview, IL: American Association of Neuroscience Nurses; 2005

[3] Bader MK. Gizmos and gadgets for the neuroscience intensive care unit. J Neurosci Nurs. 2006; 38 (4):248–260

[4] Bader MK. Recognizing and treating ischemic insults to the brain: the role of brain tissue oxygen monitoring. Crit Care Nurs Clin North Am. 2006; 18(2):243–256, xi

[5] Binder DK, Horton JC, Lawton MT, McDermott MW. Idiopathic intracranial hypertension. Neurosurgery. 2004; 54(3):538–551, discussion 551–552

[6] Bota DP, Lefranc F, Vilallobos HR, Brimioulle S, Vincent JL. Ventriculostomy-related infections in critically ill patients: a 6-year experience. J Neurosurg. 2005; 103(3):468–472

[7] Fan JY. Effect of backrest position on intracranial pressure and cerebral perfusion pressure in individuals with brain injury: a systematic review. J Neurosci Nurs. 2004; 36(5):278–288

[8] Hickey JV. The Clinical Practice of Neurological and Neurosurgical Nursing. Philadelphia, PA: Lippincott Williams & Wilkins; 2009

[9] Inoue K. Caring for the perioperative patient with increased intracranial pressure. AORN J. 2010; 91(4):511–515, quiz 516–518

[10] Key CB, Rothrock SG, Falk JL. Cerebrospinal fluid shunt complications: an emergency medicine perspective. Pediatr Emerg Care. 1995; 11(5):265–273

[11] Mcilvoy L. The impact of brain temperature and core temperature on intracranial pressure and cerebral perfusion pressure. J Neurosci Nurs. 2007; 39(6):324–331

[12] Noble KA. Traumatic brain injury and increased intracranial pressure. J Perianesth Nurs. 2010; 25 (4):242–248, quiz 248–250

[13] Nyholm L, Steffansson E, Fröjd C, Enblad P. Secondary insults related to nursing interventions in neurointensive care: a descriptive pilot study. J Neurosci Nurs. 2014; 46(5):285–291

[14] Olson DM, Lewis LS, Bader MK, et al. Significant practice pattern variations associated with intracranial pressure monitoring. J Neurosci Nurs. 2013; 45(4):186–193

[15] Open Anesthesia. Intracranial Pressure/Nervous System/Critical Care Manual. 2015; https://www .openanesthesia.org/intracranial_pressure__nervous_system__critical_care_manual/#ICP_vs._CPP. Accessed September 14, 2015

[16] Posner JB, Saper CB, Schiff ND, Plum F. Plum and Posner's Diagnosis of Stupor and Coma. 4th ed. Oxford: Oxford University Press; 2007

[17] Raichle ME, Plum F. Hyperventilation and cerebral blood flow. Stroke. 1972; 3(5):566–575

4 Hydrocephalus

Donna C. Wallace and Michele M. Grigaitis

Abstract

Hydrocephalus affects many patients with neurologic conditions. It is a result of dilatation of the ventricles in the brain, usually caused by blockage of the cerebrospinal fluid pathways. Because hydrocephalus can occur with many neurologic disorders, recognition of its symptoms and knowledge of its treatment are essential for nurses and all health care providers.

Keywords: cerebrospinal fluid, endoscopic third ventriculostomy, intracranial pressure, lumboperitoneal shunt, normal pressure hydrocephalus, ventriculoperitoneal shunt

4.1 Hydrocephalus

Hydrocephalus is a condition that results in dilatation of the cerebral ventricles, usually after blockage of the cerebrospinal fluid (CSF) pathways in the brain (Video 4.1). It was recognized early on by the Greeks, who treated it by puncturing the swollen ventricles with reeds or by banding the skull to prevent it from expanding further. The Greek physician Galen (129–200 AD) theorized that the cerebral ventricles communicated with one another and posited that the ventricles were the vessels that transported waste products through the pituitary gland. Centuries later, Vesalius (1514–1564) was able to describe the mechanisms of hydrocephalus more clearly.

In patients with hydrocephalus, CSF does not travel from its point of production in the ventricles to its point of absorption in the systemic circulation. Hydrocephalus is generally classified according to its point of obstruction; however, this classification system is the subject of much debate.

Hydrocephalus is often considered to primarily affect children, but it also occurs in adults with certain neurologic conditions or diseases. Because this handbook addresses neurologic concerns in adult patients only, our discussion on hydrocephalus and its implications will be limited to the adult population (Box 4.1 Conditions Associated with Hydrocephalus).

Box 4.1 Conditions Associated with Hydrocephalus

- Traumatic brain injury
- Tumor
- Subarachnoid hemorrhage
- Meningitis
- Encephalitis
- Congenital anomaly
- Arnold-Chiari malformation
- Clotting disorder
- Blood cancer

4.1.1 Classification of Hydrocephalus

Hydrocephalus is sometimes divided into two distinct types: obstructive and communicating (► Fig. 4.1).

Obstructive Hydrocephalus

- Also referred to as noncommunicating hydrocephalus (► Fig. 4.2)
- Caused by tumors, congenital abnormalities of the brain, cysts, inflammation resulting from infection, or other conditions that interfere with patency of the CSF pathways.

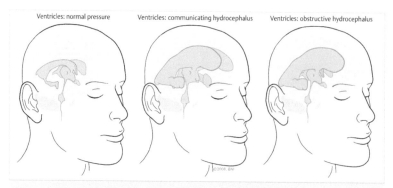

Ventricles: normal pressure   Ventricles: communicating hydrocephalus   Ventricles: obstructive hydrocephalus

Fig. 4.1 Depiction of ventricle size for each type of hydrocephalus.

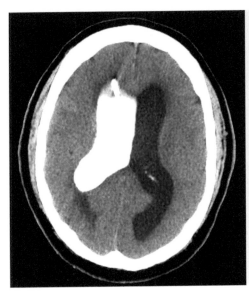

Fig. 4.2 Injected contrast agent in only one lateral ventricle, suggestive of obstructive hydrocephalus.

Communicating Hydrocephalus

- Occurs when the arachnoid villi can no longer adequately absorb CSF (▶ Fig. 4.3)
- Caused by intraventricular or subarachnoid hemorrhage or by some infections

Idiopathic Normal Pressure

- Type of communicating hydrocephalus
- Etiology unknown

4.1.2 Pathophysiology of Hydrocephalus

- Most CSF is produced by the choroid plexus in the ventricles, but it is also produced in other areas along the neuraxis (▶ Fig. 4.4). In adults, CSF is replaced several times each day, and roughly 400 to 500 mL of CSF is produced daily. The total amount of CSF in the ventricles, brain, and along the neuraxis is about 150 mL at any given time
- CSF flow occurs as follows
  - CSF travels from the lateral ventricles through the two foramina of Monro to the third ventricle and then through the aqueduct of Sylvius to the fourth ventricle (▶ Fig. 4.5)

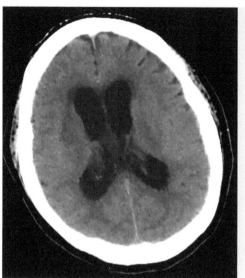

Fig. 4.3 Symmetric enlarged ventricles demonstrate possible communicating hydrocephalus.

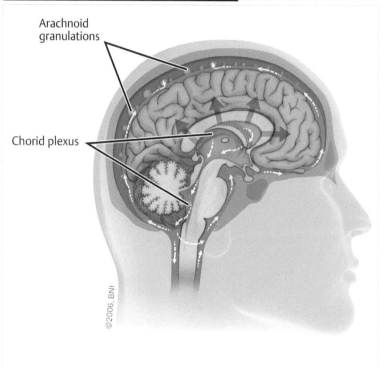

Arachnoid granulations

Chorid plexus

©2006, BNI

Fig. 4.4 Flow of cerebrospinal fluid.

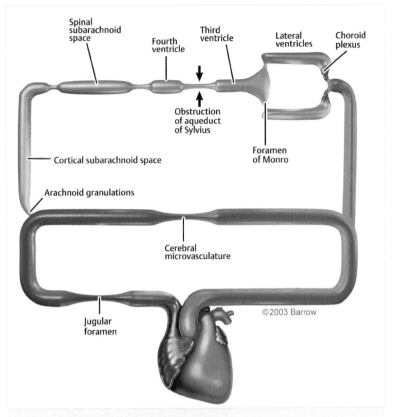

Fig. 4.5 Cerebrospinal fluid pathway.

- ○ CSF continues down the spinal canal in the posterior portion of the spinal sac and returns to the brain
- ○ As CSF circulates over the cerebral hemispheres, it is absorbed into the sagittal sinus via the arachnoid villi
- Hydrocephalus results from
  - ○ Failure of the CSF absorption mechanism
  - ○ Obstruction of the CSF pathway
  - ○ Overproduction of CSF (rare)

Epidemiology

- The rate of persons born with congenital hydrocephalus is 0.5 to 4 per 1000 persons

- The actual number of people living with hydrocephalus is hard to determine
- Approximately 25,000 shunting procedures are performed annually in the United States, but some believe this number may be as high as 50,000

Etiology

Congenital

- Neonatal developmental anomaly
- Genetic disorders
- Intracranial abnormalities
  ○ Dandy–Walker malformation (occurs when the roof of the fourth ventricle does not develop and the ventricle therefore becomes enlarged)
  ○ Aqueductal stenosis (▶ Fig. 4.6)
  ○ Choroid plexus papilloma (resulting in the overproduction of CSF)
  ○ Spina bifida

Acquired

- Aqueductal stenosis (may not show symptoms until older, or may be acquired after infection or bleeding)
- Subarachnoid, intraventricular, or intracranial hemorrhage (Box 4.2 Hydrocephalus in Patients with Subarachnoid Hemorrhage)
- Bacterial, viral, fungal, or parasitic infection (after which the pathways on the arachnoid villi are blocked)
- Tumor, cyst, or other obstruction
- Arnold-Chiari malformation
- Traumatic brain injury or swelling of the brain
- Thrombosis of the superior sagittal sinus

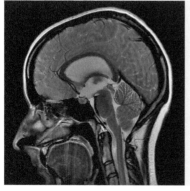

Fig. 4.6 Hydrocephalus resulting from aqueductal stenosis.

Clinical Manifestations

- Visual changes, especially diplopia
- Cognitive changes
- Change in personality
- Changes in vital sign, including bradycardia and hypertension; see also Chapter 3: Principles of Intracranial Pressure
- Pathologic reflexes
- Upward gaze palsy
- Headache
- Seizures (rare)

Idiopathic Normal Pressure Hydrocephalus

- Insidious onset, usually after the age of 40 years. The average age of persons who develop idiopathic NPH is over 60 years (Box 4.3 Pain Management in the Elderly)
- Minimum duration is 3 to 6 months
- No evidence of antecedent event (e.g., traumatic brain injury and stroke)
- Progresses over time
- Symptom triad
  - Gait disturbance
  - Cognitive deficit
  - Urinary incontinence

4.1.3 Diagnosis of Hydrocephalus

History

- Patient's chief complaint
- History of shunt placement (i.e., when shunt was placed, what type of shunt the patient received, and previous valve settings) (Box 4.4 Shunt Failure)
- Any other neurological history (e.g., tumor)

Box 4.4 Shunt Failure

- Clinical manifestations of shunt failure are identical to symptoms of hydrocephalus

---

Assessment

The classic symptom triad in patients with hydrocephalus includes dementia, urinary incontinence, and abnormal gait. An adequate assessment should include each of the following components:

- Level of consciousness (LOC)
- Cranial nerve assessment
- Motor, sensory, cognitive, and gait assessment
- Visual acuity
- Incontinence
- Cognitive testing (specifically for NPH)
  - Folstein's Mini–Mental State Examination

Diagnostic Tools

Health care practitioners may use various tools to diagnose hydrocephalus (▶ Table 4.1).

Computed Tomography

- A computed tomography (CT) scan is the imaging study of choice in patients with suspected or confirmed hydrocephalus. It shows
  - Ventricular size
  - Position of an existing intraventricular catheter

Magnetic Resonance Imaging

- Magnetic resonance imaging (MRI) shows more detail than CT scan
- No radiation

Table 4.1 Diagnostic tests associated with hydrocephalus

Diagnostic study	Expected findings	Nursing implications
CT	Ventricle size Location of existing catheter Bleeding Hemorrhage in subarachnoid space Midline shift	N/A
MRI	Same as for CT More detailed imaging than CT Catheter not visible on MRI	No radiation Patient may require sedation if claustrophobic; if fast-spin echo MRI or "one bang" MRI is used, sedation may be unnecessary
Cine MRI	Depicts CSF flow	Same as for MRI
Lumbar puncture	Measurement of pressure Observation of CSF qualities; provides CSF for culture	Requires patient cooperation; nurse may need to assist with patient positioning Patient must remain flat for designated period after examination
Venogram	Measures ICP and venous pressures in the heart; can help identify pressure gradients (blockage)	Same as for any operative procedure Patient will be anesthetized
Shuntogram	Radionuclide injected to follow CSF flow through the shunt to determine its patency	Preparation of site Assisting in sterile removal of CSF for diagnostic procedure No special precautions

Abbreviations: CSF, cerebrospinal fluid; CT, computed tomography; ETV, endoscopic third ventriculostomy; ICP, intracranial pressure; MRI, magnetic resonance imaging; N/A, not applicable.

- Fast-spin echo or "one bang" MRI is a rapid scan (approximately 3 minutes in duration) that does not require sedation
- Programmable shunts may require plain radiographs to check settings after MRI, because the magnet in MRI may change valve settings

Shuntogram

- Shuntogram, also called *radionuclide cisternography*, shows CSF flow through the shunt, recording emptying time and demonstrating possible obstruction
- Used to determine shunt function if the patient is not responding to therapy

Cine MRI

- A video-style MRI that shows the movement of CSF flow

Lumbar Puncture

- May be used to obtain CSF cultures
- Contraindicated until a space-occupying lesion has been ruled out, because lumbar puncture could cause herniation in the presence of a space-occupying lesion; see also Chapter 3: Principles of Intracranial Pressure
- A large-volume tap is used to assess NPH (patient's condition may improve after removal of large volume of CSF)

4.1.4 Treatment of Hydrocephalus

Medical/Conservative

- Observation
- Acetazolamide may be tried in some circumstances

Surgical

- Serial lumbar punctures
- Shunts (discussed later) and shunt taps (Box 4.5 Focus On: Shunt Taps)
- Endoscopic third ventriculostomy (ETV)
  - An endoscope is used to create a hole in the floor of the third ventricle, thereby creating a diversion for CSF around the obstruction

---

Box 4.5 Focus On: Shunt Taps

Definition
- To enter a reservoir of a shunt, using a needle under sterile conditions to obtain a CSF sample

Indications
- To obtain sample to test for infection
- To measure pressure to assess shunt function
- To introduce intrathecal medication

Preparing the patient
- If possible, explain the procedure
- Obtain patient consent
- Obtain equipment (varies depending on institution)
- Obtain vital signs

Preparing for urgent tap
- Protect airway
- Call Neurosurgery
- Monitor vital signs and perform neurologic assessment
- Gather equipment

Equipment
- Adult lumbar puncture tray, including manometer
- Betadine or chlorhexidine
- 23-gauge butterfly needle
- Sterile gloves
- Signed patient consent form

Sending sample
- Gram's stain
- Culture
- Glucose
- Protein
- Cell count (and differential)
- Anaerobes (usually done automatically)
- Medication levels, as necessary

Shunts

A shunt is a diversion device that includes three main parts: a proximal catheter implanted into the ventricular system or subarachnoid space, a valve, and a catheter distal to the absorption site (e.g., the peritoneum).
- Indication
  - Used to divert CSF around obstruction, thereby preventing the accumulation of excess CSF
- Examples of shunt systems include (▶ Table 4.2)
  - Ventriculoperitoneal shunt (VPS)
  - Ventriculoatrial shunt (VAS)
  - Lumboperitoneal shunt (LPS)
  - ETV
- Shunt valves
  - Valves work by regulating the flow of CSF
  - Many different types and brands of valves are available, and there is much debate regarding which one is most effective (▶ Table 4.3)
  - The consensus is that the best valve is the one that the surgeon is most comfortable implanting
  - In selecting the valve, the surgeon should take into account the patient's diagnosis, age and frailty, and other diagnostic criteria

Complications Associated with Shunts

- Overshunting, which occurs when the valve drains too much CSF and causes intracranial hypotension

Table 4.2 Types of shunts

Type of shunt	Indication	Nursing implications
VPS	Drains CSF from ventricles to peritoneal cavity	Abdominal pain may indicate infection or a dislodged catheter
VAS	Can be used when patient is unable to absorb CSF in peritoneum CSF is drained directly into blood stream	Be aware of potential for cardiac arrhythmias or catheter migration into the superior vena cava
LPS	Drains CSF from subarachnoid space to peritoneum Used to treat patients with conditions such as PTC and slit ventricle syndrome	Leg pain or back swelling may indicate shunt failure or malposition of catheter
Cisterna magna—VPS	Drains CSF from inside the ventricles and from the subarachnoid space May be needed if LP shunt alone cannot be used, as in cases of blockage or scar tissue	May be used for patients with PTC
Other	When scar tissue or another obstruction prevents drainage of CSF to peritoneum or heart, catheters may instead terminate in the gallbladder or pleural space	Learn shunt catheter termination site from surgeon and assess patient for gallbladder pain or pleuritis, as appropriate

Abbreviations: CSF, cerebrospinal fluid; LP, lumbar puncture; LPS, lumboperitoneal shunt; PTC, pseudotumor cerebri; VAS, ventriculoatrial shunt; VPS, ventriculoperitoneal shunt.

Table 4.3 Types of shunt valves

Valve type	Examples	Advantages	Disadvantages
Programmable	Codman Hakim Programmable Valve System	Possible long life	More expensive
	Strata Valve	Can fine tune tolerances to meet requirements for individual patients	Requires user practice
	proGAV Sophysa Polaris Valve	Compatible with MRI; no imaging required to read shunt setting	
Non-programmable	Delta Valve Codman Hakim Precision Fixed Pressure Valve	Less expensive No programming required	Cannot change range without surgery

Abbreviation: MRI, magnetic resonance imaging.

- Subdural hematoma
  ○ Caused by tearing of bridging veins
  ○ Relatively common in elderly patients
  ○ May result from overshunting
- Infection
- Shunt failure
  ○ Improper positioning or breakage of shunt catheter
  ○ Obstruction of catheter or valve
- Bowel perforation (applies only to VPS and LPS)
- Hearing loss (applies only to patients with NPH)

4.1.5 Conditions and Terms Associated with Hydrocephalus

Pseudotumor Cerebri

Pseudotumor cerebri (PTC) is a syndrome that leads to increased intracranial pressure (ICP) that is not associated with hydrocephalus or an intracranial lesion. It is thought to result from a problem with absorption in the venous system due to actual blockage or an idiopathic cause resulting from elevated venous pressures, but its cause may also be exogenous (Box 4.6 Clinical Alert: Exogenous Causes of Pseudotumor Cerebri).

- Venous outflow abnormalities
- Most often seen in young, obese women
- May be idiopathic

Box 4.6 Clinical Alert: Exogenous Causes of Pseudotumor Cerebri

- Excessive ingestion of vitamin A
- Antibiotics
- Some chemotherapies
- The exact mechanism of action in PTC is unclear

Pathophysiology

- Cerebrospinal fluid is absorbed into the venous system after traveling passively through the arachnoid villi
- A blockage (e.g., a thrombus) somewhere in the veins prevents CSF absorption
- Medications such as vitamin A and some oral antibiotics alter venous pressures by altering the absorption of CSF at the cellular level
- Elevated pressure in the right ventricle of the heart may also increase the pressure in the cerebral venous system
- In women, obesity is a common cause of elevated right-heart pressure

Clinical Manifestations

- Increased ICP
- Headaches
- Impaired vision (may progress to blindness)

Diagnosis

- Assessment
  - Papilledema
  - Ophthalmologic examination to test visual acuity
- History
  - Recent weight gain and morbid obesity should be considered possible indicators of PTC
  - Use of certain medications, especially some oral antibiotics and vitamins
- Lumbar puncture to obtain an opening pressure, which in some patients with PTC can be ≥ 40 cm H_2O (normal opening pressure is between 10 and 20 cm H_2O)
- Retrograde venography
  - Measures venous pressures in the heart and inside the skull
  - The gold standard for diagnosis and for possible identification of the cause of PTC
  - Ventricles can appear normal on MRI or CT, so retrograde venography may facilitate the diagnosis of PTC

Treatment

- Medical/conservative
  - If the patient is obese and has elevated right-heart pressure, weight loss is recommended
  - Cessation of possible offending medications may be indicated
  - Acetazolamide
- Surgical
  - Shunt placement, usually LPS (VPS is not as effective because the ventricles in patients with PTC are typically small, and the absorption problem is outside the brain)
  - Fenestration of optic nerve sheath may be performed to preserve vision
  - Both shunting and optic nerve sheath fenestration are the methods used for redirecting CSF
  - Bariatric surgery may be indicated in morbidly obese patients to secondarily reduce ICP

Ventriculomegaly

- Enlargement of the ventricles, usually due to pressure

Hydrocephalus Ex Vacuo

- A condition that occurs when brain tissue has atrophied (i.e., after stroke), leaving empty space in the cranium; the ventricles compensate by producing more CSF to fill this space

Slit Ventricle Syndrome

- So named because of the slit-like appearance that the ventricles have on MRI or CT; this condition results from overshunting
- May have gradual onset
- The skull may not have been able to grow appropriately; thus, ICP is elevated
- Causes cyclical intermittent negative pressures, especially when the patient is upright; proximal obstruction of the shunt catheter can lead to elevated ICP
- Also called *noncompliant ventricle syndrome*

4.2 Nursing Management for Patients with Hydrocephalus

Patients with hydrocephalus often present a host of challenges to caregivers. Hydrocephalus may result from a congenital defect or from a neurologic condition or disorder, and it can worsen if a shunt intended to treat it fails (▶ Table 4.4 and **Appendix A2: Nursing Management of Patients with Hydrocephalus and Shunt Failure**).

This chapter is intended as a basic reference for bedside care of patients with hydrocephalus. For more information, the reader is urged to consult the references included at the end of this chapter.

4.2.1 Neurologic Assessment

- Evaluate LOC; see also Chapter 2: Assessment
- Perform cranial nerve assessment, including vision testing
- Conduct motor, sensory, and gait assessments
- Document urinary symptoms, noting the presence of urinary incontinence
- Evaluate for cerebellar dysfunction

4.2.2 Respiratory Assessment

- The patient's LOC may affect the results of respiratory assessment
- Tachypnea, or hyperventilation, may be associated with pain
- Cheyne–Stokes respiration may indicate increased ICP

Table 4.4 Shunt failure/hydrocephalus: what to watch for

Problem	Action	Nursing implication/rationale
Headache	Neurologic assessment Vital signs	Assessing for possible increased ICP caused by shunt failure
	Headache diary	Diary helps determine whether headache onset is related to the time of day or a specific activity It may also reveal causative or alleviating activities
	Consider shunt tap	Shunt tap will allow accurate measurement of ICP
Vomiting	Neurologic assessment	Assessing for possible increased ICP caused by shunt failure
Fever	If shunt was placed more than 6 months ago, look for cause of fever other than shunt	Likelihood of shunt infection decreases with time Shunt infection is most common within 3 months of surgery
	Consider laboratory tests such as CBC and C-reactive protein	
	Shunt tap with CSF sent for culture, if other source is not found	Obtain CSF to rule out infection (Gram's stain, culture, glucose, protein, and cell count)
	If patient has a VAS, obtain blood cultures and 24-h urine to assess total protein	Complications of VAS infection include endocarditis and shunt nephritis
Redness or swelling along shunt tract or operative wound	Vital signs, CBC, and possible shunt tap	Look for signs of infection
Other signs of increased ICP	Visual changes, irritability, personality changes, and decline in work or school performance	Assessing for shunt failure
Exposed hardware	Cover with sterile dressing and call or consult Neursurgery	Exposed hardware is a source of infection and needs to be surgically repaired
Seizures	Rarely result from shunt failure	Patients with seizure disorders may experience increase in seizures with shunt failure

Abbreviations: CBC, complete blood cell count; CSF, cerebrospinal fluid; ICP, intracranial pressure; VAS, ventriculoatrial shunt.

4.2.3 Cardiovascular Assessment

- The patient's LOC may affect the results of cardiovascular assessment
- Bradycardia may indicate increased ICP
- Document elevated blood pressure or widened pulse pressure

4.2.4 Integumentary Assessment

- Check soft tissue for redness, swelling, or pain along the shunt tract
- Monitor incision sites for signs of infection

4.2.5 Fever Management

- Document and report the presence of fever
- Administer antipyretics, if warranted
- Fever may necessitate a shunt tap for CSF culture
- Obtain a complete blood call count (CBC) and C-reactive protein test to assess for infection

4.2.6 Pain Assessment

- Assess the location and quality of pain
- Medicate, as needed
- Note abdominal pain if the patient has VPS
- Document whether pain changes with position (e.g., low-pressure headache when the patient is sitting or standing; the headache is relieved when the head of the bed is flat)

4.2.7 Patient and Family Teaching

- Educate the patient and family on the type of shunt that the patient has received and on its settings (if it is a programmable shunt)
- Encourage the patient and family to consult resources such as the Hydrocephalus Association website (www.hydroassoc.org)
- Ensure that the patient and family fully understand discharge instructions (**Appendix B1: Sample Discharge Instructions after Placement of a Ventriculoperitoneal Shunt**)

4.2.8 Collaborative Management

- Nursing
- Neurosurgery
- Neurology

- Internal medicine
- Therapy specialties
  - Physical therapy
  - Occupational therapy
  - Speech therapy/cognition
- Physiatry/rehabilitation
- Neuropsychology
- Case management or social work

Video

Video 4.1 Enlargement of the ventricles associated with hydrocephalus.

Suggested Reading

[1] Agamanolis DP. Neuropathology: An Illustrated Course for Medical Students and Residents. Rootstown, OH: Northeastern Ohio University of Medicine; 2008

[2] Bergsneider M, Black PM, Klinge P, Marmarou A, Relkin N. Surgical management of idiopathic normal-pressure hydrocephalus. Neurosurgery. 2005; 57(3) Suppl:S29–S39, discussion ii–v

[3] Bondurant CP, Jimenez DF. Epidemiology of cerebrospinal fluid shunting. Pediatr Neurosurg. 1995; 23(5):254–258, discussion 259

[4] Brazis PW. Surgery for idiopathic intracranial hypertension. J Neuroophthalmol. 2009; 29(4): 271–274

[5] Brean A, Eide PK. Prevalence of probable idiopathic normal pressure hydrocephalus in a Norwegian population. Acta Neurol Scand. 2008; 118(1):48–53

[6] Cartwright CC, Wallace DC. Nursing Care of the Pediatric Neurosurgery Patient. 3rd Ed. Heidelberg: Springer; 2017

[7] Drake J, Sainte-Rose C. The Shunt Book. Cambridge, MA: Blackwell Science; 1995

[8] Hydrocephalus Association. About Hydrocephalus: A Book for Families. San Francisco, CA: University of California; 2011

[9] Hydrocephalus Association. http://www.hydroassoc.org. Accessed June 8, 2017

[10] Jaraj D, Rabiei K, Marlow T, Jensen C, Skoog I, Wikkelsø C. Prevalence of idiopathic normal-pressure hydrocephalus. Neurology. 2014; 82(16):1449–1454

[11] Jones RW, Wallace DC. Hydrocephalus. In: Bader MK, Littlejohns LR, eds. AANN Core Curriculum for Neuroscience Nursing. 6th ed. Philadelphia, PA: WB Saunders; 2016

[12] Klinge P, Marmarou A, Bergsneider M, Relkin N, Black PM. Outcome of shunting in idiopathic normal-pressure hydrocephalus and the value of outcome assessment in shunted patients. Neurosurgery. 2005; 57(3) Suppl:S40–S52, discussion ii–v

[13] McLone DG. Pediatric Neurosurgery: Surgery of the Developing Nervous System. 4th ed. Philadelphia, PA: WB Saunders; 2001

[14] Neilsen N, Breedt A. Hydrocephalus. In: Cartwright CC, Wallace DC, eds. Nursing Care of the Pediatric Neurosurgery Patient. Heidelberg: Springer; 2017

[15] Passero C, McCaffery M. Pain Assessment and Pharmacologic Management. St. Louis, MO: Mosby Elsevier; 2011

[16] Rekate HL. The definition and classification of hydrocephalus: a personal recommendation to stimulate debate. Cerebrospinal Fluid Res. 2008; 5:2

[17] Saito M, Nishio Y, Kanno S, et al. Cognitive profile of idiopathic normal pressure hydrocephalus. Dement Geriatr Cogn Dis Extra. 2011; 1(1):202–211

[18] Satzer D, Guillaume D. Hearing loss in hydrocephalus: a review, with focus on mechanisms. Neurosurg Rev. 2016; 39(1):13–24–, discussion 25

[19] Sirven J, Malamut B. Clinical Neurology of the Older Adult. Philadelphia, PA: Wolter Kluwer; 2008

[20] Torsnes L, Blåfjelldal V, Poulsen FR. Treatment and clinical outcome in patients with idiopathic normal pressure hydrocephalus–a systematic review. Dan Med J. 2014; 61(10):A4911

[21] Uretsky S. Surgical interventions for idiopathic intracranial hypertension. Curr Opin Ophthalmol. 2009; 20(6):451–455

[22] van Veelen-Vincent ML, Delwel EJ, Teeuw R, et al. Analysis of hearing loss after shunt placement in patients with normal-pressure hydrocephalus. J Neurosurg. 2001; 95(3):432–434

5 Electrolyte Disturbances

Denita Ryan

Abstract

Electrolyte disturbances affect many patients with neurologic conditions. The most common electrolyte disturbances in these patients are an imbalance of sodium or glucose. Such disturbances can have serious negative effects on neurologic function; therefore, it is important for nurses to understand the causes, signs, and treatment of these abnormalities.

Keywords: antidiuretic hormone, cerebral salt wasting, diabetes insipidus, hypernatremia, hyponatremia, syndrome of inappropriate antidiuretic hormone

5.1 Electrolyte Balance

Sometimes, brain injury can cause electrolyte imbalances. Any electrolyte (sodium, potassium, chloride, or carbon dioxide) can be thrown out of balance, but in nerologic disorders, a patient's level of sodium is most likely to be affected.

Another type of metabolic disorder that is commonly found in conjunction with electrolyte imbalance is impaired glucose tolerance or excessively high or low serum concentrations of glucose. Glucose, a simple sugar, is measured as part of the metabolic panel that includes the electrolyte panel. Although glucose is not an electrolyte per se, patients with neurologic conditions often have glucose imbalance along with electrolyte imbalances.

Electrolyte and glucose imbalances can exacerbate neurologic injury, causing further decline. The best way to manage these imbalances is to detect and treat them early.

5.2 Sodium

The definition of the normal sodium level may vary slightly by institution. Sodium levels within the "normal" or laboratory "reference" range of 135 to 145 mEq/L are generally considered acceptable.

5.2.1 Antidiuretic Hormone

Antidiuretic hormone (ADH), also called *vasopressin*, is a peptide hormone that is active in the blood vessels and kidneys. It causes more absorption of water into the blood. In turn, this dilution reduces the concentration of serum sodium.

- Produced by the posterior portion of the pituitary gland, called the *hypothalamus*, and released into systemic circulation
- Release of ADH is regulated by
  - Baroreceptors in the carotid sinus (and aortic arch)
  - Plasma osmolality (Box 5.1 Osmolality)
- Prompts decreases in blood pressure and blood volume

Box 5.1 Osmolality

- Osmolality is defined as the number of particles present per kilogram weight of solvent
- Normal serum osmolality is 275 to 295 mOsm/kg

Functions of Antidiuretic Hormone

- Increases rate of water reabsorption
  - Dilutes circulating blood
  - Reduces and concentrates urine
- Plays a key role in maintaining osmolality and serum–urine sodium levels
- Deficiency of ADH can lead to diabetes insipidus (DI), discussed later in this chapter

5.2.2 Hyponatremia

Hyponatremia is a condition in which the level of serum sodium is too low. In most institutions, hyponatremia is diagnosed in patients whose level of serum sodium is less than 135 mEq/L. There may be several causes of hyponatremia. It can be

- Relatively common in patients with neurologic disorders
- Associated with cerebral edema, which increases intracranial pressure (ICP); see Chapter 3: Principles of Intracranial Pressure (Box 5.2 Clinical Alert: Hyponatremia)
- Caused by volume overload (then referred to as *hypervolemic hyponatremia*), as seen in congestive heart failure

In neurosurgical patients, hyponatremia usually manifests as a syndrome of inappropriate ADH (SIADH) or as cerebral salt wasting. The etiologies of these two types of hyponatremia and their respective treatments differ vastly (Box 5.3 Conditions Associated with Hyponatremia and ▶ Table 5.1).

Table 5.1 Comparison of syndrome of inappropriate antidiuretic hormone and cerebral salt wasting

Comparative factor	SIADH	Cerebral salt wasting
Serum sodium value	Below 134 mg/dL	Below 134 mg/dL
Urine sodium value	Normal or increased	Increased
Serum osmolality	Decreased	Normal or increased
Urine osmolality	Increased	Normal or increased
Intravascular volume	Normal or increased	Decreased
Fluid restriction	Restrict free water, approximately 1 L every 24 h	Never
Treatment	Fluid restriction; may add salt supplements, such as salt tablets and hyperosmolar saline solution (3%). May also add demeclocycline or furosemide (Lasix)	Volume replacement, salt supplements, or hyperosmolar saline solutions (3%)
Associated neurologic disorder	Could be related to any neurologic disorder, including brain tumor, stroke, trauma, and infectious process	Subarachnoid hemorrhage

Abbreviation: SIADH, syndrome of inappropriate antidiuretic hormone.

Box 5.2 Clinical Alert: Hyponatremia

- Hyponatremia is associated with cerebral edema
- Patients with cerebral edema or those at risk for it may be maintained at a higher serum sodium level

---

Box 5.3 Conditions Associated with Hyponatremia

- Most disorders of the central nervous system, including
  - Cerebral trauma
  - Tumors
  - Strokes
  - Infectious processes (e.g., abscess, meningitis, and encephalitis)
- Pulmonary disease, including
  - Carcinoma
  - Chronic obstructive pulmonary disease
  - Pneumonia
- Some drugs, including
  - Anesthesia

○ Selective serotonin reuptake inhibitors (e.g., Paxil [paroxetine hydrochloride], Zoloft [sertraline hydrochloride], and Celexa [citalopram hydrobromide])
○ Some opiates
○ Carbamazepine (prescribed for epileptic patients or for those with nerve pain)

Syndrome of Inappropriate Antidiuretic Hormone

- Electrolyte imbalance caused by excessive ADH release from the pituitary gland
- Hyponatremia with high urine osmolality
- Can occur in hypervolemic patients (patients with elevated blood volume) or in normovolemic patients (patients with normal blood volume)
- Associated with intracranial trauma, abnormalities, or malignancies

Clinical Manifestations of Syndrome of Inappropriate Antidiuretic Hormone

- Confusion
- Lethargy
- Seizures
- Decreased level of consciousness (LOC)
- Cerebral edema and signs of increased ICP
- Signs of fluid overload
- Possible weight gain

Cerebral Salt Wasting

- Manifests as hyponatremia with hypovolemia (decreased blood volume)
- Associated with subarachnoid hemorrhage, with or without vasospasm

Clinical Manifestations of Cerebral Salt Wasting

- Confusion
- Lethargy
- Seizures
- Decreased LOC
- Cerebral edema and signs of increased ICP
- Possible orthostatic hypotension
- Possible weight loss
- Symptoms may range from vague to severe (Box 5.4 Hyponatremia)

Box 5.4 Hyponatremia

- In the presence of intracranial disease or trauma, even mild hyponatremia may cause symptoms
- Patients with chronic hyponatremia may not have symptoms right away

Treating Hyponatremia

- Treatments for SIADH and cerebral salt wasting differ significantly
- The cause of hyponatremia must be determined before initiating treatment
- Fluid restriction could be extremely harmful for a patient with cerebral salt wasting

Treating Syndrome of Inappropriate Antidiuretic Hormone

- The treatment of choice for SIADH is fluid restriction, especially the restriction of free water
- Salt supplements, including hyperosmolar saline solution, may also be effective

Treating Cerebral Salt Wasting

- Fluid replacement
- Salt tablets and hyperosmolar saline
- Fluid restriction is absolutely contraindicated because it could trigger vasospasm (Box 5.5 Clinical Alert: Correction of Hyponatremia)

Box 5.5 Clinical Alert: Correction of Hyponatremia

- Hyponatremia should be corrected cautiously; serum sodium level should not be increased more than 10 mEq/L in 24 hours
- Rapid correction could cause a rare but serious neurologic condition called *central pontine myelinolysis*, which has been indicated in cases of neurologic deterioration or death

---

5.2.3 Hypernatremia

Hypernatremia is a condition in which the patient's serum sodium level is too high. Most institutions diagnose hypernatremia as levels of serum sodium exceeding 150 mEq/L. In neurosurgical settings, hypernatremia is often associated with DI, which is caused by a deficiency of ADH.

Diabetes Insipidus

- Characterized by hypernatremia and low urine specific gravity
  - A urine specific gravity test measures the concentration of solutes in urine
  - The density of urine is compared to the density of water
- In patients with DI, the kidneys are unable to concentrate urine, resulting in a high output of dilute urine
- Associated thirst and dehydration
- Various potential causes
  - Most commonly results from decreased ADH secretion
  - Often occurs in conjunction with pituitary tumors due to altered pituitary function or traumatic brain injury; see also Chapter 7: Tumors (Box 5.6 Causes of Diabetes Insipidus)

Box 5.6 Causes of Diabetes Insipidus

- Impairment of the hypothalamic–hypophyseal portal system, which transports hormones from the hypothalamus to the anterior pituitary gland
- Primary or metastatic lesions in the sella turcica (i.e., pituitary tumors)
- Infections
- Vascular lesions (e.g., aneurysms in the anterior system and stroke)
- Trauma involving the sellar region
- Familial (hereditary)

Clinical Manifestations of Diabetes Insipidus

- Polydipsia (extreme thirst)
- Polyuria (high urine output, more than 300 mL/h for at least three consecutive hours)
- Low urine specific gravity (≤ 1.004)
- Dehydration (▶ Table 5.2).

Table 5.2 Characteristics of diabetes insipidus

Comparative factor	Diabetes insipidus
Serum sodium value	Greater than 150 mEq/L
Urine sodium value	Normal
Serum osmolality	Normal or increased
Urine osmolality	Increased
Urine specific gravity	Decreased (1.000–1.005)
Intravascular volume	Decreased
Treatment	Volume replacement with desmopressin acetate (DDAVP)
Associated neurologic disorders	Pituitary lesions and intracranial trauma

Table 5.3 Pharmacology for management of patients with electrolyte disorders

Treatment	Indication	Nursing implications
Salt supplement	Sodium supplement, SIADH, and cerebral salt wasting	Monitor sodium levels Never give on an empty stomach (may cause nausea) Document intake and output
Hyperosmolar saline	Sodium supplement, SIADH, and cerebral salt wasting	Assess sodium and serum osmolality (usually every 6 h) to ensure that levels are within acceptable reference range Ensure patency of IV access because solution is irritating to vein; large-bore IV or central line is best Monitor strict intake and output
Demeclocycline	ADH antagonist and SIADH	Document sodium levels and intake and output Contraindicated in patients with tetracycline allergies
Furosemide (Lasix)	Decreased fluid volume (the body loses more water than sodium, increasing urinary concentration of sodium) and SIADH	Monitor sodium levels Document intake and output
Desmopressin acetate (DDAVP)	Exogenous ADH and DI	Assess sodium and serum osmolality (usually every 6 h) Monitor strict intake and output Assess urine specific gravity

Abbreviations: ADH, antidiuretic hormone; DI, diabetes insipidus; IV, intravenous; SIADH, syndrome of inappropriate antidiuretic hormone.

Treating Diabetes Insipidus

- Fluid replacement
- Administration of ADH or exogenous ADH (▶ Table 5.3)

5.3 Other Common Electrolyte Imbalances

5.3.1 Calcium

- Normal range is 8.5 to 10.5 mg/dL
- Critical for regulation of neuromuscular conduction and blood coagulation
- Controlled by the parathyroid gland
- Hypocalcemia is associated with seizures, hypotension, and arrhythmias
- Hypercalcemia induces muscular weakness, confusion, and coma

5.3.2 Potassium

- Normal range is 3.5 to 5.0 mEq/L
- Necessary for protein and glucose synthesis
- Helps maintain cell membrane potential
- Potassium imbalance can cause cardiac arrhythmia

5.3.3 Magnesium

- Regulated by renal excretion
- Associated with regulation of vascular smooth muscle tone
- Increases the incidence of muscle twitching
- Increases the risk of seizure

5.4 Glucose

Although glucose is not an electrolyte, its balance in the blood is often affected after neurologic trauma or disease. It can be easily measured by a finger-stick glucose test. For patients with neurologic conditions, it is typically included in the metabolic work-up, which includes electrolyte levels. The normal glucose range is usually 70 to 150 mg/dL.

5.4.1 Hyperglycemia

Hyperglycemia is a condition in which the level of glucose in the blood is too high. In neurologically compromised patients, it can be associated with increased mortality and morbidity. It is diagnosed when the patient's blood glucose exceeds 150 mg/dL, and it is associated with

- Increased cerebral edema
- Increasing size of stroke (i.e., amount of brain affected); see Chapter 8:
  Vascular Disorders

5.4.2 Hypoglycemia

Hypoglycemia occurs when the level of glucose in the blood dips too low, usually less than 70 mg/dL.

- Can be detrimental to patients with neurologic injury or disease, because of associated cerebral hypoxia

5.5 Nursing Management for Patients with Electrolyte Imbalances

Electrolyte imbalances are common in neurosurgical patients. Their consequences may be mild, such as increased duration of hospitalization, but they can also be severe, including devastating neurologic compromise and death (▶ Table 5.4). A

Table 5.4 Electrolyte disturbances: what to watch for

Complication	Indication	Nursing action	Rationale
Confusion, decreased LOC, and seizures	Hyponatremia	Monitor laboratory values, especially serum sodium, serum osmolality, and urine sodium Check IV solution, if currently infusing (glucose solutions contraindicated) Administer salt supplements or hyperosmolar solutions as ordered Maintain fluid restriction if SIADH is suspected (contraindicated in cerebral salt wasting) Monitor strict intake and output Report new abnormal values	Hyponatremia may facilitate cerebral edema and increase ICP Fluid restriction (absolutely contraindicated) in patients with subarachnoid hemorrhage may exacerbate vasospasm May cause confusion and cerebral edema
	Hypoglycemia	Check blood glucose via fingerstick method or blood draw Administer D50 IV solution as ordered	Hypoglycemia or hyperglycemia may exacerbate cerebral edema and increase ICP
	Hyperglycemia	Monitor laboratory values Check blood glucose via fingerstick method or blood draw Administer insulin as directed	Hypoglycemia or hyperglycemia may exacerbate cerebral edema and increase ICP
Confusion, polydipsia, and polyuria	Diabetes insipidus	Monitor laboratory values, especially serum sodium and osmolality Check urine specific gravity Monitor strict intake and output Administer desmopressin acetate (DDAVP) as directed Report new abnormal test results or abnormal fluid balances as indicated	May cause confusion or cerebral edema if untreated

Abbreviations: D50, 50% dextrose solution; ICP, intracranial pressure; IV, intravenous; LOC, level of consciousness; SIADH, syndrome of inappropriate antidiuretic hormone.

more comprehensive guide on nursing management is presented in **Appendix A3: Nursing Management of Patients with Electrolyte Imbalances**.

This chapter is intended to be a basic reference for neuroscience nurses caring for patients with electrolyte disturbances. The references listed at the end of this chapter offer more information on how to provide the best care.

5.5.1 Neurologic Assessment

- Evaluate LOC; see also Chapter 2: Assessment
- Report any change in mental activity, including lethargy and confusion
- Deficits are rarely focal
- Watch for signs of increased ICP; see Chapter 3: Principles of Intracranial Pressure
- Note any changes in motor or sensory functions resulting from imbalanced calcium levels

5.5.2 Respiratory Assessment

- Perform an airway assessment
- Observe respiratory rate and rhythm
- Measure arterial blood gases, using an O_2 saturation monitor, if appropriate
- Results of respiratory assessment will be related to LOC

5.5.3 Cardiovascular Assessment

- Use hemodynamic monitoring
- Monitor electrocardiogram (ECG) for cardiac arrhythmias, especially if potassium levels are imbalanced
- Watch for signs of fluid overload or dehydration
- Results of cardiovascular assessment will be related to LOC

5.5.4 Fluid and Electrolyte Assessment

- Monitor levels of all electrolytes, especially sodium
- Monitor blood glucose level
- Report any new abnormal test results
- Measure urine specific gravity
- Administer medications as ordered
- Document accurate values for intake and output, including running totals
- Record the patient's weight daily
- Be aware of other medications and foods that the patient receives, as those may affect electrolyte levels (Box 5.7 Steroids and Glucose)

> ## Box 5.7 Steroids and Glucose
>
> • The use of steroids (dexamethasone) increases the glucose level

5.5.5 Seizures

• Administer medications, being mindful of drug interactions and levels, if indicated
• Safety

5.5.6 Patient and Family Teaching

• Teach the patient and family how to perform ongoing monitoring of electrolytes and inform them about diet and medications

5.5.7 Collaborative Management

• Nursing
• Neurosurgery
• Internal medicine
• Endocrine consult, especially for the management of sodium in patients with pituitary disorders or diabetes mellitus
• Dietary consult
• Diabetic education
• Case management or social work to facilitate home diabetic care

Suggested Reading

[1] Avanecean D, McNett MM, Villanueva NE. Neuroendocrine. In: Bader MK, Littlejohns LR, Olson DM, eds. AANN Core Curriculum for Neuroscience Nursing. 6th ed. Chicago, IL: American Association of Neuroscience Nurses; 2016, pp 217–228

[2] Chamberlain L. Hyponatremia caused by polydipsia. Crit Care Nurse. 2012; 32(3):e11–e20

[3] Greenberg MS. Handbook of Neurosurgery. 8th ed. New York, NY: Thieme Medical Publishers; 2016

[4] Hickey J. Clinical Practice of Neurological and Neurosurgical Nursing. 7th ed. Philadelphia: Lippincott Williams and Wilkins; 2013

[5] Keane M. Recognising and managing acute hyponatraemia. Emerg Nurse. 2014; 21(9):32–36, quiz 37

[6] McGrail A, Kelchner LN. Adequate oral fluid intake in hospitalized stroke patients: does viscosity matter? Rehabil Nurs. 2012; 37(5):252–257

[7] Mentes JC, Kang S. Hydration management. J Gerontol Nurs. 2013; 39(2):11–19

[8] Nelson JM, Robinson MV. Hyponatremia in older adults presenting to the emergency department. Int Emerg Nurs. 2012; 20(4):251–254

[9] Thomason C. Dehydration in stroke patients admitted to hospital. Nurs Times. 2012; 108(42):23

[10] Yuan W. Managing the patient with transsphenoidal pituitary tumor resection. J Neurosci Nurs. 2013; 45(2):101–107, quiz E1–E2

[11] Zygun DA, Steiner LA, Johnston AJ, et al. Hyperglycemia and brain tissue pH after traumatic brain injury. Neurosurgery. 2004; 55(4):877–881, discussion 882

6 Seizures

Madona Plueger

Abstract

Seizures are a complication that can arise in patients with neurologic conditions. There are many different types of seizures, and each type is associated with different presentations, symptoms, and treatment. Effective care for patients with seizures requires the health care team to know about different seizure types, their presentation, and their available treatments, which include pharmacologic and nonpharmacologic options, surgery, and specialty monitoring units.

Keywords: epilepsy, epilepsy monitoring unit, partial seizures, primary generalized seizures, psychogenic nonepileptic seizures, seizure semiology, status epilepticus

6.1 Seizures

A seizure is a single, temporary event that occurs when uncontrolled electrical neuronal discharges of the brain interrupt normal brain function. Seizures are a relatively common occurrence associated with most neurologic disorders, including tumors, trauma, and infectious processes such as meningitis. They may also occur with nonneurologic disorders, such as dehydration and other metabolic problems. Seizures can occur at any age, but they are most common in children and in people older than 60 years. The prevalence of seizures in the developed world is 0.5 to 1% (Box 6.1 Conditions Associated with Seizures).

In patients with epilepsy, seizures are spontaneous and may recur. Epilepsy may be idiopathic, or it can result from an underlying condition. It is one of the most common disorders of the central nervous system, affecting almost 2.9 million people in the United States alone. In 2010, the International League Against Epilepsy categorized epilepsy as a "disease." Individuals with epilepsy commonly face obstacles to appropriate health care, and epilepsy is often misunderstood by the public, which gives rise to stigma directed at persons with the condition.

- Neurodevelopmental abnormalities (e.g., cerebral palsy)
- Brain infections (e.g., meningitis, encephalitis, and abscess) from bacterial, viral, fungal, parasitic, or aseptic sources
- Cerebrovascular disorders (e.g., stroke—ischemic or hemorrhagic—and vascular malformation)
- Brain tumors
- Trauma
- Hypoxic insults
- Genetic and chromosomal abnormalities
- Alzheimer's disease
- Metabolic abnormalities (e.g., hyponatremia, hypoglycemia, and dehydration)
- Idiopathy

6.2 Types of Seizures

There are many different types of seizures, and a person who has epilepsy can have more than one type. Epilepsy is classified not only by seizure type (▶ Table 6.1) but also by other important distinguishing characteristics. These characteristics may include the following:

- Precipitating factors of the seizure
- Clinical features (e.g., behavior and type of movement)
- Abnormal brain wave recordings (e.g., spikes and sharp waves)
- Genetic features
- Expected course of the disorder
- Expected response to the treatment

6.2.1 Generalized Seizure

- The only type of seizure seen in idiopathic generalized epilepsy
  - Has a genetic component
  - Affects a younger population
  - Affects both cerebral hemispheres
  - Results in loss of consciousness
  - Symptoms include
    - Blank stare
    - Falling to the floor
    - Sudden muscle jerking
    - Repetitive stiffening and relaxing of muscles

Table 6.1 Types of epilepsy

Type	Partial[a]	Features	Generalized[a]	Features
Idiopathic (genetic)	Benign focal epilepsy of childhood	Seizures are infrequent and usually nocturnal; usually only span 1–3 y after onset	Childhood absence epilepsy (also called *pyknolepsy*)	Seizures occur several times a day; girls are more frequently affected than boys
			Juvenile myoclonic epilepsy (also called *Janz's syndrome*)	Occurs in the morning or in cases of stress or fatigue. No associated mental decline
			Epilepsy with seizures that occur on awakening	Grand mal seizures
Symptomatic (known cause)	Temporal lobe epilepsy	Accounts for 60% of all epilepsy cases; auras are common	West's syndrome	Infantile spasms
	Frontal lobe epilepsy	Brief recurring seizures that often occur while the patient is asleep	Lennox–Gastaut syndrome	Atypical absence epilepsy
Cryptogenic (unknown cause)				

[a]These lists are not definitive and include only the most common types of epilepsy.

Secondarily generalized seizures, which are partial seizures that include loss of consciousness, are particularly common.

6.2.2 Partial Seizure

- Affects a specific area of one cerebral hemisphere
- May evolve into prolonged seizures
- Results from structural disruption in a specific part of the brain (type of symptoms indicate which area of the brain is affected)

- May evolve into a condition called *status epilepticus*, or repeated (i.e., continuous) epileptic seizures, in which the patient does not regain consciousness between episodes

Simple Partial Seizure

- This brief sensation of abnormality is also called an *aura*; it can, but does not necessarily, progress to a more serious seizure
- Does not result in loss of consciousness
- Depending on the part of the brain in which the seizure originates, simple partial seizures may include
  - Motor symptoms (e.g., muscle stiffening or jerking on one or both sides of the body)
  - Visual, auditory, olfactory, and gustatory abnormalities
  - Vertiginous sensation
  - Effects of autonomic involvement (e.g., pallor, sweating, flushing, pupil dilation, and abnormal epigastric sensation)

Complex Partial Seizure

A complex partial seizure usually starts in the temporal or frontal lobe of the brain before spreading to other areas of the brain. It may begin with motor impairment and typically culminates in impaired awareness. This type of seizure may be preceded by an aura. Common characteristics include

- Loss of consciousness and several minutes of unresponsiveness
- Blank stare and impaired awareness (e.g., confusion and unfocused mental state)
- Unusual sensations (e.g., memory flashbacks, depersonalization of surroundings, a reported "out-of-body" experience, visual or auditory distortions, and strong emotional responses, such as rage, terror, elation, and sadness)
- Automatisms (e.g., smacking of lips, chewing, picking up objects, walking aimlessly, disrobing in public, and repeating words and phrases)
- Poor safety awareness (e.g., unaware of the dangers of traffic, fire, or heights)

The period of time after a seizure is referred to as the *postictal period*. After a complex partial seizure, the patient may experience confusion and may not even remember the event.

Psychogenic Nonepileptic Seizure

A psychogenic nonepileptic seizure is an involuntary seizure triggered by stress that often occurs without evidence of psychopathology. In other words, the patient may show signs of having had a seizure, but there is no evidence of abnormal activity in the brain. Sometimes, it is referred to as a *pseudoseizure*, but this term should be avoided because it implies that the seizure is feigned and the patient is malingering for secondary gain. Psychogenic nonepileptic seizures may mask actual undiagnosed disorders, such as

- Anxiety disorders
- Posttraumatic stress disorder
- Conversion disorder
- Psychosis
- Somatization disorders
- Reinforced behavior patterns (in cognitively impaired patients)

Nonepileptic Seizures of Physiologic Origin

- Metabolic abnormalities
- Cardiac dysfunction
- Movement disorders
- Migraines
- Side effects of drugs

Seizure Semiology

Seizure semiology is a way to describe the clinical manifestations (i.e., symptoms) of a seizure. It can help the care team understand more about the seizure by determining the location of its focus, that is, the area of the brain from which the seizure originated (▶ Fig. 6.1 and ▶ Table 6.2).

6.2.3 Diagnosing Epilepsy

History

A thorough history of the patient's past experience with seizures is critical to help diagnose epilepsy (Box 6.2 International League Against Epilepsy 2014 Diagnostic Criteria). This history should include

- Types of seizures
- Frequency of seizures
- Age of patient at first seizure
- Family history of seizures
- Precipitating events
- Antiepileptic drug (AED) usage

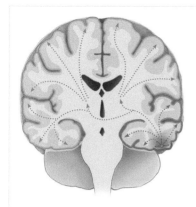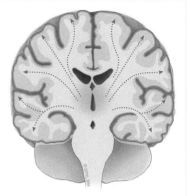

Partial onset (75%)

Simple partial
Complex partial
Secondary generalized

Generalized from onset (25%)

Absence, Myoclonic,
Tonic, Clonic,
Tonic-clonic, Atonic

Fig. 6.1 Seizure semiology.

Table 6.2 Seizure semiology

Location of seizure	Clinical manifestation
Dominant hemisphere	Delayed recovery of language and transient aphasia
Frontal lobe	Occurs without warning, while the patient is sleeping Restlessness or bilateral limb movements
Parietal lobe	Least common May have sensory aura May mimic characteristics of frontal lobe seizures Often occurs in patients with vascular malformations and cortical dysplasia Patients usually respond well to surgical therapy
Temporal lobe	Auras accompany approximately 80% of temporal lobe seizures Auras may be classified by symptom type (i.e., somatosensory, special sensory, autonomic, or psychic symptoms)
Occipital lobe	Occurs with visual aura Electrical spread may cause seizure to progress to a seizure with the characteristics of a temporal or frontal lobe seizure

- A person is considered to have epilepsy if any of the following criteria are met:
  - At least two unprovoked seizures occurring more than 24 hours apart
  - One unprovoked seizure and a probability of additional seizures
  - Diagnosis of an epilepsy syndrome
- Epilepsy is considered to be resolved for persons who have been free of seizures for 10 years and who have not been taking AEDs for the last 5 years

Imaging Studies and Noninvasive Diagnostic Tests

The imaging studies and noninvasive diagnostic tests described in the following sections can help physicians determine the type and focus of seizures that the patient is having, so that they can diagnose or rule out epilepsy (▶ Table 6.3).

Imaging Studies

- Magnetic resonance imaging (MRI)
  - Identifies structural lesions or areas of sclerosis to locate seizure focus
- Positron emission tomography scan
  - Identifies areas of hypometabolism to identify seizure focus
- Ictal single-photon emission computed tomography
  - Radioactive tracer injected intravenously (IV) during a seizure helps locate the focus of the seizure by tracking blood flow in the brain

Other Diagnostic Tests

- Electroencephalogram (EEG)
  - Noninvasive; records 20 minutes of brain wave activity (▶ Table 6.4)
  - Lateralization (determining whether the seizure originates from the left or the right hemisphere) and localization (identifying the focus within a specific region of one hemisphere) begin with standard scalp EEG recordings
  - The presence of interictal (between seizures) epileptiform discharges (sharp waves or spikes) in a single location is highly suggestive of the onset of seizure in that region
  - Ictal scalp EEGs during complex partial or secondarily generalized seizures usually show a lateralized rhythmic discharge that increases in frequency and amplitude as it spreads to the postictal stage and that varies in location

Table 6.3 Diagnostic testing for seizures

Diagnostic test	Testing procedure	Expected findings	Nursing implications
EEG	Electrodes are applied to the scalp with a thick paste and can be removed by washing after the EEG is completed The EEG takes about 1 h	Seizure/epileptiform activity	Procedure should be carefully explained, stressing the importance of the patient's cooperation Certain food, fluids, and medications (including AEDs) may stimulate or depress brain waves and therefore should be withheld
MRI	Magnetic field and radio frequency pulses show internal body structures, including organs and soft tissue	Structural lesion, which may be seizure focus	Monitors, telemetry units, nerve stimulators, or IV pumps cannot be present in the MRI suite
PET	Patient must lie still during the procedure Patient will receive an injection of radioactive glucose, which will take approximately 45 min to distribute throughout the body	Areas of hypometabolism, which may be seizure focus	Diabetic patients must have insulin doses adjusted
Ictal SPECT	Radioactive tracer injected into the patient IV during a seizure tracks the blood flow in the brain	Radioactive tracer will help identify seizure focus	Not commonly used
Brain mapping	Electrodes placed directly on the brain help care team map brain activity	Mapping may reveal the area of the brain from which the seizure originates	Patient is likely in an EMU
Depth wires (depth electrodes)	Stereotactically placed through burr holes, usually for suspected medial temporal lobe epilepsy	Electrodes may reveal the area of the brain from which the seizure originates	Patient must be in an EMU Surgical procedure

Table 6.3 (*continued*)

Diagnostic test	Testing procedure	Expected findings	Nursing implications
Wada test	Neuroradiologist puts one side of the brain to sleep for a short period by injecting an anesthetic into the internal carotid artery to confirm that the injected side of the brain is asleep EEG recordings are done at the same time	Determines hemisphere dominance and localizes speech and motor centers	Cerebral angiography is done before Wada testing
Subdural electrodes	Craniotomy must be done to place electrodes on the brain	Electrodes may reveal the area of the brain from which the seizure originates	Patient must be in an EMU after initial stay in an intensive care unit
Video EEG monitoring	Continuous EEG with concurrent video camera monitoring to observe the patient's behavior when the seizures occur	Patient's behavior during seizure may reveal the type of seizure being experienced	Patient must be in an EMU

Abbreviations: AED, antiepileptic drug; EEG, electroencephalogram; EMU, epilepsy monitoring unit; IV, intravenously; MRI, magnetic resonance imaging; PET, positron emission tomography; SPECT, single-photon emission computed tomography.

Table 6.4 Brain waves seen on electroencephalogram

Wave type	Hertz range	Location	Normal	Pathologic
Delta	0–4 Hz	Frontal lobe	Slow-wave sleep in adults	Diffuse lesions Metabolic encephalopathy Hydrocephalus
Theta	4–7 Hz	Both sides symmetrical if normal or focal if abnormal	Normal drowsiness	Posterior dominant rhythm in awake adult Metabolic encephalopathy or deep midline disorders
Alpha	7–14 Hz	Posterior region of head on both sides; amplitude is higher on dominant side	Relaxed or reflecting, closing the eyes	Coma
Beta	15–30 Hz	Both sides, symmetrical distribution, most evident frontally; low-amplitude waves	Alert or working Active, busy, or anxious thinking and active concentration	Absent in patients with cortical damage Benzodiazepine use

Abbreviation: Hz, hertz.

133

- Two forms of provocative tests are used during a standard EEG
  - Hyperventilation: In this test, patients are asked to hyperventilate for 3 to 5 minutes; this lowers the level of intracerebral carbon dioxide and elicits epileptic and other abnormal neuronal activity
  - Photic stimulation: In this test, a strobe light is used to trigger a convulsion; the light elicits epileptic activity in 5% of patients with epilepsy
  - The EEG may not capture seizure activity, unless it is being recorded during the seizure
  - Simple partial seizures, including auras, often do not appear on scalp EEG studies
- EEG–video monitoring
  - Cornerstone of epilepsy surgery evaluation; involves continuous EEG with concurrent video camera monitoring to observe the patient's behavior when the seizures occur
  - Patients undergoing this type of testing are transferred to an epilepsy monitoring unit (EMU) until they have a typical seizure spell
  - AEDs are often withheld to elicit spells more quickly
  - EEG–video monitoring can confirm whether the patient's spells are in fact epileptic
  - Roughly 25% of patients who are referred to an EMU for an epilepsy presurgical evaluation do not have epileptic seizures (most have psychogenic nonepileptic seizures)
- Wada test
  - Helps establish which hemisphere houses language and memory centers
  - During this test, the conscious patient undergoes a cerebral angiogram after unilateral injection of amybarbital into the internal carotid artery; amybarbital anesthetizes the entire contralateral hemisphere of the brain
  - The patient is asked to remember various words
  - Language is tested by recording the patient's ability to speak after injection (the patient is unable to speak or understand language when the language-dominant hemisphere has been anesthetized)
  - Memory is tested by asking the patient to recall the words after the effect of the anesthetic wears off

Invasive Diagnostic Procedures and Invasive Monitoring

Patients for whom medical treatment has failed are usually candidates for epilepsy surgery. For these procedures, as described in the following sections, electrodes are placed directly on or in the brain during a presurgical evaluation to ensure accurate localization of the seizure focus. The two most common types of electrodes are depth electrodes and subdural electrodes.

Depth Electrodes

- A cable with cylindrical contacts along its distal end, primarily used in cases of suspected medial temporal lobe epilepsy
- Placed in hippocampus and amygdala for medial temporal lobe epilepsy; see also Chapter 1: Anatomy
- Stereotactically placed through burr holes in the skull; see also Chapter 15: Neurosurgical Interventions
- May be used in combination with subdural strip electrodes, described in the following section

Subdural Electrodes

- A platinum or stainless steel disk embedded in a thin plastic cover
- Can be used to record the area of seizure onset and to perform extraoperative stimulation mapping of cortical function in underlying brain tissue
- Records activity from the surface of the brain
- Most commonly used in neocortical epilepsy or suspected medial temporal lobe epilepsy to delineate the region of seizure onset (▶ Fig. 6.2 and ▶ Fig. 6.3)
- Requires a craniotomy for placement

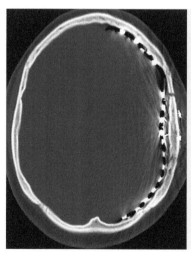

Fig. 6.2 Axial computed tomogram showing subdural electrodes.

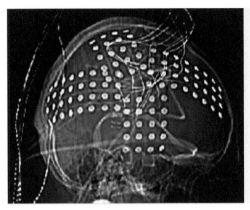

Fig. 6.3 Sagittal computed tomogram showing subdural electrodes.

Brain Mapping

- This procedure may be done with the patient awake
- A grid is placed on the surface of brain, and various areas of the brain are electrically stimulated through the contacts of the grid
- Neurologic assessment of the patient during this stimulation helps determine the function of different areas of the brain under the grid; this allows the surgeon to determine the safety of resecting specific areas of the brain (► Fig. 6.4 and ► Table 6.5)

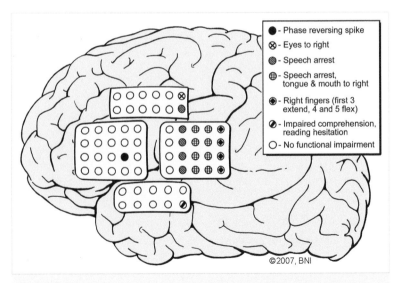

- Phase reversing spike
- Eyes to right
- Speech arrest
- Speech arrest, tongue & mouth to right
- Right fingers (first 3 extend, 4 and 5 flex)
- Impaired comprehension, reading hesitation
- No functional impairment

©2007, BNI

Fig. 6.4 Brain mapping.

Table 6.5 Advantages and disadvantages of invasive monitoring techniques

Type of device	Advantages	Disadvantages	Complications
Depth wires	Require small burr holes; no craniotomy needed Lower complication rate Offer snapshot of different, distinct areas of brain Identify the specific region of the brain where seizures originate	Not useful in patients whose seizures originate from eloquent areas Do not facilitate "tailored" resections Not used for stimulation to map critical areas	Infection Pain Pneumonia Deep vein thrombosis Bleeding Swelling
Strips or grids	Smooth silicone and plastic surface embedded with electrodes Different designs are available Can stimulate the brain and record its activity Placed directly on the surface of the brain Essential when no lesion is evident	Require open craniotomy for insertion and removal Postoperative swelling increases complication rate Damage to vital structures is possible in postlesionectomy patients Infection is more likely with this type of device	Infection Pain Pneumonia Deep vein thrombosis Bleeding Swelling Accidental removal of grids or strips

6.2.4 Treatment of Seizures

Medical Management

- AEDs may be prescribed; however, if a patient has only had one seizure, he or she may not be prescribed an AED (▶ Table 6.6)
- Patients may be kept under observation on an EMU (Box 6.3 Focus on Epilepsy Monitoring Units)

Table 6.6 Pharmacology for management of epilepsy

Drug/dosage	Type of seizure	Side effects	Nursing implications
Dilantin (phenytoin) 300–600 mg/d	Partial Generalized	Sedation Gingival hypertrophy Rash Nausea Confusion Nervousness Slurred speech Decreased coordination	Monitor patient for allergic reaction IV phenytoin or fosphenytoin may be effective in treating status epilepticus IV phenytoin must be given slowly, through large-bore catheter Monitor patient's drug levels during seizure episodes Toxicity indicated by lethargy, nystagmus, and ataxia
Tegretol (carbamazepine) 600–1,200 mg/d, divided doses	Partial Not used for absence seizures (i.e., brief lapses of consciousness)	Sedation Dizziness Nausea Blurred vision Nystagmus	Should be taken with food Avoid generic versions of this drug in patients who have intractable seizures; older AEDs (i.e., Dilantin, Tegretol, and Depakote) alter metabolism and can alter drug levels, affecting seizure threshold May lower serum sodium levels
Luminal (phenobarbital) 60–250 mg/d, divided or single dose	Partial Generalized	Sedation May cause difficulty with memory or cognition May exacerbate depression	Do not discontinue abruptly because this may increase the frequency of seizures
Depakote (valproic acid or divalproex sodium) 15–60 mg/kg/d, divided doses	Generalized	Tremor Weight gain	May increase phenytoin levels Monitor patient's drug levels during seizure episodes
Lamictal (lamotrigine) 300–500 mg/d	Partial Generalized	Rash Headache Dizziness Blurred vision	Risk of rash is higher in patients who are also taking valproic acid Dosage titrated to effect, not to blood level

Table 6.6 (continued)

Drug/dosage	Type of seizure	Side effects	Nursing implications
Neurontin (gabapentin) 900–3,600 mg/d, divided doses	Partial	Sedation Dizziness Ataxia Decreased coordination Nystagmus	Should not be taken within 2 h of taking antacid May also be used for neuropathic pain
Topamax (topiramate) 200–400 mg/d	Partial, as adjunct therapy	Sedation Mood disturbances Possible weight loss Kidney stones in male patients Psychomotor slowing Vision problems Decreased coordination	Patients should increase fluid intake; start low and slowly increase with titration May decrease estrogen levels in female patients on oral contraceptives and may cause menstrual changes or menstrual pain
Felbatol (felbamate) 600–3,600 mg/d	Partial Generalized	Insomnia Weight loss Aplastic anemia and hepatic failure in severe cases Chest pain Confusion	Multiple adverse drug interactions with other AEDs Monitor complete blood cell count and obtain liver function tests
Zonegran (zonisamide) 100–400 mg/d, divided or single dose	Partial, as adjunct therapy	Sedation Anorexia Irritability Kidney stones Depression	May be contraindicated in patients with sensitivity to sulfonamides

Table 6.6 (continued)

Drug/dosage	Type of seizure	Side effects	Nursing implications
Keppra (levetiracetam) 1,000–3,000 mg/d, divided dose	Partial	Sedation Behavioral abnormalities	Associated with increased upper respiratory infections
Vimpat (lacosamide) 10–400 mg/d, divided dose	Partial, as adjunct therapy in patients older than 17 y	Dizziness Headache Diplopia Shakiness	Metabolized in the kidneys
Fycompa (perampanel) Start at 2 or 4 mg/d, depending on other AEDs being taken	Partial	Blurred vision Balance problems Aggression or anger	May cause serious behavioral or psychiatric reactions, so close monitoring during titration is absolutely essential
Aptiom (eslicarbazepine) 400–800 mg/d	Partial	Dizziness Drowsiness Double vision Fatigue Loss of coordination Nausea Vomiting	Be aware of potential interactions with older AEDs Contraindicated in patients who are taking oxcarbazepine

Abbreviation: AED, antiepileptic drug; IV, intravenous.

Box 6.3 Focus on Epilepsy Monitoring Units

What is an epilepsy monitoring unit?

An EMU is a hospital unit or area that specializes in caring for patients with epilepsy. In an EMU, seizure identification and diagnosis are managed by a group of professionals who are specially trained to identify, diagnose, and manage epilepsy.

Purpose

The health care team in an EMU can assist with
- Proper diagnosis of epilepsy through seizure induction
- Identification of seizure focus
- Treatment recommendations

Phase 1
- Video and EEG recordings are performed to exclude nonepileptic spells
- Distinguish between generalized-onset epilepsy and localization-related epilepsy
- Confirm appropriateness of vagal nerve stimulation for patients who cannot undergo surgical resection

Phase 2
- Patient returns to the EMU for monitoring with intracranial electrodes
- Depth electrodes, placed through burr holes, extend into mesial structures such as the hippocampus and amygdala

Patients should proceed directly to surgery if
- Phase 1 monitoring indicates that seizure focus is at the site of a radiographically identified lesion
- Neuropsychologic testing, including the Wada test, indicates that surgical resection will not result in unacceptable disability

Staff of an epilepsy monitoring unit includes
- Nurses trained in clinical recognition of seizure presentation and EEG recognition
- EEG technicians
- Physicians specially trained in epilepsy management

Staffing needs depend on
- Number of EMU beds
- Procedures performed (i.e., invasive diagnostic tests)
- Level of observation available (e.g., video monitoring)
- Training and expertise of staff

Nursing in an epilepsy monitoring unit

Nurses in an EMU must be skilled in the following aspects of seizure management

- Medication management
- Basic seizure first aid
- Emergency seizure management, including methods of seizure abortion, use of rescue seizure medications, and seizure recognition and reporting
- Ongoing training in epilepsy and seizure management

Surgical Intervention

Surgery is considered only when all other treatment options have failed to resolve the patient's symptoms of epilepsy. There are two main categories of surgery for the treatment of epilepsy: resective and palliative.

Resective Surgery

The goal of resective surgery is to cure patients of epilepsy. Types of resective surgery include the following

- Selective amygdalohippocampectomy
  - ○ Removal of the hippocampus, which is a region of the brain responsible for memory, spatial awareness, and navigation, and removal of the amygdala, which helps regulate the processing and memory of emotional reactions (▶ Fig. 6.5). Both structures are part of the limbic system; see also Chapter 1: Anatomy
- Hemispherectomy
  - ○ Resection of one cerebral hemisphere (▶ Fig. 6.6)
  - ○ A hemispherectomy is performed when seizures affect most or all of one cerebral hemisphere

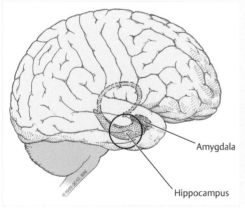

Fig. 6.5 Selective amygdalohippocampectomy.

Amygdala

Hippocampus

○ Severe seizures that necessitate hemispherectomy usually also severely damage the involved hemisphere early in the individual's development and have likely already imparted severe clinical impairment such as contralateral hemiparesis or hemianopsia. Therefore, hemispherectomy does not worsen the patient's deficits or introduce new deficits

• Anterior temporal lobectomy
  ○ An anterior temporal lobectomy is used to treat medial temporal lobe epilepsy (▶ Fig. 6.7 and Box 6.4 Medical Temporal Sclerosis)

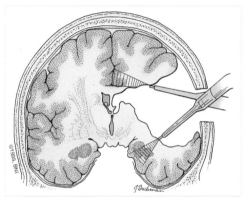

Fig. 6.6 Hemispherectomy.

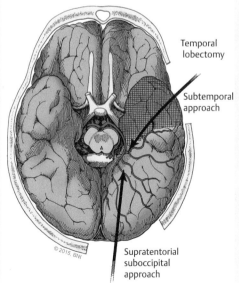

Fig. 6.7 Anterior temporal lobectomy.

Temporal lobectomy

Subtemporal approach

Supratentorial suboccipital approach

- Lesionectomy
  - In a lesionectomy, structural brain lesions are surgically resected. These usually include medial temporal sclerosis, low-grade neoplasms, vascular malformations, and malformations of cortical development

---

Box 6.4 Medial Temporal Sclerosis

- Medial temporal sclerosis is the pathologic hallmark of medial temporal lobe epilepsy
- It involves the loss of neurons and scarring of the deepest portion of the temporal lobe and is associated with certain brain injuries
- Brain damage from traumatic injury, infection, tumor, insufficient oxygen supply to the brain, or uncontrolled seizures is thought to lead to the formation of scar tissue, particularly in the hippocampus

---

Palliative Surgery

The aim of palliative surgery is to reduce the frequency of seizures, not necessarily to cure them. Types of palliative surgery include the following:

- Vagal nerve stimulators
  - A wire placed beneath the skin is attached to the left vagal nerve in the neck and is linked to an electrical stimulator (▶ Fig. 6.8)
  - The stimulator produces regular pulses of electrical signals, which can reduce the intensity or duration of seizures over time in some patients
  - Most patients do not become free of seizures after implantation of a vagal nerve stimulator
- Corpus callosotomy
  - Surgical procedure that disrupts the nerve fibers of the corpus callosum, which is the band of tissue that allows the hemispheres of the brain to communicate with one another (▶ Fig. 6.9)
  - The goal of corpus callosotomy is to keep each side of the brain from transmitting messages to the other and to thwart the spread of seizures
  - This procedure is typically used to treat atonic (i.e., drop) seizures, which involve a loss of muscle control and are associated with a high risk of injury
  - Corpus callosotomy is indicated in patients whose seizures affect most or all of one hemisphere

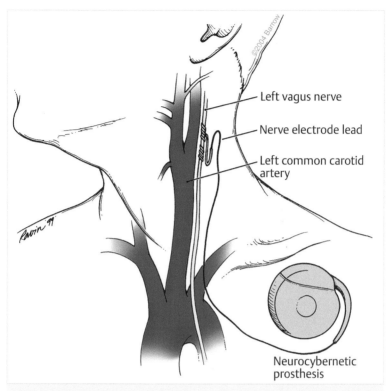

Left vagus nerve

Nerve electrode lead

Left common carotid artery

Neurocybernetic prosthesis

Fig. 6.8 Vagal nerve stimulator.

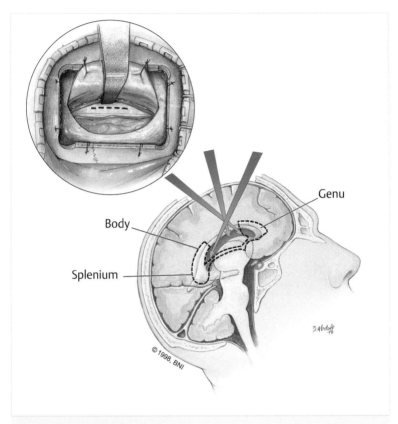

Fig. 6.9 Corpus callosotomy.

6.3 Special Considerations

6.3.1 Status Epilepticus

Status epilepticus, or repeated seizures exceeding 5 minutes in duration without recovery of consciousness between episodes, is dangerous and constitutes a medical emergency (Box 6.5 Medical Emergency: Status Epilepticus).

Box 6.5 Medical Emergency: Status Epilepticus

- A patient in status epilepticus requires immediate intervention to preserve neurologic function
- Status epilepticus refers to repeated seizures exceeding 5 minutes in duration without recovery of consciousness between episodes
- The first priority of the health care team should be to abort the seizure

---

Generalized Convulsive Status Epilepticus

- Generalized convulsive status epilepticus (GCSE) (tonic–clonic seizure, formerly known as grand mal seizure) is a continuous seizure that lasts longer than 30 minutes or two consecutive seizures without consciousness being regained between episodes
- Half of hospital-reported cases of GCSE have been associated with subtherapeutic levels of AEDs
- Intervention begins with the ABCs—airway, breathing, and circulation management, followed by preventive measures to protect neurologic function and to avoid multisystem organ failure
- Guidelines on treating convulsive status epilepticus were published in 1993
- In the United States alone, status epilepticus is responsible for nearly 45,000 deaths annually

Nonconvulsive Status Epilepticus

- Mixed disorder with several different subcategories
- Nonconvulsive status epilepticus (NCSE), defined as a mental status change lasting at least 30 to 60 minutes, is a medical emergency
- Nonconvulsive status epilepticus is most commonly associated with partial seizures and may cause neuronal damage
- Patients with disorders involving metabolism, coma, and brain lesions can develop NCSE
- Nonconvulsive status epilepticus is diagnosed by EEG and can be fatal if not promptly diagnosed and treated (Box 6.6 Emergency Management of Status Epilepticus)

Box 6.6 Emergency Management of Status Epilepticus

At zero minutes

- Initiate general systemic support of airway (insert nasal airway or intubate, if needed).
  - Check blood pressure
  - Begin nasal oxygen
  - Monitor heart rate and respiration
  - Check temperature frequently
- Obtain medical history
- Perform neurologic examination
- Send blood sample for evaluation of electrolytes, blood urea nitrogen, glucose level, complete blood cell count, toxic drug screen, and anticonvulsant levels; check arterial blood gas values
- Start IV line containing isotonic saline at a low infusion rate
- Inject 50 mL of 50% glucose IV and 100 mg of thiamine IV or intramuscularly (IM)
- Call EEG laboratory to start recording as soon as feasible
- Administer lorazepam (Ativan) at 0.1 to 0.15 mg/kg IV (2 mg/min); if seizures persist, administer fosphenytoin (Cerebyx) at 18 mg/kg IV (150 mg/min, with an additional 7 mg/kg if seizures continue)

At 20 to 30 minutes, if seizures persist

- Intubate, insert bladder catheter, start EEG recording, and check temperature
- Administer phenobarbital in a loading dose of 20 mg/kg IV (100 mg/min)

At 40 to 60 minutes, if seizures persist

- Begin pentobarbital infusion at 5 mg/kg IV initial dose, then IV push until seizures stop, using EEG monitoring. Continue pentobarbital infusion at 1 mg/kg/h; slow infusion rate every 4 to 6 hours to determine if seizures have stopped, with EEG guidance; carefully monitor blood pressure and respiration.
- Support blood pressure
  - With vasopressors, if needed, or
  - Begin midazolam (Versed) at 0.2 mg/kg and then at a dosage of 0.75 to 10 mg/kg/min, titrated to EEG monitoring, or
  - Begin propofol (Diprivan) at 1 to 2 mg/kg loading dose, followed by 2 to 10 mg/kg/h
- Adjust maintenance dosage on tolerance of fosphenytoin and phenytoin

6.3.2 Barbiturate Coma

Barbiturate coma can be used to treat refractory status epilepticus, GCSE, or NCSE; see also Chapter 3: Principles of Intracranial Pressure.

6.3.3 Sudden Unexpected Death in Epilepsy

Sudden unexpected death in epilepsy, called *SUDEP*, is a term used when a person with epilepsy suddenly dies and the actual cause of death is unknown. In order for a death to be classified as SUDEP, it must meet the following criteria:
- Unrelated to injury or drowning during or after a seizure
- Unrelated to a prolonged or severe seizure (status epilepticus)
- No other abnormality is found on autopsy to account for death

Sudden unexpected death in epilepsy is most common in people with generalized tonic–clonic seizures, especially young adults. The most significant risk factors seem to be poor seizure control or seizures during sleep in people with frequent and severe tonic–clonic seizures. It is rare in new-onset epilepsy and in epilepsy in remission. Some authors have theorized that the reason for death in SUDEP cases is that the seizure affects the part of the brain that controls the function of the heart or respiration, causing cardiac or respiratory cessation. Most people with epilepsy have a normal life span and do not die of SUDEP.

6.4 Nursing Management for Patients with Seizures

Caring for patients with seizures or epilepsy requires meticulous attention to detail and sharp observational skills (▶ Table 6.7 **and Appendix A4: Nursing Management of Patients with Seizures or Epilepsy**). This chapter is intended to be a basic reference for bedside care of patients with seizures. The reader is urged to consult the references included at the end of the chapter to find out more about points of interest.

6.4.1 Neurologic Assessment

- Evaluate level of consciousness; see also Chapter 2: Assessment
- Document the patient's seizure history
- Perform seizure assessment as needed (Box 6.7 Nursing Assessment of Seizure Event)

Table 6.7 Nursing management for patients with seizures

Nursing goal	Rationale and nursing implications
Safety	
Assess patient to ensure an adequate airway and to make sure that the cause of the seizure is not cardiac in nature (e.g., asystole)	Start with ABC (airway, breathing, and circulation)
Place something under the patient's head and loosen restrictive clothing or bed linens	Protect the patient from being harmed by the surrounding environment
Do not restrain the patient or place anything between their teeth	Trying to restrain the patient can harm them, and placing something between their teeth can result in tooth damage
Turn patient on his or her side to allow drainage of secretions	Prevent aspiration
Assessment	
Perform assessment of the seizure event (**Box 6.7: Nursing Assessment of Seizure Event**)	Nursing observations during the event are important to treat the patient appropriately
Check and record vital signs and neurologic status	Proper documentation will help you identify patterns in symptoms or seizure events
AEDs	
A comprehensive medical history should include information on the patient's AEDs and their dosage	Many AEDs have significant interactions with other drugs and foods
Be aware of drug levels	Drug may be ineffective if the dosage is subtherapeutic
Drug toxicity may also occur, which can trigger dangerous medical difficulties
Be mindful of the common side effects associated with AEDs, including allergies	Side effects of AEDs may be problematic to the patient and may require a change in medication
Some allergic reactions can lead to serious, even fatal medical complications
Patient and family teaching	
Teach patients and families about seizure safety (described above)
Ensure that patients and families understand the dosage, side effects, and drug or food interactions of their prescribed AEDs
Give patients and families the information about the legality of driving while taking AEDs	Educating patients and their families on their care after they leave the hospital is a critical step in ensuring your patient's continued health and safety
Prevention	
Provide patients and families with the information on strategies to reduce the possibility or frequency of seizures	Many seizures can be prevented by compliance with prescribed AEDs

Abbreviation: AEDs, antiepileptic drugs.

Box 6.7 Nursing Assessment of Seizure Event

- Was the seizure witnessed? If so, by whom?
- Was there a precipitating event?
- Was the patient responsive?
- In which body part did the seizure start? Did it progress to other areas of the body?
- What type of movement was involved?
- Were there pupillary changes?
- Was there gaze deviation? If so, in which direction?
- Was there bowel or bladder incontinence?
- What was the patient's mental status?
- How long did the seizure last?
- What was the patient's mental status after the seizure?
- Was there any motor weakness after the seizure?
- Was any medication given to the patient (e.g., lorazepam)? If so, what, when, and how much?

6.4.2 Respiratory Assessment

- Protect the airway during seizure events

6.4.3 Cardiovascular Assessment

- A history of cardiovascular disease may precipitate seizure
- Understand risk factors and comorbidities of cardiac disease
- Seizures may result from poor cerebral perfusion and lower seizure threshold

6.4.4 Safety

- Patients need comprehensive instructions and training on how to safely deal with seizures if they occur at home
- Advise the patient that slight changes at home and small modifications to daily activity will keep the patient safe in the event of a seizure at home

6.4.5 Patient and Family Teaching

- Discuss the appropriate safety precautions to keep the patient out of harm's way when a seizure occurs
- Provide an overview of the pharmacologic treatment, with detailed instructions for all prescribed medications, including dosage, side effects, drug interactions, and half-life of drugs

- Review discharge instructions and safety at home (**Appendix B2: Sample Discharge Instructions After Observation or Treatment in the Epilepsy Monitoring Unit, Appendix B3: Sample Discharge Instructions After Craniotomy for Treatment of Epilepsy, and Appendix B4: Sample Handout with Seizure Information and Safety Instructions**)
- Explain different types of seizures
- Differentiate between standard patient floor and EMU
- Effects of craniotomy for the treatment of epilepsy

6.4.6 Collaborative Management

Although every institution is different, treating patients with epilepsy often requires collaboration from many different health care specialties (Box 6.8 Epilepsy Management). These specialties may include

- Nursing
- Neurology or epileptology, for seizure and AED management
- Neuropsychology, to help anticipate any postoperative deficits that the patient may encounter
- Neurosurgery, for patients in which surgery is indicated
- Pharmacy, to offer dosing service for phenytoin, if appropriate

---

Box 6.8 Epilepsy Management

- Determine pathology
- Etiology: infectious, autoimmune, metabolic, or related to drugs or alcohol
- Optimize seizure control as promptly as possible to prevent SUDEP
- Reevaluate epilepsy diagnosis and treatment if AEDs fail or if generalized seizures are frequent despite the use of AEDs; consider epilepsy surgery as an alternative
- Maximize compliance with AEDs
- Use the least number of AEDs needed to control seizures
- Add an AED with the goal of replacing the current AED in a timely fashion
- Educate patients and families and help them understand what to expect

---

Suggested Reading

[1] Berg AT, Berkovic SF, Brodie MJ, et al. Revised terminology and concepts for organization of seizures and epilepsies: report of the ILAE Commission on Classification and Terminology, 2005–2009. Epilepsia. 2010; 51(4):676–685

[2] Center for Disease Control and Prevention. Epilepsy fast facts. 2016; http://www.cdc.gov/epilepsy/basics/fast-facts.htm. Accessed June 16, 2017

[3] DeLorenzo RJ, Hauser WA, Towne AR, et al. A prospective, population-based epidemiologic study of status epilepticus in Richmond, Virginia. Neurology. 1996; 46(4):1029–1035

[4] Engle J Jr. Seizures and Epilepsy. 2nd ed. New York, NY: Oxford University Press; 2012

[5] Epilepsy Foundation. http://www.epilepsy.com. Accessed July 14, 2017

[6] Fisher RS, Uthman BM, Ramsay RE, et al. Alternative surgical techniques for epilepsy. In: Engle JJ, ed. Surgical Treatment of the Epilepsies. 2nd ed. New York, NY: Raven Press; 1993: 549–564

[7] Gates JR, Mercer K. Nonepileptic events. Semin Neurol. 1995; 15(2):167–174

[8] Gilbert K. An algorithm for diagnosis and treatment of status epilepticus in adults. J Neurosci Nurs. 1999; 31(1):27–29, 34–36

[9] Gilliam F, Kuzniecky R, Faught E, Black L, Carpenter G, Schrodt R. Patient-validated content of epilepsy-specific quality-of-life measurement. Epilepsia. 1997; 38(2):233–236

[10] Hausman SV, Luckstein RR, Zwygart AM, Cicora KM, Schroeder VM, Weinhold OM. Epilepsy education: a nursing perspective. Mayo Clin Proc. 1996; 71(11):1114–1117

[11] Institute of Medicine. Epilepsy Across the Spectrum: Promoting Health and Understanding. Washington, DC: National Academies Press; 2012

[12] Karceski S, Morrell M, Carpenter D. The expert consensus guideline series: treatment of epilepsy. Epilepsy Behav. 2001; 2(6):A1–A50

[13] Krumholz A. Nonepileptic seizures: diagnosis and management. Neurology. 1999; 53(5) Suppl 2: S76–S83

[14] Long L, McAuley JW. Epilepsy: a review of seizure types, etiologies, diagnosis, treatment, and nursing implications. Crit Care Nurse. 1996; 16(4):83–92

[15] Long L, Reeves AL. The practical aspects of epilepsy: critical components of comprehensive patient care. J Neurosci Nurs. 1997; 29(4):249–254

[16] McKeon A, Vaughan C, Delanty N. Seizure versus syncope. Lancet Neurol. 2006; 5(2):171–180

[17] Nashef L. Sudden unexpected death in epilepsy: terminology and definitions. Epilepsia. 1997; 38 (11) Suppl:S6–S8

[18] Treatment of convulsive status epilepticus. Recommendations of the Epilepsy Foundation of America's Working Group on Status Epilepticus. JAMA. 1993; 270(7):854–859

Part III

Disorders of the Central Nervous System

7 Tumors

Denita Ryan and Estelle Doris

Abstract

Tumors of the central nervous system often trigger feelings of fear and concern in patients and their families. These tumors may originate within the central nervous system (primary) or may have migrated from another area of the body (metastatic). Tumors may become symptomatic in a multitude of different presentations, and degrees of malignancy and treatment options will vary. Nurses and other health care providers must know about types of tumors, possible symptoms, and treatments available for each tumor category.

Keywords: lymphoma, meningioma, metastatic tumors, nerve sheath tumors, pituitary tumors, primary tumors

7.1 Tumors of the Central Nervous System

The American Brain Tumor Association estimates that, in 2017, roughly 80,000 patients in the United States will be diagnosed with new tumors of the central nervous system (CNS) and there will be roughly 10 times as many people living with a CNS tumor. Although not all tumors are malignant, many are. In 2017, approximately 17,000 people will die from brain or spinal cord malignancies (Box 7.1 Tumor Statistics).

Box 7.1 Tumor Statistics

- Gliomas represent 30% of all brain tumors
- Glioblastoma multiforme (GBMs) represent 17% of all primary brain tumors
- Oligodendrogliomas represent 2% of all primary brain tumors
- Nearly 80,000 primary brain tumors will be diagnosed in 2017
- Most primary brain tumors are located in the meninges (37%)

Note: Data from the Central Brain Tumor Registry of the United States (CBTRUS) 2017.

7.1.1 Classification of Tumors

Benign

- Benign tumors are composed of microscopic cells that are well differentiated and not aggressive
- Complete surgical resection may be curative
- Histologically benign tumors located in surgically inaccessible and eloquent areas of the brain may cause neurologic symptoms and can result in death if allowed to grow and left untreated (Video 7.1)
- May become malignant if left untreated

Malignant

- Malignant tumors have poorly differentiated cells and may be both aggressive and invasive (▶ Table 7.1)
- Surgical resection may remove the tumor or reduce its size, but resection may not be curative because of the aggressive nature of these cells
- Prognosis is usually poor but depends on many factors, such as extent of resection
- The most commonly used grading scale for tumors is from the World Health Organization (WHO)

Primary

- Primary tumors originate in the brain or elsewhere in the CNS
- Rarely travel to other areas of the body

Metastatic

- Metastatic tumors originate in other areas of the body
- Travel to organs such as the brain and spinal cord

7.2 Primary Tumors

7.2.1 Tumors of Neuroepithelial Tissue

Glial Tumors

- These tumors arise from glial cells, which are the nourishing or supportive cells of the brain; they are referred to as *gliomas*
- There are several types of glial cells, including astrocytes, oligodendrocytes, and ependymal cells

Table 7.1 Malignant brain tumors: what to watch for

Complication	Indication	Nursing action	Rationale
Decreased LOC/ neurologic function	Cerebral edema Hemorrhage	Perform accurate and thorough neurologic assessment	An accurate initial assessment will determine the patient's neurologic status and provide a baseline for future assessments
		Compare most recent assessment to baseline assessment	Proper documentation will allow caretakers to detect improvement or decline in the patient's neurologic status
		Protect patient's airway (e.g., from aspiration), such as by keeping his head elevated	A patient with decreased LOC is at risk for respiratory failure and must have the airway protected if this cannot be done independently
		Note any sedating medications	Use of sedating drugs may be the reason for a change in LOC
		If patient is on steroids, determine the present dose and whether dosage has recently been changed	A decrease in dose of dexamethasone, especially an abrupt decrease, could cause increased vasogenic edema and decreased neurologic function
		Report changes in LOC immediately	Patient could be at risk for herniation
Seizure	If new, seizure may indicate hemorrhage or edema	Report seizure if it is a new occurrence for the patient Ensure patient's safety	Many patients with malignant tumors have seizures
Respiratory distress	PE	Perform respiratory assessment, including oxygen saturation level, arterial blood gases, pulmonary function tests, and auscultation Check other vital signs, including blood pressure and heart rate Prevent PE with Lovenox, sequential compression devices, and, most importantly, ambulation	Patients with malignant tumors may be at risk for atelectasis (i.e., incomplete expansion of the lung) and pneumonia, but PE is a life-threatening risk for all patients with malignant tumors

Abbreviations: LOC, level of consciousness; PE, pulmonary embolism.

- Different types of glial tumors are named for the type of cells from which they originate; some gliomas exist in pure form, while others have mixed cell types
- Graded according to the degree of malignancy (▶ Table 7.2)

Astrocytomas

- Arise from astrocyte cells
- Vary in degree of differentiation and malignancy
- Graded according to degree of malignancy
- Do not spread outside the CNS (▶ Fig. 7.1)

Grades of Astrocytoma

- Pilocytic astrocytoma (WHO grade I)
  - Slow-growing, benign
  - Many different types of grade I tumors exist, but pilocytic is the most common
  - Mostly occur in pediatric patients
- Low-grade astrocytoma (WHO grade II)
  - Low-grade tumor, but not benign
  - Heterogeneous
  - Treatment depends on the age of the patient and the extent of resection possible
- Anaplastic astrocytoma (WHO grade III)
  - Malignant
  - Mean age at onset is 35 to 55 years.
  - May progress to higher grade (Box 7.2 Prognostic Factors for Malignant Gliomas)
- Glioblastoma multiforme (GBM) (WHO grade IV)
  - Highly malignant and aggressive
  - Associated with vasogenic edema
  - Necrosis present within tumor
  - Complete resection impossible because of microscopic proliferation
  - Poor prognosis (▶ Fig. 7.2)

Box 7.2 Prognostic Factors for Malignant Gliomas

- The most important prognostic factors for malignant gliomas are
  - Histologic grade of tumor
  - Patient's age (survival is much greater in patients younger than 40 years)
  - Extent of resection
  - Neurologic deficits

Table 7.2 Classification of tumors: gliomas

Tumor type	Average age at onset	Clinical manifestation	Treatment	Prognosis
WHO grade I astrocytoma	Mostly in children	Varies by location and size	Observation Surgery	Excellent
WHO grade II low-grade astrocytoma	May occur at any age; in adults, average age is 30 y	Varies by location and size	Surgery Radiotherapy Chemotherapy	Depends on size, extent of resection, patient's age, and recurrence
WHO grade III anaplastic astrocytoma	Between 35 and 50 y	Varies by location and size	Surgery Radiotherapy Chemotherapy	Mean survival of 22 mo with treatment (shorter for patients aged 40 y and older, and longer for patients younger than 40 y)
WHO grade IV GBM	May occur at any age, but most commonly the onset occurs in the 50s; the incidence of this type of tumor declines thereafter	Varies by location and size Hemorrhage into tumor bed is not uncommon, but neurologic decline is more prevalent	Surgery Radiotherapy Chemotherapy	Mean survival of 14 mo with treatment (shorter for patients aged 40 y and older, and longer for patients younger than 40 y) Important prognostic factors include extent of resection, tumor size, multifocality, and whether the tumor crosses the midline
Oligodendroglioma	Between 40 and 60 y	Frequent seizures Symptoms vary by the lesion's size and location Patients may present with frontal lobe anomalies given these tumors commonly occur in the frontal lobe	Surgery Radiotherapy for higher grades Chemotherapy for higher grades	5 to more than 10 y with treatment Deletion of chromosome 1p19q is a favorable prognostic indicator
Ependymoma	Can occur at all ages, but 60% of people diagnosed with ependymomas are children	Signs and symptoms of increased ICP Hydrocephalus	Surgery Radiotherapy or chemotherapy for recurrence Shunt may be required	7 to more than 8 y with surgical treatment Poor prognostic indicators include subtotal resection, recurrence, and CSF dissemination (seeding)

Abbreviations: CSF, cerebrospinal fluid; GBM, glioblastoma multiforme; ICP, intracranial pressure; WHO, World Health Organization.

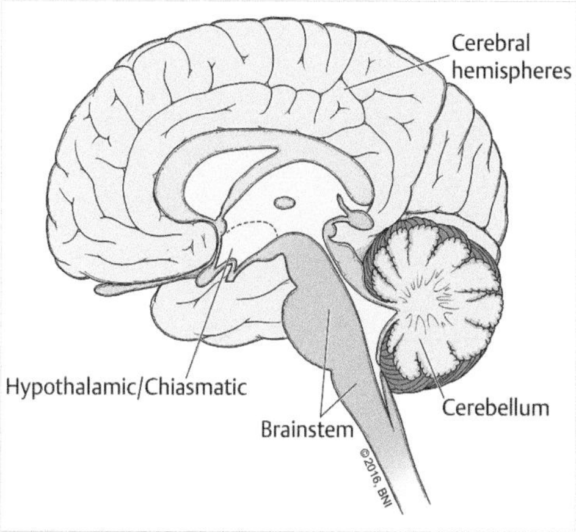
Cerebral
hemispheres
Hypothalamic/Chiasmatic
Brainstem
Cerebellum
©2016, BNI

Fig. 7.1 Common locations of intracranial astrocytomas.

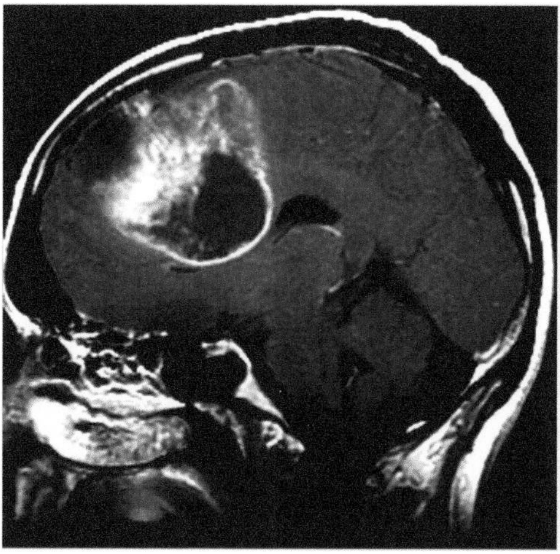

Fig. 7.2 Glioblastoma multiforme.

Oligodendrogliomas

- Arise from oligodendrocyte cells
- Categorized as grade I, II, or III by degree of malignancy

Ependymomas

- Arise from ependymal cells, which line the ventricles and spinal cord (▶ Fig. 7.3)

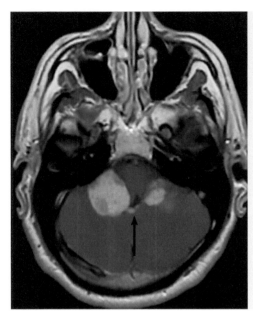

Fig. 7.3 Ependymoma.

- Account for approximately 1.7% of all primary brain tumors
- Categorized as grade I, II, or III by degree of malignancy

Gangliogliomas

- Variant of glial neoplasms, but also contain neuronal tissue
- Usually benign but may grow
- Account for fewer than 1% of all glial neoplasms
- Occur in patients of all ages
- Associated with seizures

Pineal Tumors

- Benign (▶ Fig. 7.4)
- May obstruct the aqueduct and third ventricle, causing hydrocephalus
- Headaches and visual disturbances are common symptoms
- Excellent prognosis with total resection

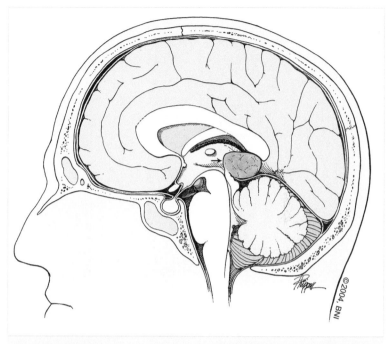

Fig. 7.4 Pineal tumor.

Choroid Plexus Papillomas

• Originate in the choroid plexus
• Can be found in any ventricle but most commonly occur in the fourth ventricle
• Hydrocephalus with increased intracranial pressure (ICP) is the most common presentation
• Occur in patients of all ages
• May be low-grade or anaplastic

7.2.2 Tumors of the Meninges

Meningiomas

• Arise from the meninges (▶ Fig. 7.5)
• Seldom invade the brain tissue

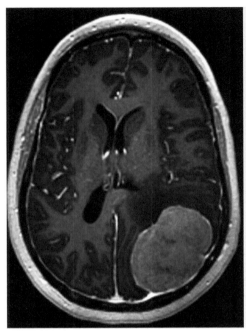

Fig. 7.5 Meningioma.

- Categorized as grade I, II, or III, depending on degree of malignancy (▸ Table 7.3)
- Grow very slowly
- Rarely malignant, but malignant meningiomas can be aggressive
- May be located in eloquent areas of the brain, causing neurologic deficits
- Histologically benign meningiomas may have features that can result in neurologic deficit (Box 7.3 Benign Tumors **and** Box 7.4 When Benign Is Not: Meningiomas)

Box 7.3 Benign Tumors

- The term *benign* may be misleading; a benign tumor in an eloquent area such as the brainstem or the speech center may be composed of benign tissue but can still cause significant neurologic deficits because of its location
- Benign histology does not necessarily mean benign disease

Table 7.3 Classification of tumors: meningiomas

Tumor type	Average age at onset	Clinical manifestation	Treatment	Prognosis
WHO grade I benign	Between 40 and 60 y	Varies by location and size Seizures Headaches	Depends on size and symptoms Observation recommended for small, asymptomatic lesions Surgery recommended for symptomatic lesions Radiotherapy recommended for progression, recurrence, or residual tumor	Excellent with complete resection
WHO grade II atypical	Between 40 and 60 y	Varies by location and size Signs mirror those for grade I tumors but have more rapid onset	Surgery Radiotherapy/ radiosurgery	Variable
WHO grade III malignant	Between 40 and 60 y	Varies by location and size Signs mirror those for grade I tumors but have more rapid course	Surgery Radiotherapy Chemotherapy (experimental)	Mean survival is 2-9 y with treatment

Abbreviation: WHO, World Health Organization.

Box 7.4 When Benign Is Not: Meningiomas

Although most meningiomas are histologically benign, they can still have adverse implications. Situations in which these tumors can be troublesome include

- Subtotal resection (because of size or location)
- Recurrence
- More than one meningioma
- Location in an eloquent area (e.g., the cerebellopontine angle) may cause neurologic deficits, such as cranial nerve deficits (e.g., dysphagia)
- Very large tumors (may require resection in several stages)
- May trigger vasogenic edema
- Malignant meningiomas

Table 7.4 Classification of tumors: sellar tumors

Tumor type	Average age at onset	Clinical manifestation	Treatment	Prognosis
Pituitary adenoma	Variable	Hormone abnormalities depend on the area of pituitary affected Visual disturbances Headaches	Medical Surgical possible Radiotherapy possible	Excellent
Craniopharyngioma	Variable	Visual disturbances Diabetes insipidus Obesity Hypopituitarism	Surgery Radiotherapy	Excellent with resection High recurrence rate
Rathke's cleft cyst	Variable	Potential site for pituitary apoplexy May be none	Surgical drainage	Excellent

7.2.3 Tumors of the Sella

Sellar tumors are rarely malignant. There are several different types (▶ Table 7.4).

Pituitary Adenomas

- These tumors occur most frequently in the anterior lobe of the pituitary gland (▶ Fig. 7.6)
- Mostly benign
- Classified by whether they are nonfunctioning (do not secrete hormones) or functioning (hormone-secreting). Functioning pituitary adenomas can be further classified by the type of hormone secreted
  ○ Prolactin. Increased levels may result in
    – Amenorrhea
    – Galactorrhea
  ○ Adrenocorticotropic hormone. Increased levels may result in
    – Cushing's disease
  ○ Growth hormone. Increased levels may result in
    – Acromegaly
  ○ Thyroid-stimulating hormone. Increased levels may result in
    – Increased heart rate
    – Anxiety
    – Weight loss

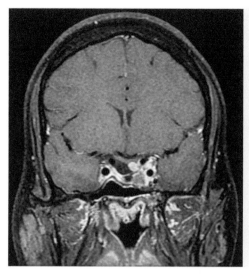

Fig. 7.6 Pituitary adenoma.

- Pituitary adenomas are also classified by size
  - Microadenoma: < 10 mm
  - Macroadenoma: ≥ 10 mm
  - Giant ≥ 40 mm
- Symptoms may be caused by hormone secretion or triggered by the pressure that a tumor exerts on the tissues that surround it; see Table 1.1 in Chapter 1
- Visual loss may be the first symptom
- May cause pituitary apoplexy (Box 7.5 Pituitary Apoplexy)
- Treatment may be medical or surgical (▶ Table 7.5)
- Prognosis is usually excellent

Box 7.5 Pituitary Apoplexy

- Pituitary apoplexy results from hemorrhage or infarction of a pituitary adenoma; it may occur in normal pituitary gland or in other areas of the sella (e.g., a Rathke's cleft cyst)
- Clinical manifestations include rapid neurologic decline, especially visual loss, headache, and decreased level of consciousness
- Pituitary apoplexy is best treated by rapid assessment and management of hormonal anomalies, including administration of steroids; surgical decompression may be warranted to preserve visual acuity and treat possible hydrocephalus

Table 7.5 Pituitary tumors: what to watch for

Complication	Indication	Nursing action	Rationale
Polydipsia and polyuria	DI	Monitor laboratory test results, especially serum sodium, serum osmolality, and urine sodium Strict intake and output Test urine specific gravity Administer desmopressin acetate (DDAVP) as directed	DI is a frequent complication of pituitary tumors; it may result from altered levels of ADH secretion, surgical trauma to the posterior pituitary gland, or possible trauma to hypothalamus
Hypotension	Adrenal crisis resulting from cortisone deficiency	Monitor serum cortisol levels Report new abnormal findings Administer steroids (e.g., prednisone, dexamethasone, and hydrocortisone)	Adrenal glands may not produce enough cortisone to maintain blood pressure or to respond to the stress of surgery, so appropriate levels must be achieved with medication
Decreased visual acuity	Cerebral edema or optic nerve atrophy Pituitary apoplexy	Perform visual acuity assessment Report new abnormal findings immediately	Decreased visual acuity may result from pressure on an optic nerve from a tumor, or postoperative edema, infarction, or hemorrhage (apoplexy)
CSF leak	CSF leak resulting from surgery	Monitor patient for rhinorrhea, ask the patient if dripping in the back of the throat is felt or if the patient has a salty taste in the mouth	Risk of infection or meningitis
		Instruct patient to refrain from drinking through a straw, nose blowing, sneezing, and using an incentive spirometer Report new findings, including increased positional headache and meningeal signs	Drinking through a straw, nose blowing, sneezing, and use of an incentive spirometer increase the risk of displacing the fat pad used to close the dura and can, in turn, cause pneumocephalus or CSF leak

Abbreviations: ADH, antidiuretic hormone; CSF, cerebrospinal fluid; DI, diabetes insipidus.

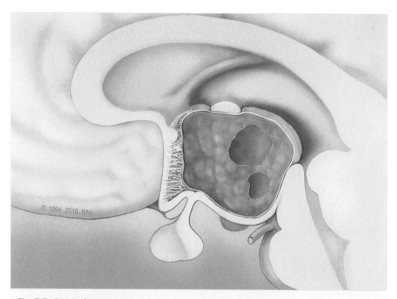

Fig. 7.7 Craniopharyngioma.

Craniopharyngiomas

Patients with a craniopharyngioma should be monitored for diabetes insipidus (DI) given that craniopharyngiomas frequently affect levels of antidiuretic hormone secretion.

- Congenital
- Benign
- Cystic
- May occur near the third ventricle and result in obstruction or hydrocephalus (▶ Fig. 7.7)
- Can be resected surgically, although they often occur in eloquent locations
- Excellent prognosis with resection

Rathke's Cleft Cyst

- A cyst, not a neoplasm
- Comprises remnants of the Rathke's pouch, which is located within the sella
- Interior of cyst resembles motor oil in color and consistency
- Optimal treatment is drainage

7.2.4 Developmental Tumors

Dermoid and Epidermoid Tumors

- Congenital
- Cystic
- Often contain epithelial tissue, teeth, and hair
- Prognosis is excellent with resection

7.2.5 Tumors of the Cranial and Spinal Nerves

Nerve Sheath Tumors

Schwannomas

- Composed of Schwann's cells, which surround every nerve, including cranial nerves (▶ Fig. 7.8)
- Usually benign
- Most common schwannomas are called *acoustic neuromas*
- Cranial nerve deficits may be the initial symptom

Acoustic neuromas most often cause deficits related to the function of the facial and vestibulocochlear nerves (cranial nerve [CN] VII and CN VIII, respectively) (▶ Table 7.6 and ▶ Table 7.7).

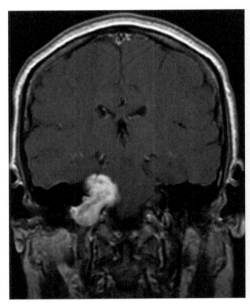

Fig. 7.8 Schwannoma.

Table 7.6 Classification of tumors: acoustic neuromas

Tumor type	Average age at onset	Clinical manifestation	Treatment	Prognosis
Acoustic neuroma	Between 40 and 60 y	Hearing loss Facial nerve weakness Vestibular symptoms (e.g., dizziness and loss of balance)	Observation, if tumor is small and asymptomatic Surgery Radiotherapy for residual tumor Gamma Knife for small tumor or for residual tumor	Excellent

Table 7.7 Acoustic neuromas: what to watch for

Complication	Indication	Nursing action	Rationale
Hearing loss	Cerebral edema	Perform bilateral assessment of hearing function	Hearing loss is often the presenting symptom of acoustic neuroma
		Report new postoperative abnormal findings	Postoperative hearing loss is not unusual, but report to the surgeon immediately if the patient did not have preoperative hearing loss
Facial weakness	Cerebral edema	Assess facial weakness and function bilaterally	Imperative to determine whether the patient experienced weakness before surgery
		Administer protection to the affected eye if it does not close completely	Eye protection (i.e., plastic bubble patch) is extremely important to avoid drying of the cornea, which may cause irreparable damage
		Determine whether the patient is receiving steroids; if so, record type, dose, and duration Report new abnormal findings	If weakness is a new finding, the patient may benefit from dexamethasone to reduce edema

Neurofibromas

- Composed of Schwann's cells
- Differentiated from schwannomas by the presence of axons within the lesion
- Usually benign peripheral nerve sheath tumors
- Associated with neurofibromatosis 1 (NF1) (see section 7.6 on Familial Tumor Syndromes)
- May become malignant

7.2.6 Primary Central Nervous System Lymphoma

- Arises from nonneural tissue
- Confined to the CNS; does not metastasize from systemic lymphoma
- Occurs in immunocompetent patients but is more common in immunocompromised patients
- Diagnosed by biopsy
- Primary CNS lymphoma represents 3.3% of all primary brain tumors
- Median age at diagnosis is 59 years (▶ Table 7.8)
- When left untreated, primary CNS lymphoma is a high-grade tumor that rapidly spreads throughout the CNS
- Poor prognosis without treatment (survival is about 3 months)
- Chemotherapy is an appropriate treatment for these radiosensitive tumors; surgery is seldom recommended
- Use of steroids after diagnosis can be beneficial

Table 7.8 Classification of tumors: primary central nervous system lymphoma

Tumor type	Median age at onset	Clinical manifestation	Treatment	Prognosis
Primary CNS lymphoma	59 y	Varies depending on location	Surgery is not usually recommended Radiotherapy (whole brain) Chemotherapy (methotrexate) Steroids (after diagnosis)	Remission is possible if treated rapidly and aggressively Prognosis is poor if not treated

Abbreviation: CNS, central nervous system.

7.2.7 Other Primary Tumors and Cysts

Chordomas and Chondrosarcomas

- Both chordomas and chondrosarcomas are malignant tumors that occur in the bones of the skull and spine (▶ Fig. 7.9); their clinical manifestations are similar, but they differ in response to treatment and in prognosis
- Most common symptoms include visual disturbance, lower cranial nerve deficits, and headaches
- Treatment is surgical, followed by radiotherapy
- Prognosis is better for chondrosarcoma than for chordomas given that chondrosarcomas are more responsive to radiation
- Five-year survival rate for chondrosarcomas is nearly 100%
- Mean survival for patients with chordomas who do not undergo treatment is about 2 years, and mean survival of patients who undergo treatment is 4 to 6 years
- Both chordomas and chondrosarcomas are characterized by a high rate of recurrence

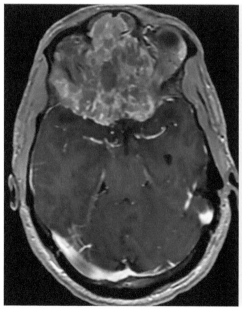

Fig. 7.9 Chordoma.

Germinomas

- Occur in the pineal region
- Usually found in young male patients, typically aged 10 to 21 years
- Treated with radiotherapy
- Excellent prognosis with treatment
- In a small percentage of patients, dissemination of the disease because of nontreatment or failed radiotherapy may be fatal

7.3 Metastatic Tumors

- Originate elsewhere in the body and travel to the brain via the venous system (Box 7.6 Common Primary Cancers that Metastasize to the Brain)
- May be solitary, but about 50% of patients have more than one tumor (▶ Fig. 7.10)
- Metastatic tumors are the most common type of tumor found in the brain (▶ Table 7.9)

Box 7.6 Common Primary Cancers that Metastasize to the Brain

- Lung cancer
- Breast cancer
- Kidney cancer
- Liver cancer
- Colon cancer
- Melanoma

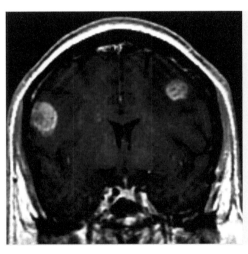

Fig. 7.10 Multiple cerebral metastases.

Table 7.9 Classification of tumors: metastatic tumors

Tumor type	Average age at onset	Clinical manifestation	Treatment	Prognosis
Metastatic tumor	May occur at any age	Varies by location, size, and number of tumors	Surgery for solitary metastasis or if tumor is symptomatic Radiotherapy Gamma Knife Chemotherapy	Usually poor Depends on the number of tumors; number of single and multiple lesions; and the type, identification, and extent of the primary disease

7.4 Tumors of the Spinal Cord

Tumors can also originate in the spinal cord (▶ Fig. 7.11). For information on other disorders related to the spine or spinal cord, see Chapter 11: Spine Disorders.

7.4.1 Intradural Intramedullary Tumors

- This type of tumor occurs within the spinal cord.
- There are many variations of intradural intramedullary tumors

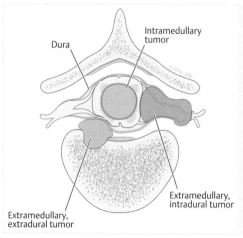

Fig. 7.11 Tumors of the spinal cord.

Astrocytomas

- Like intracranial astrocytomas, these are graded according to their degree of malignancy
- Spinal astrocytomas are usually low-grade tumors
- Treatment is always surgical, followed by chemotherapy or radiotherapy, depending on tumor grade

Ependymomas

- Ependymomas are the most common type of intradural intramedullary lesion, accounting for 37 to 60% of these lesions in adults
- Most common clinical manifestations are pain and motor deficits, which correspond to the level of the lesion
- Treatment is surgical, and radiotherapy may follow in cases of recurrence

Hemangioblastomas

- Benign, vascular lesions
- Derived from cells that are precursors to erythrocytes
- Can be found almost anywhere in the body but are most common in the spinal cord and posterior fossa
- Account for 1 to 6% of all intramedullary tumors
- Common in patients with von Hippel–Lindau disease
- Surgical intervention is the only treatment option

Metastatic Lesions

- Relatively rare in the spinal cord
- Most common primary site of metastatic lesions is the lung, but they are also found in the breast and kidney and in melanomas
- Treatment includes resection and treatment of systemic disease

7.4.2 Intradural Extramedullary Tumors

An intradural extramedullary tumor is one that occurs within the dura mater of the spinal cord but does not permeate the spinal cord.

Meningiomas

- High female-to-male ratio (4:1)
- Usually become symptomatic with pain and motor deficits
- Usually histologically benign
- Treatment is surgical

Nerve Sheath Tumors

- Usually benign
- Mostly schwannomas and neurofibromas
- Treatment is surgical if the tumor is symptomatic

Schwannomas

- Most common type of intradural extramedullary lesion
- Account for 85% of all nerve sheath tumors

Neurofibromas

- Account for 15% of all nerve sheath tumors
- Associated with NF1

7.5 Leptomeningeal Carcinomatosis

- Leptomeningeal carcinomatosis, also referred to as *neoplastic meningitis*, occurs when cancer spreads to the meninges of the brain and spinal cord
- Most common in patients with metastatic brain tumors, especially those originating in the breast or lung tissue; however, leptomeningeal carcinomatosis is also found in lymphomas and primary tumors
- Affects the entire CNS; therefore, treatment must involve the entire CNS
- Staging the cancer includes magnetic resonance imaging (MRI) of the brain and spinal cord, with and without contrast, as well as examination of cerebrospinal fluid (CSF), including cytology
- Clinical manifestations include symptomatology from the cerebral hemispheres, the cranial nerves, and the spinal cord
- Treatment includes surgery (for placement of an intraventricular catheter, such as an Ommaya reservoir), chemotherapy (including intrathecal), and radiotherapy
- Treatment is palliative in nature, as the prognosis of leptomeningeal carcinomatosis is grim

7.6 Familial Tumor Syndromes

Most tumors occur de novo; however, familial tumor syndromes can occur both in the CNS and elsewhere in the body. Genetic mutations can be inherited from a parent or can occur de novo prenatally. In almost every case, the disease is autosomal dominant, with 50% of offspring being affected (Box 7.7 Clinical Alert: Familial Tumor Syndromes).

7.6.1 Neurofibromatosis 1

- NF1 is the most common autosomal dominant genetic tumor syndrome, affecting approximately 1 in every 3,000 people
- Clinical manifestations include café au lait spots, which are flat, tan spots on the skin; subcutaneous neurofibromas; and various neoplasms

7.6.2 Neurofibromatosis 2

- Classic finding of NF2 is bilateral acoustic schwannomas
- It has fewer cutaneous symptoms than NF1
- Less common than NF1

7.6.3 von Hippel–Lindau disease

- Autosomal dominant
- Characteristic lesions are hemangioblastomas of the CNS or other areas of the body, such as the retina and kidneys
- Usually involves multiple lesions
- Treatment is surgical

7.7 Clinical Manifestations and Implications of Tumors of Central Nervous System

Clinical manifestations of tumors depend on several factors, including the tumor's location, size, and histology. Some tumors, such as meningiomas, grow slowly and may have been present for decades. A slow-growing tumor allows the brain the time to adjust to it and accommodate it, so it may become symptomatic with mild or delayed symptoms. Conversely, a fast-growing, aggressive tumor such as a high-grade glioma becomes symptomatic earlier.

The location of a tumor is extremely significant; see Chapter 1: Anatomy. Tumors that occur in less eloquent areas of the brain may produce more subtle symptoms than those located in eloquent areas (e.g., the brainstem and speech center).

7.7.1 Diagnosis

- History
- Imaging studies
  - Magnetic resonance imaging with and without gadolinium
- Pathology (Box 7.8 Clinical Alert: Diagnosis)

Box 7.8 Clinical Alert: Diagnosis

- Imaging studies can confirm the presence of a lesion presumed to be a tumor; however, definitive diagnosis is possible only after pathologic examination

---

7.7.2 Risk Factors

The existence of risk factors for primary brain tumors is highly controversial. Many factors have been evaluated, including environmental factors, occupational factors, diet, and medical history. Significant risk factors include

- Radiation exposure: Exposure to ionizing radiation in childhood yields a higher incidence of developing a meningioma later in life
- Certain familial or genetic factors: These may increase the risk of certain types of tumor syndromes, as described earlier (Box 7.9 Genesis of Neuroepithelial Tumors)

Box 7.9 Genesis of Neuroepithelial Tumors

The cancer stem cell hypothesis states that neural stem cells that undergo a defective differentiation process become glial tumors. These neural stem cells are thought to

- Originate from the subventricular zone of the lateral ventricles and from the subgranular layer of the hippocampal dentate gyrus
- Have a long life expectancy and divide frequently; this makes them susceptible to genetic mutations and errors during cell division
- Become cancer stem cells (stem cells that acquire the ability to generate tumors after genetic mutation or environmental alterations)

Potential areas of defect in these cells include

- Errors in molecular signaling pathways, which become dysregulated, leading to tumor initiation, progression, and tumor cell spread
- Transcription factors that may induce tumor cells to behave like stem cells
- Microenvironment: molecular pathways that contribute to tumor maintenance, growth, and transformation

---

7.7.3 Treatment

Appropriate treatment for a brain tumor depends on
- Tumor histology, location, and extent of resection
- History of previous tumors and treatment
- Patient's age and symptoms

For most suspected tumors, treatment includes surgical resection, but there are exceptions to this general rule. Small, asymptomatic meningiomas may simply require observation with serial MRI. In some cases, a tumor may be in a location considered too dangerous to attempt resection (e.g., the brainstem or speech center). In these cases, biopsy may be an option, because optimal treatment depends on pathologic analysis.

Surgical Resection

The goal of surgical resection is to
- Debulk (reduce) the size of the tumor
- Obtain tissue sample for pathologic diagnosis
- Alleviate symptoms

Medical Management

Depending on the size and location of the tumor, medical management may be an adjuvant treatment to surgical resection (▶ Table 7.10).

Chemotherapy

- Intended to destroy tumor cells
- May be administered intravenously, orally, or intrathecally (usually into an implanted reservoir, such as an Ommaya reservoir)
- Type, dosage, and route of administration of drug depend on type of tumor (Box 7.10 Common Chemotherapeutic Drugs for Brain Tumors)
- Chemotherapeutic drugs also may damage normal cells (Box 7.11 Side Effects of Chemotherapeutic Drugs)
- Usually used concurrently with radiotherapy

Table 7.10 Pharmacology for management of brain tumors

Drug	Category	Tumor type	Purpose	Nursing implications
Dexamethasone	Steroid	Malignant tumors, especially GBMs Some metastatic tumors Any tumor with significant vasogenic edema	Decrease vasogenic edema	Ensure that the patient does not miss doses May cause hyperglycemia and leukocytosis May cause steroid psychosis
Phenytoin (Dilantin) Levetiracetam (Keppra) Carbamazepine (Tegretol)	Antiepileptics	Any tumor with associated seizures	Decrease seizure threshold	Monitor drug levels if appropriate; see also Chapter 6: Seizures
Oxycodone (OxyContin) Hydrocodone (Vicodin) Hydromorphone (Dilaudid) Morphine (Kadian) Tramadol (Ultram)	Opioids	Any	Pain control	Monitor patient for pain, administer medication as ordered, and evaluate effectiveness Avoid overmedication
Enoxaparin (Lovenox) Heparin	Anticoagulants	Any, especially GBM	Decrease risk of deep vein thrombosis	Must be withheld before invasive procedures
Desmopressin acetate/ vasopressin (DDAVP)	Pituitary hormone replacement	Pituitary, in the presence of DI	Decreases serum sodium	Available in many forms Monitor laboratory values, especially serum sodium and serum and urine osmolality Monitor urine specific gravity Strictly monitor intake and output

181

Table 7.10 (*continued*)

Drug	Category	Tumor type	Purpose	Nursing implications
Hydrocortisone	Steroid	Pituitary	Replaces steroid deficiencies Protects until the presence of endogenous steroids is confirmed Protects against Addisonian crisis (hypotension, shock, and death)	Ensure that patient does not miss dose, coordinate with ordered laboratory draws

Abbreviations: DI, diabetes insipidus; GBM, glioblastoma multiforme.

- Temozolomide (Temodar)
- Nitrosoureas
- Carmustine (BiCNU)
- Lomustine (CCNU)
- Bevacizumab (Avastin)

Temozolomide and nitrosoureas have been approved by the Food and Drug Administration for the treatment of malignant gliomas.

- Decreased white blood cell count, increasing the risk of infection
- Hair loss
- Nausea and/or vomiting
- Fatigue
- Mouth sores
- Decreased appetite
- Constipation

Radiotherapy

Radiotherapy, or the use of high-energy X-rays to treat tumors, is often used after resective surgery or for tumors that cannot be resected safely or completely. It may serve as the first line of treatment for lesions that are radiosensitive or are located in an eloquent area of the brain. Radiotherapy is discussed in greater detail in Chapter 16: Radiotherapy.

Stereotactic Radiosurgery

Stereotactic radiosurgery is a type of surgery in which many radiation beams are aimed at the tumor from different directions. At their point of intersection, the beams deliver a powerful dose of localized radiation; see also Chapter 16: Radiotherapy.

- May include Gamma Knife or linear accelerator (i.e., LINAC)–based stereotactic radiosurgery
- May be effective for several types of tumors, including
  - Small tumors that are not candidates for surgical resection
  - Residual tumors
  - Tumor bed of metastatic tumors

Magnetic Resonance Imaging-Guided Stereotactic Laser-Induced Thermotherapy

- Laser-induced thermotherapy can be used in several scenarios, including
  - Small tumor recurrences
  - Initial treatment of small, deep lesions
  - Radiation necrosis
- Performed under general anesthesia
- Requires rigid head fixation in an MRI-compatible head holder
- Laser energy is delivered to the target area, guided by intraoperative MRI
- Approach allows for tissue biopsy, followed by ablation
- Typically requires 24-hour admission but does not require a stay in an intensive care unit
- Dexamethasone, used intraoperatively, is tapered off over the course of 1 to 2 weeks

7.7.4 Ethical and End-of-Life Issues

The diagnosis of a brain tumor, especially a malignant one, evokes a host of emotions in patients and their families. Common feelings are fear, shock, disbelief, and helplessness. Brain cancer is not just neoplastic; it is often neurodegenerative. For patients with malignant brain tumors, the prognosis may involve steady, unrelenting neurologic decline. Caring for these patients is not always straightforward and may involve consideration of many ethical issues.

Quality of Life

Quality of life (QOL) is a conceptual assessment of the perceived sense of well-being regarding health, happiness, and satisfaction with life. To achieve the highest possible QOL, patients need to be able to make educated decisions about their care, including how much burden of disease they are willing to accept. Successful neurosurgic resection of a brain tumor does not always equate to a successful outcome by the patient's standards (Box 7.12 Ethical Concerns).

Box 7.12 Ethical Concerns

- For many people diagnosed with a malignant brain tumor, QOL is more meaningful than length of survival
- Remember that end-of-life issues are often influenced by ethnic or cultural values, and healthcare providers must be able to separate personal views or values from those of patients and families
- The patient's autonomy and dignity should be considered and respected in all health care decisions

Advance Directive

An advance directive (i.e., a living will) is a written statement that outlines patients' wishes for treatment in the event they are unable to speak for themselves. Ideally, an advance directive should be created before hospitalization, but all too often, this is not the case. If possible, patients should fill out an advance directive that outlines their specific wishes regarding the continuation of care in the event of severe decline.

Withdrawal of Care and End of Life

Sometimes, patients and families ask for support or advice as they ponder the implications of withdrawal of care or other end-of-life issues such as organ donation. Helping patients and their families with these decisions is an important element of caring for patients with tumors. It is a tremendous responsibility that should not be taken lightly.

Patients with malignant tumors may undergo multiple surgical procedures, radiotherapy, and chemotherapy. At some point, the decision to stop active therapeutic treatment may be made. This is usually a difficult time for the patient, the family, and the nursing and medical staff (Box 7.13 Spiritual Support).

Box 7.13 Spiritual Support

- Spiritual support should be considered when patients and their families are faced with difficult health care decisions, such as the decision to withdraw care or to deal with other end-of-life issues.
- It is important to address the spirituality of the patient and family. Although the patient's religious affiliation should be addressed and honored, spirituality encompasses more than religion
- If appropriate, a consultation with chaplain, clergy, or other spiritual service should be offered

---

7.8 Nursing Management for Patients with Tumors of the Central Nervous System

Suggestions for managing patients with tumors of the CNS are interspersed throughout this chapter. Below, you will find generalized implications that are appropriate for most patients with tumors of the CNS. A more comprehensive nursing management table is presented in **Appendix A5: Nursing Management of Patients with Brain Tumors**.

This chapter is meant to be a basic reference for bedside care of patients with tumors of the CNS. For more information, the reader may consult the references included at the end of this chapter. They offer a wealth of information and will help the reader become more knowledgeable on this complex topic.

7.8.1 Neurologic Assessment

- Level of consciousness (LOC); see also Chapter 2: Assessment
- Motor, sensory, and cranial nerve function
- Cognitive testing (Karnofsky Performance Scale)
- Nursing interventions to maintain normal ICP, and ICP monitoring if appropriate; see Chapter 3: Principles of Intracranial Pressure
- Knowing the location of the tumor is important because location helps determine what neurologic deficits to expect in the patient
- If craniotomy is part of the patient's treatment, knowing the planned surgical approach will heighten the awareness of complications associated with that approach (e.g., the transsphenoidal approach for pituitary tumors may result in CSF leakage); see also Chapter 15: Neurosurgical Interventions for more information on this subject

7.8.2 Respiratory Assessment

- Perform assessment of the patient's airway
- Observe respiratory rate and rhythm
- Measure arterial blood gases, including O_2 saturation if appropriate
- Respiratory assessment will be related to LOC

7.8.3 Cardiovascular Assessment

- Perform hemodynamic monitoring, if appropriate
- Monitor electrocardiogram for signs of cardiac arrhythmia
- Cardiovascular assessment will be related to LOC

7.8.4 Fluid and Electrolyte Assessment

- Monitor intake and output strictly, especially in patients with pituitary tumors
- Track serum sodium level, observe patient for signs of hyponatremia, and report new or abnormal results
- Monitor glucose levels if the patient is on steroids, and administer any required medications to keep glucose at the appropriate level
- See also Chapter 5: Electrolyte Disturbances

7.8.5 Seizures

- Document any history of seizures, including type, onset, and frequency
- Indicate whether the patient is taking any medications for seizure, being mindful of drug interactions and appropriate levels, if indicated
- Educate patients and families on safety precautions in the event of a seizure
- See also Chapter 6: Seizures

7.8.6 Immobility

- Administer an anticoagulant such as enoxaparin (Lovenox), unless contraindicated
- Obtain sequential compression devices for the patient
- Remember that early ambulation is key for patients who have undergone surgery for tumors of the CNS
- Observe the patient for signs and symptoms of deep vein thrombosis, and report these immediately (Box 7.13 Clinical Alert: Deep Vein Thrombosis in Patients with Glioblastoma Multiforme)

Box 7.14 Clinical Alert: Deep Vein Thrombosis in Patients with Glioblastoma Multiforme

- Patients with GBM are more likely to develop deep vein thrombosis and pulmonary emboli. You should administer an anticoagulant such as enoxaparin as soon as possible and ensure that they ambulate early

---

7.8.7 Patient and Family Teaching

- Provide appropriate educational materials to the patient and family, as needed (**Appendix B5: Sample Discharge Instructions after Resection of a Pituitary Tumor**)
- Refer the patient and family to helpful websites of support groups
- Consult clergy and palliative care, if appropriate
- Ensure that the patient has discharge instructions (**Appendix B5: Sample Discharge Instructions After Resection of a Pituitary Tumor, Appendix B6: Sample Discharge Instructions After Craniotomy for Acoustic Neuroma, and Appendix B7: Sample Discharge Instructions After Craniotomy for Resection of a Brain Tumor**)

7.8.8 Collaborative Management

Management of patients with tumors of the CNS requires a multifaceted approach. A neuroscience nurse plays a pivotal role in the care of these patients, including coordinating and facilitating consultations from the many specialties that are essential to these unique patients. Below is a list of some services that may collaborate to offer the best possible care to these patients

- Nursing
- Neurosurgery
- Radiation oncology
- Neuro-oncology or medical oncology
- Radiosurgery
- Neurology for seizure management
- Ophthalmology for visual disturbances and/or loss
- Therapies as appropriate, including
  - Physical therapy
  - Occupational therapy
  - Speech, including swallowing evaluation, if appropriate
  - Rehabilitation consult, if appropriate
- Neuropsychology
- Clergy, chaplain, or other spiritual support
- Palliative care or hospice, if appropriate

Video

Video 7.1 Acoustic neuroma tumor growth.

Suggested Reading

[1] American Association of Neuroscience Nurses. Care of the Adult Patient with a Brain Tumor. AANN Clinical Practice Guideline Series. Chicago, IL: American Association of Neuroscience Nurses; 2014

[2] American Brain Tumor Association. http://www.abta.org. Accessed June 20, 2017

[3] American Cancer Society. http://www.cancer.org. Accessed June 20, 2017

[4] Burger PC. Classification and biology of brain tumors. In: Youmans J, ed. Neurological Surgery: A Comprehensive Reference Guide for the Diagnosis and Management of Neurosurgical Problems. 3rd ed. Philadelphia, PA: WB Saunders; 1990: 2967–2999

[5] Carpentier A, Chauvet D, Reina V, et al. MR-guided laser-induced thermal therapy (LITT) for recurrent glioblastomas. Lasers Surg Med. 2012; 44(5):361–368

[6] Central Brain Tumor Registry of the United States. http://www.cbtrus.org. Accessed June 20, 2017

[7] Chamberlain MC. Diagnosis and treatment of neoplastic meningitis. In: Prados M, ed. Atlas of Clinical Oncology: Brain Cancer. London: BC Decker, Inc.; 2002: 391–405

[8] House JW, Brackmann DE. Facial nerve grading system. Otolaryngol Head Neck Surg. 1985; 93(2): 146–147

[9] Huttner A. Overview of primary brain tumors: pathologic classification, epidemiology, molecular biology, and prognostic markers. Hematol Oncol Clin North Am. 2012; 26(4):715–732

[10] Illerhaus G, Marks R, Ihorst G, et al. High-dose chemotherapy with autologous stem-cell transplantation and hyperfractionated radiotherapy as first-line treatment of primary CNS lymphoma. J Clin Oncol. 2006; 24(24):3865–3870

[11] Kalkanis SN, Rosenblum ML. Malignant gliomas. In: Bernstein M, Berger M, eds. Neuro-oncology: The Essentials. 3rd ed. New York, NY: Thieme; 2014: 254–265

[12] McDermott MW, Quinones-Hinojosa A, Bollen FW, Larson M. Meningiomas. In: Prados M, ed. Atlas of Clinical Oncology: Brain Cancer. London: BC Decker; 2002: 333–364

[13] National Brain Tumor Society. http://www.braintumor.org. Accessed June 20, 2017

[14] National Cancer Institute. https://www.cancer.gov. Accessed June 20, 2017

[15] Rao MS, Hargreaves EL, Khan AJ, Haffty BG, Danish SF. Magnetic resonance-guided laser ablation improves local control for postradiosurgery recurrence and/or radiation necrosis. Neurosurgery. 2014; 74(6):658–667, discussion 667

[16] Roonprapunt C, Silvera VM, Setton A, Freed D, Epstein FJ, Jallo GI. Surgical management of isolated hemangioblastomas of the spinal cord. Neurosurgery. 2001; 49(2):321–327, discussion 327–328

[17] Sanai N, Polley MY, McDermott MW, Parsa AT, Berger MS. An extent of resection threshold for newly diagnosed glioblastomas. J Neurosurg. 2011; 115(1):3–8

[18] Schiestel C, Ryan D. Quality of life in patients with meningiomas: the true meaning of "benign." Front Biosci (Elite Ed). 2009; 1:488–493

[19] Taylor MD, Nakahara Y. Familial tumor syndromes. In: Bernstein M, Berger M, eds. Neuro-oncology: The Essentials. 3rd ed. New York, NY: Thieme; 2014: 418–428

8 Vascular Disorders

Denita Ryan

Abstract
Vascular disorders of the central nervous system encompass a variety of conditions that affect the brain and spinal cord. These conditions include ischemic and hemorrhagic stroke, aneurysms, and other neurovascular malformations such as cavernous malformations and arteriovenous malformations. Patients with vascular disorders require skillful, knowledgeable care. Nurses and the rest of the health care team should be aware of different types of vascular disorders and their associated symptoms, complications, and treatments.

Keywords: aneurysm, arteriovenous malformation, carotid stenosis, cavernous malformation, ischemic cascade, reperfusion injury, stroke

8.1 Vascular Disorders

Vascular disorders of the central nervous system (CNS) include cerebrovascular malformations such as cavernous malformations and arteriovenous malformations (AVMs), aneurysms, and stroke. These disorders comprise a challenging set of conditions that can be life-changing for patients and their families. Patients with vascular disorders often present with a vast array of coexisting medical conditions, such as subarachnoid hemorrhage, seizures, hydrocephalus, sodium abnormalities, and cardiac and respiratory challenges.

8.2 Cerebrovascular Malformations

Malformations of the cerebrovascular system are believed to be embryonic anomalies. The most common types are cavernous malformations and AVMs. They can be located anywhere within the CNS.

8.2.1 Cavernous Malformations

Cavernous malformations are clusters of abnormal sinusoidal vascular channels. Their characteristics include
- Dense fibrous tissue with little or no intervening brain parenchyma
- Variable size
- Blood in various amounts and stages of thrombus and degradation
- Well-circumscribed dimensions
- Color varying from dark red to purple
- Multilobulated masses described as having a "mulberry-like" appearance (▶ Fig. 8.1; ▶ Fig. 8.2)

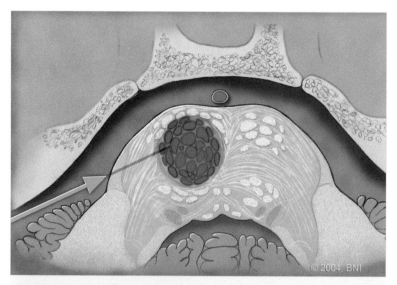

Fig. 8.1 Cavernous malformation.

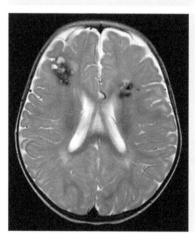

Fig. 8.2 Magnetic resonance image of cavernous malformation.

Historically, cavernous malformations were often misinterpreted as neoplastic lesions, such as hemangioblastomas, instead of malformations. They are also known as

• Cavernous angiomas
• Cavernous hemangiomas
• Capillary hemangiomas
• Cavernomas

There are two types of cavernous malformations: sporadic and hereditary (familial). Multiple genes that are linked to both types of cavernous malformations have been identified.

Epidemiology of Cavernous Malformations

Both types of cavernous malformations have certain characteristics in common. These commonalities are as follows:
- Account for 1% of all intracranial mass lesions
- Account for 5 to 10% of all cerebrovascular lesions
- Found at autopsy or on routine imaging studies in about 0.4% of the population
- Hemorrhage rate is between 0.1 and 22.3% per lesion per year
- Hemorrhage rate for deep-seated lesions or lesions in the brainstem is higher
- Rehemorrhage rate is about 5% per year
- Found in patients of all ages but are most common between the second and fifth decades of life
- Most are asymptomatic
- Cavernous malformations usually hemorrhage in small amounts, because they are low-pressure lesions
- Episodes of hemorrhage may be separated by months or years
- For each episode, the patient may experience neurologic deficits that are worse at the onset and gradually improve as blood is reabsorbed, but the patient may never quite return to neurologic baseline

Location of Cavernous Malformations

Most cavernous malformations occur in the brain, but they can also occur in the spine. The breakdown of common locations is as follows:
- Supratentorial, 80%
- Infratentorial, 15%
  - Evenly divided between the brainstem and the cerebellum
- Spine, 5%

Clinical Manifestations of Cavernous Malformations

Symptoms associated with cavernous malformations depend on the size and location of the lesion. Patients with cavernous malformations commonly present with symptoms similar to those of patients with other neurologic disorders, including
- Seizure
- Headache
- Motor or sensory disturbances
- Cranial nerve deficits

Depending on the location of the cavernous malformation, patients with hemorrhages present with varying degrees of neurologic deficits. A patient with a small frontal hemorrhage may present with subtle neurologic complaints, such as headache, whereas one with a hemorrhage in the cervical cord or brainstem may present with devastating neurologic deficits; see also Chapter 2: Assessment.

Diagnosis of Cavernous Malformations

History

- Family history
- Recent and past medical history, including seizures

Imaging Studies

- Magnetic resonance imaging (MRI) is the most definitive type of imaging study (▶ Fig. 8.2)
- Imaging may be negative in up to 50% of MRI scans
- Computed tomography (CT) may show the presence and location of a lesion but does not indicate the type of lesion (i.e., cavernous malformation or tumor)
- Angiograms are not diagnostic, because cavernous malformations are low-flow lesions that do not image well with angiography

Treatment of Cavernous Malformations

Medical

- Observation may be appropriate for patients with small cavernous malformations if the lesions are asymptomatic; however, they should undergo serial MRI scans to monitor the growth of the lesion
- Associated seizures may be treated with antiepileptic drugs; see also Chapter 6: Seizures

Surgical

The goals of surgery are to obliterate the lesion to prevent rebleeding and to manage neurologic symptoms such as seizures (Box 8.1 Hemorrhage of Cavernous Malformations and Neurologic Function). Radiosurgery is not a standard treatment for cavernous malformations. Indications for surgery include

- Refractory or worsening seizures
- Neurologic deterioration
- Hemorrhage or rehemorrhage
- Mass effect

Box 8.1 Hemorrhage of Cavernous Malformations and Neurologic Function

- Neurologic function after hemorrhage from a cavernous malformation or postoperatively may be worse than prehemorrhage or preoperative status
- Improvement is expected, but it rarely returns to baseline

Familial Cavernous Malformations

- Genetics appear to play a part in the incidence of familial cavernous malformations
- Autosomal dominant pattern of inheritance
- Familial cavernous malformations are associated with multiple lesions and a family history of seizures
- More prevalent in families of Mexican American heritage

Treatment

- Serial monitoring of family members with annual MRI
- Genetic counseling of children and siblings of patients with familial cavernous malformations
- Surgical indications for single and multiple lesions are the same, but in patients with multiple lesions, the symptomatic lesion is usually surgically targeted

8.2.2 Arteriovenous Malformations

An AVM is a mass of abnormal blood vessels in which arterial blood flows directly into the venous system through a nidus (central portion), with no intervening capillary bed (▶ Fig. 8.3).

- AVMs appear as tangled mass of vessels
- The nidus is the center or focus of the AVM
- Blood vessels within an AVM do not have normal characteristics
- AVMs do not contain normal brain tissue
- An AVM is a high-flow system with arterial blood flowing directly into the venous system
- Hemorrhage is often the first symptom of an AVM.

Epidemiology of Arteriovenous Malformations

- Incidence is 3 per 100,000 persons
- AVMs affect male patients slightly more often than female patients
- AVMs account for approximately 8.6% of all cases of subarachnoid hemorrhage (SAH)
- AVMs can be located anywhere within the CNS

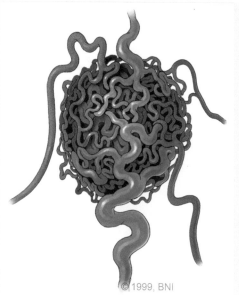

Fig. 8.3 Arteriovenous malformation.

Clinical Manifestations of Arteriovenous Malformations

- Hemorrhage is frequently the first symptom
- This space-occupying lesion displaces normal brain tissue as it grows, so symptoms may progress slowly for slow-growing lesions
- Mass effect or vascular steal may cause neurologic symptoms, even if the AVM has not hemorrhaged
- Vascular steal occurs when rapid blood flow through the AVM draws blood away from the normal brain
- The rapid-onset effects of hemorrhage may cause severe neurologic compromise, coma, or death as the presenting symptom
- Severity of associated neurologic deficits depends on size of the hemorrhage and eloquence of the affected brain
- Seizures are common

Classification of Arteriovenous Malformations

Arteriovenous malformations have three important characteristics
- Size
- Eloquence of the affected brain
- Presence of draining veins

Spetzler-Martin Grading Scale

The Spetzler-Martin Grading Scale was created to help clinicians make decisions when treating AVMs (▶ Fig. 8.4). The presence of associated aneurysms must also be taken into account when determining treatment.

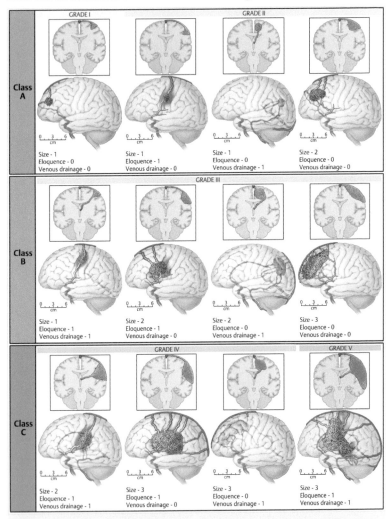

Fig. 8.4 Spetzler-Martin Grading Scale. (Reproduced with permission from Spetzler RF, Martin NA. A grading system for arteriovenous malformations. J Neurosurg 1986;65:476–483, with permission from the American Association of Neurological Surgeons.)

Table 8.1 Spetzler-Martin Grading Scale for arteriovenous malformations

Graded feature	Points
Size	
Small (< 3 cm)	1
Medium (3–6 cm)	2
Large (> 6 cm)	3
Eloquence of adjacent brain	
Noneloquent	0
Eloquent	1
Draining veins	
Superficial	0
Deep	1

Source: Used with permission from Spetzler RF, Martin NA. A proposed grading system for arteriovenous malformations. J Neurosurg 1986; 65:476–483.

- The Spetzler-Martin Grading Scale assigns points for size, eloquence, and draining veins
- Each AVM is given a grade based on those points
- Lower-grade AVMs have lower morbidity; higher-grade AVMs have higher morbidity (▶ Table 8.1)

Diagnosis of Arteriovenous Malformations

- History
- Imaging studies
  - MRI is the best method for diagnosis
  - Cerebral angiography determines the involvement of cerebral vasculature, including the presence of any associated aneurysms

Treatment of Arteriovenous Malformations

Treatment options include surgery, endovascular embolization, radiosurgery, and conservative treatment such as management of symptoms and observation. The best treatment can be determined using the Spetzler-Martin Grading Scale.

- Grades I and II: Surgical resection is the treatment of choice and should be performed at a center where large numbers of cerebrovascular procedures are routinely done
- Grade III: Resection, embolization, or radiosurgery, depending on analysis of the individual case (e.g., characteristics of the AVM, patient age and comorbidities, and the availability of a center where such complex procedures are routinely performed)

- Grades IV and V: Alternate treatments such as embolization, radiosurgery, and observation are preferred, as surgical resection of higher-grade AVMs has a relatively high morbidity and mortality, even if performed by the most experienced surgeon

Medical

- The goal of medical management is to treat the symptoms of the AVM
- This may include seizure control and pain management

Surgical

The goal of surgery is to occlude associated aneurysms and other high-flow areas within the AVM. It is not uncommon to treat AVMs, especially higher-grade AVMs, with more than one surgical intervention, either as a staged procedure or as surgery in conjunction with an endovascular procedure or radiosurgery.

- Craniotomy for resection of AVM (may also require clipping of associated aneurysms)
- Neuroendovascular; see also Chapter 14: Neuroradiology and Neuroendovascular Interventions
  - Coil
  - Embolization
- Gamma Knife radiosurgery; see also Chapter 16: Radiotherapy;
  - May be used to treat surgically inaccessible lesions
  - May be used in combination with surgery to treat large or higher-grade AVMs

8.2.3 Other Vascular Malformations

Arteriovenous Fistulas

- Arteriovenuous fistulas (AVFs) are dilated arterioles that connect directly to a vein (▶ Fig. 8.5)
- High-flow, high-pressure lesions
- Low incidence of hemorrhage
- Usually amenable to endovascular intervention

Dural Arteriovenous Fistulas

- Dural AVFs (DAVFs) are a type of AVF that is directly associated with the dura (▶ Fig. 8.6)
- Most AVFs are DAVFs

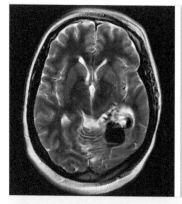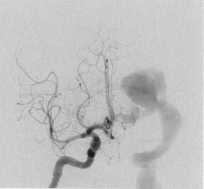

Fig. 8.5 Arteriovenous fistula.

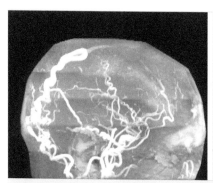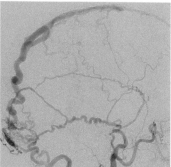

Fig. 8.6 Dural arteriovenous fistula.

Carotid Cavernous Fistulas

- Carotid cavernous fistulas are direct high-flow shunts between the internal carotid artery and the cavernous sinus
- Frequently occurs as a result of rupture in the cavernous portion of the internal carotid artery
- Most often result from trauma but may also be spontaneous
- Symptoms include eye pain, proptosis, and decreased visual acuity
- Intervention may be surgical or endovascular

Capillary Telangiectasias

- Capillary telangiectasias are small capillary lesions composed of clusters of vessels
- Most common in the pons
- Appear as dilated capillaries
- Carry little clinical significance

8.3 Intracerebral Aneurysms

The word *aneurysm* comes from the Greek *aneurysma*, which means widening. An aneurysm is an outpouching of an artery, often described as resembling a sac, blister, or balloon. The most common type of aneurysm is the saccular, or berry, aneurysm.

8.3.1 Classification of Aneurysms

- Type
  - Saccular (berry) (▶ Fig. 8.7)
    - Has a distinctive neck
    - Most common type of aneurysm
  - Fusiform (▶ Fig. 8.8)
    - A portion of the vessel wall appears to expand outward
    - Has no defined neck
- Size
  - Usually less than 10 mm
  - Can be more than 25 mm ("giant" aneurysm)

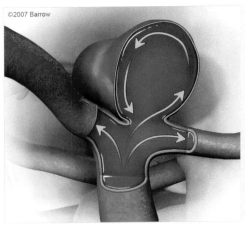

©2007 Barrow

Fig. 8.7 Saccular aneurysm.

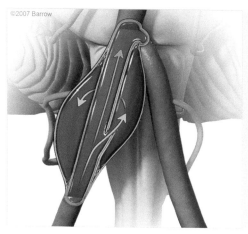

Fig. 8.8 Fusiform aneurysm.

- Location
  - Anterior circulation, 85%
  - Most anterior circulation aneurysms occur in the circle of Willis (▶ Fig. 8.9)
  - Posterior circulation, 15% (Box 8.2 Common Locations of Aneurysms)

Box 8.2 Common Locations of Aneurysms

- Anterior communicating artery
- Posterior communicating artery
- Middle cerebral artery
- Internal carotid artery
- Basilar tip
- Ophthalmic artery

8.3.2 Epidemiology of Aneurysms

- Occurs in approximately 5% of population (Box 8.3 Risk Factors for Cerebral Aneurysms)
- Mean age at diagnosis is about 50 years
- Slightly higher female prevalence
- About 7 to 20% are the familial form
- About 10 to 20% of patients with aneurysms have more than one aneurysm
- Familial aneurysms are those that occur in two first- or second-degree relatives
  - May be ruptured or unruptured
  - Incidence is about 10%
  - A genetic component is most likely involved

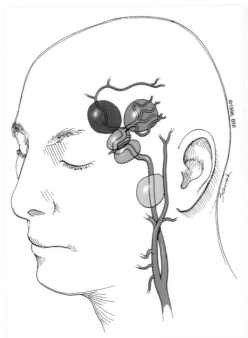

Fig. 8.9 Common locations of aneurysms.

Box 8.3 Risk Factors for Cerebral Aneurysms

- Smoking
- Hypertension
- Family history of aneurysms
- Age (more than 40 years)
- Diagnosis of connective tissue disorder
- Blood vessel injury (dissection)
- Slight female preponderance

8.3.3 Clinical Manifestations of Aneurysms

Most aneurysms do not elicit symptoms until they rupture; thus, few are found incidentally (Box 8.4 Clinical Manifestations of Aneurysms [Ruptured and Unruptured]; Video 8.1).

- Aneurysms may occasionally be found due to vague, subtle complaints (e.g., frequent headache, nausea and vomiting, and lethargy)

- Larger aneurysms may cause mass effect, with focal neurologic symptoms resulting from the pressure exerted on surrounding brain tissue
- Symptoms of ruptured aneurysms include
  - Severe headache
  - Sudden loss of function in one or more parts of the body
  - Seizures
  - Decreased level of consciousness (LOC)
  - Death

Box 8.4 Clinical Manifestations of Aneurysms (Ruptured and Unruptured)

Unruptured aneurysms
- New or unusual headache
- Unexplained nausea and vomiting
- New neurologic impairment

Ruptured aneurysms
- Headache with stiff neck
- Sudden severe neurologic impairment
- Sudden "worst headache of my life."
- New onset seizure

8.3.4 Common Complications of Aneurysms

Numerous complications are associated with cerebral aneurysms.

Subarachnoid Hemorrhage

- Blood enters the subarachnoid space after an intracerebral aneurysm has ruptured (▶ Table 8.2 and ▶ Fig. 8.10)
- Blood may extend into the ventricles (intraventricular hemorrhage)
- Amount of blood present in the subarachnoid space determines the Hunt and Hess classification scale score, discussed later
- Fatality rate of SAH is about 40 to 50%
- In the United States, 30,000 cases occur annually
- Hallmark complaint of patients at the time of SAH rupture is "worst headache of my life"

Table 8.2 Subarachnoid hemorrhage: what to watch for

Problem	Indication	Nursing action	Rationale
Decline in neurologic assessment	Hemorrhage	Perform thorough neurologic assessment, compare to baseline, and repeat at appropriate intervals Watch for signs of ICP; see also Chapter 3: Principles of Intracranial Pressure	Patients with SAH are at risk for rebleeding if aneurysm is present and not clipped or coiled
		Check laboratory values, especially serum sodium (desired parameters for serum sodium may be higher than normal [>145 mm Hg])	Hyponatremia, usually caused by cerebral salt wasting in SAH, may facilitate cerebral edema and raise ICP
	Vasospasm	May need cerebral angiogram to rule out vasospasm	Patients with SAH are at risk for vasospasm for 3–10 days after hemorrhage
	Hydrocephalus	May need CT of head	Patients with SAH are at risk for developing hydrocephalus due to poor absorption of CSF
	Seizure	Check laboratory values, especially drug levels, if appropriate Obtain EEG Report new abnormal changes in assessment	Nonconvulsive status epilepticus may appear as a decrease in LOC
Hypertension/ hypotension	Triple-H therapy	Be aware of desired blood pressure parameters for patient on triple-H therapy	Most patients with SAH benefit from blood pressure higher than their average (MAP 20–30 mm Hg above baseline)
		Vasopressors, as ordered, to maintain blood pressure parameters, as ordered	May require vasopressors and appropriate hemodynamic monitoring
		Watch for "overshoot"	Potential to "overshoot" desired target

Table 8.2 (*continued*)

Problem	Indication	Nursing action	Rationale
		Avoid hypotension at all costs	Adequate blood pressure, which may be at higher levels than usual, is needed to maintain adequate CBF Hypotension puts brain at risk for inadequate CBF and further neuronal damage
Hypervolemia	Triple-H therapy	Intravenous fluids, as ordered Strict intake and output Monitor laboratory values, especially serum sodium and osmolality Watch for signs of cardiac overload due to extra fluid	Increases CBF
Hemodilution	Triple-H therapy	Monitor laboratory values, especially complete blood count (hematocrit)	Increases CBF

Abbreviations: CBF, cerebral blood flow; CSF, cerebrospinal fluid; CT, computed tomography; EEG, electroencephalogram; ICP, intracranial pressure; LOC, level of consciousness; MAP, mean arterial pressure; SAH, subarachnoid hemorrhage.

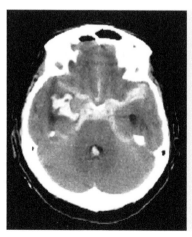

Fig. 8.10 Subarachnoid hemorrhage.

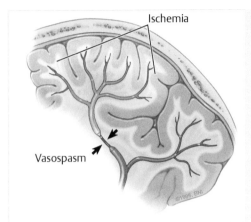

Fig. 8.11 Vasospasm.

Vasospasm

- Occurs only in arteries and is triggered by the presence of blood in the subarachnoid space
- Causes arteries to constrict, restricting blood flow (▶ Fig. 8.11)
- May result in decreased neurologic function (Box 8.5 Clinical Manifestations of Vasospasm)
- Risk for vasospasm is reflected by Fisher Grading Scale score (see next section); greater amount of blood present represents higher risk for vasospasm
- Greatest risk of vasospasm is 4 to 14 days after SAH
- Accounts for about 20% of morbidity and disability in patients with SAH
- Detected by angiography or transcranial Doppler study
- Triple-H therapy is gold standard for prevention of vasospasm
  - Hypertension
    - Vasopressors increase mean arterial pressure to about 20 to 30 mm Hg above baseline
  - Hemodilution
    - Accomplished by increasing fluids
  - Hypervolemia
    - Increases volume by use of fluids

- May be asymptomatic
- Confusion
- Decreased LOC
- Focal neurologic deficits, including aphasia and motor deficits, depending on the location of vessel in spasm
- May appear as stroke

Rehemorrhage

- All ruptured aneurysms are at risk for rehemorrhage
- Risk increases over time
- Risk is highest within 24 hours of initial hemorrhage; 4 to 10% of aneurysms rebleed within 24 hours of initial hemorrhage
- A total of 20 to 25% rebleed within 2 weeks of initial hemorrhage
- Hypertension increases the risk
- Potentially life-threatening
- Likelihood of survival is reduced when aneurysms rehemorrhage
- Early treatment, aimed at aneurysm obliteration, is essential to prevent rehemorrhage

Hydrocephalus

- Occurs when blood in the subarachnoid space causes poor absorption of cerebrospinal fluid (CSF) by the arachnoid granulations; see also Chapter 4: Hydrocephalus
- May initially require an external ventricular drain to control and monitor hydrocephalus
- One-third of patients with SAH will develop hydrocephalus
- Most patients with hydrocephalus will require a permanent shunt

Seizures

- Occur in about 20 to 40% of patients with SAH
- May be temporary
- Treated with antiepileptic drugs; see also Chapter 6: Seizures

Hyponatremia

Hyponatremia occurs when the amount of sodium in blood is too low (Box 8.6 Hyponatremia in Subarachnoid Hemorrhage). See also Chapter 5: Electrolyte Disturbances.

- Cerebral salt wasting
  - Most commonly seen in patients with SAH
  - Occurs when levels of natriuretic peptide are increased, resulting in leakage of salt and water from the body
  - Depletes fluid and sodium stores in the body
  - Treatment is administration of sodium (oral or intravenous [IV])
- Syndrome of inappropriate antidiuretic hormone
  - Caused by oversecretion of antidiuretic hormone
  - Results in dilution of sodium in blood
  - Treatment is fluid restriction

Box 8.6 Hyponatremia in Subarachnoid Hemorrhage

- Confusion, lethargy, or seizure may be the sign of hyponatremia
- Monitor serum sodium level
- Monitor intake and output, as well as which IV fluids are running, if any
- Report sodium level of less than 135 mg/L or desired parameter
- Patients with hyponatremia are at risk for seizures
- Cerebral salt wasting is more common than syndrome of inappropriate antidiuretic hormone; see also Chapter 5: Electrolyte Disorders

---

Cardiac Stunning

- Occurs in about 5% of patients with SAH
- May present as transient disturbance on electrocardiogram (ECG), life-threatening arrhythmia, or myocardial infarction
- Mechanism of cardiac stunning is unclear

8.3.5 Diagnosis of Aneurysm and Subarachnoid Hemorrhage

- History
- Lumbar puncture to determine the presence of SAH
- Imaging studies
  - CT or MRI will reveal a large aneurysm or SAH
  - Cerebral angiogram is gold standard to determine the exact artery on which the aneurysm is located and whether the aneurysm is ruptured or unruptured (▶ Fig. 8.12 and ▶ Fig. 8.13)

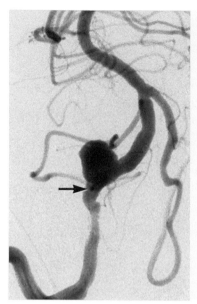

Fig. 8.12 Unruptured aneurysm. Arrow indicates base of aneurysm where it arises from the V4 segment of the vertebral artery.

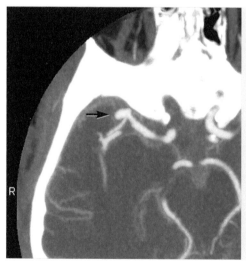

Fig. 8.13 Ruptured aneurysm (arrow) within a focus of subarachnoid hemorrhage.

Table 8.3 Hunt and Hess classification of subarachnoid hemorrhage

Grade	Description
0	Unruptured
I	Asymptomatic, or mild headache and slight nuchal rigidity
II	Cranial nerve palsy, moderate to severe headache, and nuchal rigidity
III	Mild focal deficit, lethargy, or confusion
IV	Stupor, moderate to severe hemiparesis, and decerebrate rigidity
V	Deep coma, decerebrate rigidity, and moribund

Source: Used with permission from Hunt WE, Hess RM. Surgical risk as related to time of intervention in the repair of intracranial aneurysms. J Neurosurg 1968;28(1):14–20.

8.3.6 Grading Scales

The grading scales discussed below provide common classification systems to facilitate communication among health care professionals and standardize diagnostic terminology.

- Fisher Grading Scale
  - Predicts risk of vasospasm
  - Grade is based on the amount and location of blood seen on CT scan
  - Higher grade indicates higher risk for vasospasm
- Hunt and Hess classification of SAH
  - Grade is based on neurologic assessment
  - Higher grade indicates severity of SAH
  - Useful as guidelines for treatment (▶ Table 8.3)

8.3.7 Treatment of Aneurysms

The treatment of aneurysms depends on several factors. The most important factor when deciding on the appropriate treatment is whether the aneurysm is ruptured or unruptured. Other factors to consider are as follows:

- Patient's age
- Patient's medical condition
- Physical characteristics of aneurysm
  - Size
  - Type (saccular or fusiform)
  - Location
  - Number of aneurysms (single or multiple)

Unruptured Aneurysms

- May be found incidentally
- May be symptomatic due to mass effect (because an aneurysm is a space-occupying lesion)

- Has several treatment options, including
  - Observation, with serial MRI to monitor the size of the aneurysm
  - Surgical clipping
  - Endovascular coiling or embolization (Video 8.2)

Ruptured Aneurysms

- Because of the risk of rehemorrhage, time is usually important
- Surgical clipping
- Endovascular coiling or embolization
- Some aneurysms (because of size or other physical attributes) are more amenable to one intervention than the other
- Total obliteration of the aneurysm is the goal

Surgical Treatment

The International Study of Unruptured Intracranial Aneurysms (ISUIA) found that SAH mortality (66%) far outweighed the risk of surgery (mortality 2.6%; morbidity 10.9%). The recommendations of the ISUIA are that surgery to obliterate an unruptured aneurysm is the best therapeutic option. Surgical treatment of cerebral aneurysms is achieved by craniotomy and must be performed by a specially trained cerebrovascular surgeon.

- Direct clipping (Video 8.1)
  - Most common method
  - Surgical clip is placed directly across the aneurysm neck (► Fig. 8.14)
  - Usually results in complete destruction of the aneurysm
  - Preferred treatment for patients with large or giant aneurysms

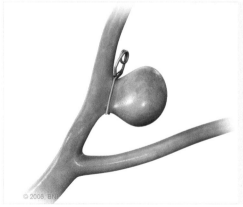

Fig. 8.14 Clipped aneurysm.

- Trapping
  - Surgical clip is placed across the artery feeding the aneurysm to "trap" the aneurysm and cause it to clot
- Reconstruction
  - Some aneurysms require reconstruction of the aneurysmal portion of the artery because of unusual anatomy
  - This procedure may be complicated and extensive
- Cardiac standstill
  - In extreme situations, cardiac standstill may be instituted to allow the surgeon to obliterate the aneurysm safely
  - Performed only under extreme circumstances by a surgical team specifically trained in this procedure

Endovascular Treatment

Several methods may be used to treat aneurysms endovascularly. These methods involve the insertion of a catheter through the femoral artery, with navigation to the involved artery in the brain. See also Chapter 14: Neuroradiology and Neuroendovascular Interventions.

- Coils, usually made of platinum, are introduced into the aneurysm, filling it to slow the flow of blood (Video 8.2)
- The goal is to clot the aneurysm and remove it from the blood flow of the parent artery
- Stents can be placed across the aneurysmal portion of the artery to cut off blood flow to the aneurysm
- Occasionally, a combination of these methods is used (▶ Fig. 8.15)

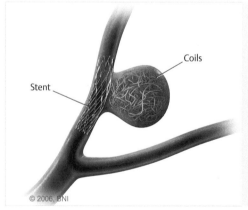

Fig. 8.15 Coiled aneurysm.

Coils

Stent

© 2006, BNI

Endovascular versus Surgical Treatment

Sometimes, the best way to obliterate an aneurysm is a combination of open surgical treatment and endovascular coiling.

• Endovascular treatment does not require open surgery, which avoids the risks associated with open craniotomy

• Endovascular treatment may reduce the length of hospital stay for some patients

• Aneurysms may recur after endovascular treatment and require additional treatment

• Endovascular treatment is generally reserved for smaller aneurysms and is not the best treatment for all types of aneurysms

8.4 Stroke

Stroke is a brain attack (▶ Table 8.4). The phrase "time is brain" conveys the need for health care professionals and the general public to treat symptoms of

Table 8.4 National Stroke Association Prevention Guidelines

Guideline	What you can do
Have your blood pressure checked annually	Be compliant with antihypertensive medication, if prescribed A diet low in salt and low in fat will help lower your blood pressure Start and maintain an exercise program
Find out if you have atrial fibrillation	Atrial fibrillation is diagnosed by an electrocardiogram Blood thinners such as warfarin or aspirin can decrease risk of stroke
Cease smoking	Smoking cessation lowers risk of stroke by half
Consume alcohol in moderation	If you drink, consume no more than 2 drinks per day If you do not drink, do not start
Know your cholesterol level	High cholesterol can be controlled by diet and exercise Be compliant with medication that lowers cholesterol, if prescribed
Learn how to manage your diabetes, if diagnosed	Diabetes may be controlled by diet or medication, or both Maintain an exercise program
Exercise regularly	A well-balanced exercise regimen will help prevent stroke
Adhere to a diet low in sodium and fat	Limit consumption of sodium, added sugars, and solid fats
Manage circulation problems	Consult your doctor if you experience circulatory symptoms or if you have a history of anemia or sickle-cell anemia
Know symptoms of stroke	Know the signs and symptoms of stroke, and call emergency personnel immediately if stroke is suspected

stroke as a medical emergency. Timely treatment may mean the difference between functional recovery and lifelong neurologic disabilities.

Stroke is defined as a decline in neurologic function associated with a specific location within the brain. This decline can be either rapid or gradual. Stroke occurs when blood flow to a specific vascular territory is restricted to the point that the brain tissue no longer receives the blood that it requires to function.

8.4.1 Epidemiology of Stroke

- Stroke is the fifth leading cause of death in the United States
- Approximately 795,000 cases of stroke are reported per year
- Prevalence of stroke is almost twice as high for African Americans as for Caucasians
- Approximately 10% of all strokes occur in individuals between the ages of 18 years and 50 years
- Roughly 4 million people are stroke survivors
- Women are more likely than men to die from stroke (about 60% vs. 40%)

8.4.2 Types of Stroke

Stroke can occur in one of two ways
- Ischemic stroke
  - An obstructed blood vessel interrupts the flow to a specific area of the brain
  - Embolic
  - Thrombotic
- Hemorrhagic stroke
  - Occurs when an artery bleeds, interrupting the flow to a specific area of the brain

Both types result in cerebral ischemia, with neurologic deficits related to the specific area of the brain affected.
- Brain cells that are deprived of oxygen for an extended period of time begin to die (infarct)
- As the brain becomes deprived of oxygen, it loses function, depending on the area of the brain affected
- Impaired functions may include motor, sensory, speech, and cognition

Ischemic Stroke

Ischemic stroke is the most common type of stroke (▶ Fig. 8.16). It accounts for about 80 to 87% of all strokes. Atherosclerosis is the main contributing

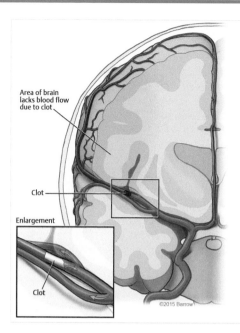

Fig. 8.16 Ischemic stroke.

factor to ischemic stroke. Ischemic stroke is further classified according to mechanism.

- Cardioembolic (20%)
  - Blood clot from faulty heart valve or atrial fibrillation
  - Results when a clot dislodges and travels to an area of decreased circulation
- Thrombotic (20%)
  - Arterial plaque as a result of atherosclerosis
- Lacunar (25%)
  - Small-vessel disease
  - A vessel is coated with a lipid compound, a process known as *lipohyalinosis*, that causes the lumen to thicken and restricts blood flow
  - Associated with hypertension
- Cryptogenic (30%)
  - No cause found for stroke
- Other (5%)
  - Coagulopathies
  - Vasculitis
  - Drug abuse
  - Infections

Specific Terms Associated with Ischemic Stroke

Carotid Stenosis

- Narrowing of the carotid artery due to atherosclerotic plaques
- Narrowing of the arterial lumen occurs; this may restrict blood flow and cause cerebrovascular insufficiency
- May result in transient ischemic attacks (TIAs) or stroke, if left untreated
- Occluded carotid artery may find collateral flow, occasionally avoiding neurologic compromise
- Carotid occlusions of more than 70% may benefit from surgical intervention

Transient Ischemic Attacks

Transient ischemic attacks are temporary focal neurologic deficits associated with a specific location of the brain.

- Known as brain attacks
- Caused by vascular disease
- Most TIAs resolve within an hour
- Many patients have one or more TIAs before having a complete stroke
- Nearly half (40%) of all patients with TIA will go on to have a complete stroke
- Transient ischemic attack may be temporary, but the vascular disease that causes them is not temporary
- Transient ischemic attacks are often warning signs for impending stroke (Box 8.7 National Stroke Association Guidelines for Management of Transient Ischemic Attacks)

Box 8.7 National Stroke Association Guidelines for Management of Transient Ischemic Attacks

- Hospital admission within 24 to 48 hours of initial event
- Specialized clinical evaluation within 24 to 48 hours of diagnosis
- Medical assessment within 24 to 48 hours with imaging
  - Imaging includes CT, computed tomography angiography (CTA), MRI, magnetic resonance angiography (MRA) and transcranial Doppler
  - Carotid imaging (ultrasonography, MRA, or CTA of the head and neck)
  - Cerebral angiography
- Cardiac evaluation
  - Includes echocardiogram when patient is younger than 45 years and neck and brain imaging shows no cause for TIA
- Noncardioembolic TIA
  - Antiplatelet therapy immediately (clopidogrel)
- Cardioembolic TIA (with atrial fibrillation)

○ Oral anticoagulation (warfarin) with target international normalized ratio of 2.5
○ Aspirin
• No anticoagulants for patients in sinus rhythm, unless other risk is present (recent myocardial infarction or valve replacement)

Penumbra

• Silent (nonfunctional) area of the brain that is not infarcted (dead) and could be restored with timely perfusion (▶ Fig. 8.17)
• Neurologic damage caused by oxygen deprivation of specific brain tissue
  ○ Brain tissue becomes infarcted when deprived of oxygen for a certain length of time
  ○ Dead tissue is referred to as necrotic
• Penumbra exists around the necrotic core

Ischemic Cascade

• Series of events occurring in response to cellular hypoxia (Box 8.8 Ischemic Cascade)

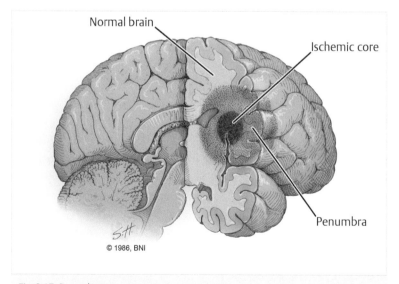

Fig. 8.17 Penumbra.

- Events are due to impaired electrolyte activity and intracellular swelling
- Cerebral ischemia follows, with further increase in cerebral edema and intracranial pressure (ICP)
- Cerebral edema is a major cause of death after ischemic stroke

---

Box 8.8 Ischemic Cascade

- The ischemic penumbra surrounds the necrotic core
- The ischemic penumbra receives low blood flow, low oxygen, and low metabolites, such as glucose
- Local autoregulation is impaired due to low metabolic factors
- Results in decreased production of adenosine triphosphate
- Cell membrane permeability is increased, causing intake of sodium and potassium
- Results in intracellular swelling
- Ischemic area increases
- Area of infarction increases

Reperfusion Injury

- Activated oxygen-free radicals cause further injury to the damaged cells after the blood supply is reestablished to a previously oxygen-deprived area of the brain (Box 8.9 Reperfusion Injury)
- Results in cerebral edema and increased ICP

Box 8.9 Reperfusion Injury

Reperfusion injury may occur after many neurosurgical procedures, including
- Carotid endarterectomy
- Resection of AVMs
- Bypass procedures, such as superficial temporal artery to middle cerebral artery (STA-MCA)

Clinical Manifestations of Ischemic Stroke

- Depend on location of involved vessel and extent of occlusion (▶ Table 8.5)
- Symptoms that resolve completely are likely TIAs
- "Completed" strokes result in irreversible damage

Table 8.5 Clinical manifestations of stroke or occluded arteries related to specific ischemic vascular territories

Vascular territory	Clinical manifestations
Anterior circulation	
Anterior cerebral artery	Contralateral paresis and/or sensory deficits of lower extremities Impaired gait Incontinence Cognitive deficits Blunted affect Memory deficits
Internal carotid artery	Contralateral motor and sensory deficits Aphasia (if dominant hemisphere) Apraxia; neglect (if nondominant hemisphere) Visual field deficits Cranial nerve deficits
Middle cerebral artery (most common)	Contralateral motor and sensory impairment Upper extremity and face more impaired than lower extremity Aphasia (if dominant hemisphere) Homonymous hemianopsia
Posterior circulation	
Vertebral/basilar arteries	Ataxia; dyscoordination Cranial nerve deficits (eye movement disorders, dysphagia)

Diagnosis of Ischemic Stroke

- History (duration of symptoms)
- Imaging studies (▶ Table 8.6)
  - Cerebral angiography shows details of vasculature
  - CT is mandatory to rule out hemorrhagic stroke (not diagnostic for early ischemic stroke)
  - Carotid ultrasound to diagnose carotid stenosis

Treatment of Ischemic Stroke

The best treatment for stroke is prevention (Box 8.10 Risk Factors for Stroke).
- Identify risk factors
- Modify risk factors
- Educate patients

Disorders of the Central Nervous System

Table 8.6 Diagnostic tests for cerebrovascular disorders

Test	Indication	Rationale
Serum electrolytes	Hyponatremia	Risk factor for increased cerebral edema Significant in the presence of SAH and vasospasm
	Hyperglycemia	Could be indicative of steroid use (dexamethasone) Significant risk for ischemic brain
ABG	Hypoxia; hypercapnia	Depressed neurologic state may also indicate depressed respiratory drive; decreased levels of oxygen and increased levels of CO_2 may drive up ICP Hypoxia is indicator of poor neurologic outcome
Cerebral angiography	Vascular abnormalities (cerebral aneurysms and AVMs)	Angiography is gold standard for visualization of the arterial system
MRI DWI	Ischemic abnormalities Cavernous malformations	MRI will demonstrate small lesions not seen on CT scan Demonstrates ischemic areas
MRA (see also Chapter 14: Neuroradiology and Neuroendovascular Interventions)	Vascular abnormalities	Demonstrates the vascular system and large aneurysms
Lumbar puncture	Blood in CSF (SAH) Blood in CSF appears yellow with time due to blood breakdown; this indicates history of SAH	Lumbar puncture is contraindicated until space-occupying lesion can be ruled out
EEG	Seizure activity	Common in SAH and vascular malformations because of altered electrical activity in the brain
CT	Hemorrhage Hydrocephalus Edema	CT scans are appropriate as initial test to determine the presence of blood, hydrocephalus, or life-threatening cerebral edema Once SAH is confirmed, further testing is warranted

Abbreviations: ABG, arterial blood gases; AVM, arteriovenous malformation; CSF, cerebrospinal fluid; CT, computed tomography; DWI, diffusion weighed imaging; EEG, electroencephalogram; ICP, intracranial pressure; MRA, magnetic resonance angiography; MRI, magnetic resonance imaging; SAH, subarachnoid hemorrhage.

220

Box 8.10 Risk Factors for Stroke

- Modifiable
  - Hypertension
  - Atrial fibrillation
  - Hyperlipidemia
  - Diabetes mellitus
  - Valvular disease
  - Coronary artery disease
  - Excessive use of alcohol
  - Sedentary lifestyle
  - Obesity
  - Smoking
- Nonmodifiable
  - Family history
  - Age
  - Sex
  - Ethnicity

Medical Management

- Management of risk factors
- Weight management
  - Healthy diet
  - Exercise
- Smoking cessation
- Antiplatelet therapy
  - Inhibits aggregation of platelets to the wall of injured vessel
  - Current antiplatelet agents: aspirin and clopidogrel (Plavix) (▸ Table 8.7)
- Anticoagulation therapy
  - Decreases further development of thrombi
  - Causes intra-arterial thrombolysis
  - Aids patients with documented occlusion of large vessels
  - Current thrombolytic agents: tissue plasminogen activase (t-PA), prourokinase, and streptokinase (Box 8.11 Eligibility Criteria for Thrombolytic Therapy **and** ▸ Table 8.8)

Table 8.7 Pharmacology for cerebrovascular disorders

Drug	Category	Indication	Nursing Implications
Dopamine (Intropin) Dobutamine (Dobutrex) Phenylephrine (Neo-synephrine) Norepinephrine (Levophed) Epinephrine (Adrenaline)	Vasopressors Cardiac stimulants	Increase blood pressure	May result in hypertension Should have hemodynamic monitoring (central line and arterial line) Must be in ICU or monitored unit
Labetalol (Normodyne) Metoprolol (Lopressor) Hydralazine (Apresoline) Nitroglycerine Nitroprusside (Nipride) Enalapril (Vasotec)	Antihypertensives	Reduce blood pressure	May result in hypotension Must be in ICU or monitored unit for intravenous use May require hemodynamic monitoring (e.g., central line and arterial line)
Nimodipine (Nimotop) Nicardipine (Cardene)	Calcium channel blockers	Reduce blood pressure Reduce vasospasm	May result in hypotension
Clopidogrel (Plavix) Aspirin Apixaban (Eliquis) Rivaroxaban (Xarelto)	Antiplatelet agents	Reduce platelet aggregation in TIA, stroke, placement of stents, and valves	Monitor for bleeding Must be held before surgical procedure
Warfarin (Coumadin) Enoxaparin (Lovenox) Heparin Apixaban (Eliquis) Rivaroxaban (Xarelto)	Anticoagulation agents	Deep vein thrombosis/ pulmonary embolus Atrial fibrillation Thrombotic stroke	Monitor PT/INR (Coumadin) or PTT (heparin) Family teaching for home use
Tissue plasminogen activase Streptokinase	Antithrombotic agents	Recanalization of occluded arteries, restoring oxygenation and cerebral blood flow	Must meet eligibility criteria Increase risk of bleeding or reperfusion injury Monitored unit (Box 8.11 Eligibility Criteria for Thrombolytic Therapy)

Table 8.7 (continued)

Drug	Category	Indication	Nursing Implications
Mannitol	Hyperosmotic solution	Reduces vasogenic edema	Monitored unit Monitor serum sodium and osmolality levels
Famotidine (Pepcid) Ranitidine (Zantac)	H2 blockers	Reduce acid in the stomach	Thrombocytopenia
Phenytoin (Dilantin) Carbamazepine (Tegretol) Divalproex (Depakote) Gabapentin (Neurontin) Lamotrigine (Lamictal) Phenobarbital Clonazepam (Klonopin) Ethosuximide (Zarontin) Levetiracetam (Keppra) Lacosamide (Vimpat)	Antiepileptic drugs	Prevent seizures	Thrombocytopenia Allergic reactions (can be severe) Gingivitis Monitor blood levels, when appropriate Possible drug–food interactions

Abbreviations: ICU, intensive care unit; INR, international normalized ratio; PT, prothrombin time; PTT, partial thromboplastin time; TIA, transient ischemic attack.

Table 8.8 Postthrombolytic therapy: what to watch for

Problem	Indication	Nursing action	Rationale
Bleeding from catheter site	Possible hemorrhage	Monitor for bleeding at catheter insertion site	Potential for hemorrhage at insertion site
Decline in neurologic assessment	Possible hemorrhage	Monitor neurologic assessment closely Monitor for signs of increased ICP Report all new abnormal findings	Potential for ICH

Abbreviations: ICH, intracranial hemorrhage; ICP, intracranial pressure.

Box 8.11 Eligibility Criteria for Thrombolytic Therapy

Inclusion criteria
- Symptom onset: In less than 3 hours
- Age: More than 18 years
- Clinical diagnosis of ischemic stroke with measurable deficit, according to the National Institutes of Health Stroke Scale
- CT confirmation that hemorrhage has been excluded

Exclusion criteria
- Stroke or head trauma within 3 months
- Systolic blood pressure more than 185 mm Hg, or diastolic blood pressure more than 110 mm Hg
- Glucose level less than 50 mg/dL or more than 400 mg/dL
- Platelet count less than 100×10^9/L
- Rapidly improving or declining neurologic status
- Recent myocardial infarction
- Recent treatment with heparin
- Pregnancy

Endovascular Intervention

Endovascular intervention includes modalities to treat vascular lesions associated with significant neurologic compromise. These interventional radiology procedures are performed by interventional radiologists or endovascular surgeons. This is discussed in more detail in Chapter 14: Neuroradiology and Neuroendovascular Intervention.
- Percutaneous angioplasty
  - Breaks up atherosclerotic plaque by inflation of a balloon at the site of stenosis
- Intravascular stenting
  - Frequently used in conjunction with percutaneous angioplasty
  - Used to maintain vessel patency

Surgical Intervention

- Carotid endarterectomy
  - Indicated when carotid occlusion is more than 70% (▶ Table 8.9)
- Bypass (revascularization) procedures
  - Direct or indirect methods of augmenting adequate blood flow to hypoperfused areas of brain
  - Direct method
    - Extracranial-to-intracranial bypass

Table 8.9 Postoperative carotid endarterectomy: what to watch for

Problem	Indication	Nursing action	Rationale
Respiratory distress and/ or difficulty swallowing	Postoperative hemorrhage	Measure neck circumference on arrival to unit and then at least hourly for first 24 h Monitor incision for swelling and hematoma Observe patient for difficulty in swallowing Observe for tracheal deviation in presence of swelling or hemorrhage	Potential for hemorrhage from surgical site, with possible tracheal deviation and respiratory distress
Decline in neurologic function	Stroke or hemorrhage	Perform neurologic assessment at least hourly for immediate postoperative period and then as directed	Potential for embolic stroke or hemorrhage

- – Most frequently, STA-MCA anastomosis
- – Controversial procedure, but favorable results are likely when a surgeon highly specialized in revascularization techniques performs the bypass
- ○ Indirect method
  - – Encephaloduroarteriosynangiosis or encephalomyosynangiosis
  - – Autologous tissue is placed on the surface of the brain, achieving revascularization by angiogenesis from the graft into the vascular system
  - – Referred to as an *onlay procedure*
- ○ Revascularization procedures such as the STA-MCA bypass are also used in patients with large aneurysms, when certain arteries must be sacrificed to protect against possible catastrophic aneurysmal rupture (Box 8.12 Focus On: Moyamoya Disease)

Box 8.12 Focus On: Moyamoya Disease

- Relatively rare cerebrovascular occlusive disease
- Characterized by progressive occlusion of the terminal segments of the internal carotid artery and its branches
- Results in severe impairment of the arterial reserve capacity
- Clinical manifestations are consistent with TIA or stroke
- Presentation may be unilateral or bilateral
- Treatment for symptomatic moyamoya disease is revascularization surgery
- Found predominately in East Asian population but occurs in all populations
- Japanese translation is "puff of smoke"

Hemorrhagic Stroke

Hemorrhagic stroke, also referred to as intraparenchymal or intracerebral hemorrhage (ICH), is most commonly caused by rupture of a blood vessel (▶ Fig. 8.18 and ▶ Fig. 8.19).

• Accounts for approximately 15 to 20% of all strokes
• Half of all patients with ICH die within the first 2 days after hemorrhage
• Mortality is about 35 to 50% in the first 30 days after ICH

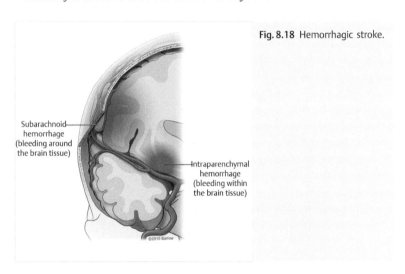

Fig. 8.18 Hemorrhagic stroke.

Subarachnoid hemorrhage (bleeding around the brain tissue)

Intraparenchymal hemorrhage (bleeding within the brain tissue)

©2015 Barrow

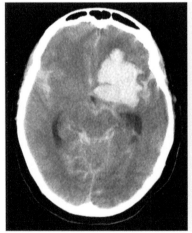

Fig. 8.19 Intracranial hemorrhage.

- Most common cause is hypertension
- Subarachnoid hemorrhage is a type of ICH; this is discussed in greater detail later
- ICH also occurs in trauma patients

Clinical Manifestations of Hemorrhagic Stroke

- Signs and symptoms usually occur rapidly, often without warning (▶ Table 8.10)

Table 8.10 Stroke: what to watch for

Problem	Indication	Nursing action	Rationale
Decline in neurologic assessment	Cerebral edema Hemorrhage	Perform complete neurologic assessment and compare with previous assessment; check vital signs (blood pressure, heart rate, and respiratory rate) Check current laboratory values, especially serum sodium and osmolarity, and CBC Check respiratory status, including oxygen saturations, arterial blood gases, and respiratory rate and pattern	Potential for patient to extend an ischemic stroke, or to rebleed from hemorrhagic stroke Hyponatremia or hyperglycemia may facilitate cerebral edema Low hemoglobin indicates low oxygen-carrying capacity of red blood cells, leading to cerebral hypoxia and edema Poor systemic oxygenation suggests cerebral hypoxia; this may lead to cerebral edema
	Seizure	EEG	Nonconvulsive status epilepticus, which is the cause for decreased LOC
	Hydrocephalus	CT	Hydrocephalus common after stroke
Respiratory distress	Respiratory failure	Perform respiratory assessment, including oxygen saturation, arterial blood gases, respiratory rate and rhythm, and auscultation of lungs Be prepared for intubation and mechanical ventilation	Patients with decreased LOC may not be able to protect airway and are at risk for aspiration, atelectasis, and pneumonia

Abbreviations: CBC, complete blood count; CT, computed tomography; EEG, electroencephalogram; LOC, level of consciousness.

- Symptoms depend on the area of brain affected
- Headache is a common presenting sign
- Common affected areas of the brain are the putamen and surrounding internal capsule (about 50% of all patients with ICH), due to hypertension
- Neurologic damage progresses rapidly, so coma or death may be the first symptom
- If ICH volume is large, symptoms may be the result of increased ICP and herniation syndromes; see also Chapter 3: Principles of Intracranial Pressure

Diagnosis of Hemorrhagic Stroke

History

- Risk factors
  - Hypertension
  - Advanced age
  - Coagulopathy
  - Alcoholism
  - Illicit drug use (e.g., amphetamines and cocaine)

Imaging Studies

- CT
- MRI

Treatment of Hemorrhagic Stroke

Medical Management

- Prevention.
  - Modification of risk factors
    - Hypertension
    - Obesity
    - Diabetes
- Hemodynamic management
- Reversal of coagulopathy may be needed in cases of anticoagulation-induced hemorrhage
- Management of increased ICP; see also Chapter 3: Principles of Intracranial Pressure
- Palliative care may be an option after catastrophic hemorrhage

Surgical Intervention

- Ventriculostomy for ICP management
- Craniotomy for evacuation of ICH; see also Chapter 15: Neurosurgical Interventions
- Craniectomy (removal of bone flap) for management of ICP

Nonaneurysmal Subarachnoid Hemorrhage

Subarachnoid hemorrhage is another form of hemorrhagic stroke.

- Nonaneurysmal, nontraumatic SAH has a very different course than aneurysmal SAH
- Accounts for approximately 10% of all SAH
- Less severe clinical manifestations, with better outcome
- The cause may never be diagnosed
- Subarachnoid hemorrhage may also occur from trauma
  - Most common form of SAH
  - Clinical course similar to other hemorrhagic stroke

8.5 Nursing Management for Patients with Vascular Disorders

This chapter contains an overview of the unique challenges associated with caring for patients with vascular disorders. Below are generalized implications appropriate for most patients with cerebrovascular disorders (Box 8.13 Clinical Alert: Medical Emergency **and** Box 8.14 Example of Acute Stroke Pathway, **and Appendix A6: Nursing Management of Patients with Stroke and Appendix A7: Nursing Management of Patients with Subarachnoid Hemorrhage**).

This chapter is intended as a basic reference for bedside care of neurologic patients with cerebrovascular disorders. For more information, the reader is urged to consult the references at the end of this chapter.

Box 8.13 Clinical Alert: Medical Emergency

- The onset of neurologic symptoms indicating stroke is a medical emergency
- Notify attending physician immediately of any new symptoms indicating possibility of stroke
- Initiate stroke protocols immediately

Box 8.14 Example of Acute Stroke Pathway

- Record time of onset of stroke (last time the patient is seen without symptoms of stroke), page the stroke team (onset of stroke symptoms < 6 hours), and notify attending physician
- Order stat CT of head and CTA of head and neck
- Start two IV lines (18-gauge): normal saline at 100 mL/h; reserve 1 line for nicardipine (Cardene)
- Stat blood draw for complete blood count, coagulation profile, and basic metabolic profile (draw blood before CT scan)
- Arterial line
- Oxygen via nasal cannula to maintain oxygen saturation level more than 95%
- Complete vital signs and neurologic assessment every 15 minutes
- Continuous ECG monitor
- Blood pressure treatment: first choice
  ○ If systolic blood pressure (SBP) > 185 mm Hg and < 200 mm Hg, begin nicardipine at 5 mg/h
  ○ If SBP > 200 mm Hg and < 220 mm Hg, begin nicardipine at 9 mg/h
  ○ If SBP > 220 mm Hg, begin nicardipine at 13 mg/h
- Adjust nicardipine by 5 mg/h every 5 minutes to maintain target range of BP, that is, < 185/110 mm Hg
- Blood pressure treatment: second choice
  ○ If SBP 200 to 220 mm Hg, apply 1 in nitroglycerine (NTG) ointment and begin either labetalol 10 mg IV every 10 minutes or hydralazine 5 mg IV every 20 minutes
  ○ If SBP > 200 mm Hg, apply 1 in NTG ointment and begin either labetalol 20 mg IV every 10 minutes or hydralazine 10 mg IV every 20 minutes

8.5.1 Neurologic Assessment

- Obtain comprehensive patient and family history
- Assess LOC; see also Chapter 2: Assessment
- Test motor, sensory, cognitive, and cranial nerve functions
- Evaluate risk factors
- Consult the NIH Stroke Scale for thorough assessment (► Table 8.11)
- Monitor the patient closely for changes from baseline neurologic examination
- Use appropriate nursing interventions to maintain ICP and perform ICP monitoring, if appropriate; consult Chapter 3: Principles of Intracranial Pressure for more information

Table 8.11 Modified National Institutes of Health Stroke Scale*

Item	Name	Response
1A	Level of consciousness	0 = Alert
		1 = Not alert, but arouses easily
		2 = Not alert, obtunded
		3 = Unresponsive
1B	Questions	0 = Answers both questions correctly
		1 = Answers one correctly
		2 = Answers neither correctly
1C	Commands	0 = Performs both tasks correctly
		1 = Performs one task correctly
		2 = Performs neither task correctly
2	Gaze	0 = Normal
		1 = Partial gaze palsy
		2 = Total gaze palsy
3	Visual fields	0 = No visual loss
		1 = Partial hemianopsia
		2 = Complete hemianopsia
		3 = Bilateral hemianopsia
4	Facial palsy	0 = Normal
		1 = Minor paralysis
		2 = Partial paralysis
		3 = Complete paralysis
5	Motor arm a. left b. right	0 = No drift
		1 = Drift before 10 seconds
		2 = Falls before 10 seconds
		3 = No effort against gravity
		4 = No movement
6	Motor leg a. left b. right	0 = No drift
		1 = Drift before 5 seconds
		2 = Falls before 5 seconds
		3 = No effort against gravity
		4 = No movement
7	Ataxia	0 = Absent
		1 = One limb
		2 = Two limbs
8	Sensory	0 = Normal
		1 = Mild loss
		2 = Severe loss

Table 8.11 (*continued*)

Item	Name	Response
9	Language	0 = Normal
		1 = Mild aphasia
		2 = Severe aphasia
		3 = Mute or global aphasia
10	Dysarthria	0= Normal
		1 = Mild
		2 = Severe
11	Extinction	0 = Normal
		1 = Mild
		2 = Severe

*From Meyer BC, Lyden PD. The Modified National Institutes of Health Stroke Scale (mNIHSS): Its time has come. Int J Stroke 2009; 4(4):267-273

8.5.2 Respiratory Assessment

• Perform airway assessment and protection
• Document and monitor respiratory rate and rhythm
• Assess arterial blood gases, using an O_2 saturation monitor, as appropriate
• Results of respiratory assessment will be relative to the patient's LOC

8.5.3 Cardiovascular Assessment

• Control blood pressure, administering medication, as needed, to maintain it within appropriate parameters
• Perform hemodynamic monitoring
• Use triple-H therapy for patients with SAH
• Monitor ECG for cardiac arrhythmias (remember cardiac stunning)
• Results of cardiovascular assessment will be relative to the patient's LOC

8.5.4 Fluid and Electrolyte Assessment

• Monitor glucose levels and administer medications as directed to maintain glucose at the target level
• Monitor strict intake and output
• Monitor serum sodium level, watch for hyponatremia, and report abnormal values
• See also Chapter 5: Electrolyte Disturbances

8.5.5 Seizure Assessment

- History (type, onset, and frequency); see also Chapter 6: Seizures
- Medications (drug interactions and levels, if indicated)
- Safety

8.5.6 Immobility Assessment

- Administer enoxaparin (Lovenox), if appropriate
- Use sequential compression devices
- Encourage mobility—early ambulation is important
- Watch for signs and symptoms of deep vein thrombosis; report immediately

8.5.7 Patient and Family Teaching

- Provide educational materials, as appropriate
- Refer patients and their families to support and educational websites
- Consult clergy or palliative care representatives, if appropriate
- Offer comprehensive discharge instructions
  - Carotid endarterectomy (Appendix B9 Sample discharge instructions after carotid endarterectomy)
  - Cerebral angiogram for aneurysm embolization or coiling (Appendix B19 Sample discharge instructions after cerebral angiogram for cerebral aneurysm embolization or coiling)
  - Craniotomy for aneurysm clipping (Appendix B8 Sample discharge instructions after craniotomy for aneurysm clipping)

8.5.8 Collaborative Management

After the initial, acute phase of stroke, the nursing staff, patient, and family must cope with some degree of neurologic compromise. Regardless of the type of vascular anomaly, neurologic deficits may range from subtle to catastrophic. Numerous adjunct services can provide assistance in the care of these challenging patients. These various specialties may include the following:

- Nursing
- Neurosurgery
- Neurology service for seizure management or stroke service
- Internal medicine or neurointensivist
- Ophthalmology for visual disturbances or loss of vision
- Therapy specialties
  - Physical therapy
  - Occupational therapy
  - Speech therapy for cognitive evaluation, including swallow evaluation, if appropriate

- Rehabilitation services
- Neuropsychology for cognitive evaluation
- Social work or case management
- Clergy, chaplain, or spiritual support
- Palliative care or hospice

Videos

Video 8.1 Development and rupture of a basilar tip aneurysm.
Video 8.2 Aneurysm treated with coiling.

Suggested Reading

[1] American Association of Neuroscience Nurses. http://www.aann.org. Accessed June 29, 2017

[2] American Association of Neuroscience Nurses. Guide to the care of the patient with ischemic stroke: AANN Reference Series for Clinical Practice. Glenview, IL: American Association of Neuroscience Nurses; 2004

[3] American Heart Association. http://www.heart.org. Accessed June 29, 2017

[4] American Stroke Association. http://www.strokeassociation.org. Accessed June 29, 2017

[5] Barrow Neurological Institute. http://www.thebarrow.org. Accessed June 29, 2017

[6] Benjamin EJ, Blaha MJ, Chiuve SE, et al, American Heart Association Statistics Committee and Stroke Statistics Subcommittee. Heart disease and stroke statistics—2017 update. A report from the American Heart Association. Circulation. 2017; 135:e146–e603

[7] Broderick JP, Brott T, Tomsick T, Miller R, Huster G. Intracerebral hemorrhage more than twice as common as subarachnoid hemorrhage. J Neurosurg. 1993; 78(2):188–191

[8] Buckley DA, Hickey JV. Cerebral aneurysms. In: Hickey JV, ed. The Clinical Practice of Neurological and Neurosurgical Nursing. 7th ed. Philadelphia, PA: Lippincott Williams & Wilkins, a Wolter Kluwer business; 2014

[9] Fisher CM, Kistler JP, Davis JM. Relation of cerebral vasospasm to subarachnoid hemorrhage visualized by computerized tomographic scanning. Neurosurgery. 1980; 6(1):1–9

[10] Frangione-Edfort E, American Association of Neuroscience Nurses. A guideline for acute stroke: evaluation of New Jersey's practices. J Neurosci Nurs. 2014; 46(6):E25–E32

[11] Hauck EF, Wohlfeld B, Welch BG, White JA, Samson D. Clipping of very large or giant unruptured intracranial aneurysms in the anterior circulation: an outcome study. J Neurosurg. 2008; 109(6): 1012–1018

[12] Herrmann LL, Zabramski JM. Nonaneurysmal subarachnoid hemorrhage: a review of clinical course and outcome in two hemorrhage patterns. J Neurosci Nurs. 2007; 39(3):135–142

[13] Jandial R, Aryan HE, Nakaji P. Neurosurgical Essentials. St. Louis, MO: Quality Medical Publishing, Inc.; 2004

[14] Johnston SC, Nguyen-Huynh MN, Schwarz ME, et al. National Stroke Association guidelines for the management of transient ischemic attacks. Ann Neurol. 2006; 60(3):301–313

[15] Juvela S. Prehemorrhage risk factors for fatal intracranial aneurysm rupture. Stroke. 2003; 34(8): 1852–1857

[16] Kaminogo M, Yonekura M, Shibata S. Incidence and outcome of multiple intracranial aneurysms in a defined population. Stroke. 2003; 34(1):16–21

[17] Khurana VG, Spetzler RF. The Brain Aneurysm: A Comprehensive Resource for Brain Aneurysm Patients, Their Families, and Physicians. Bloomington, IN: AuthorHouse; 2006

[18] Kokuzawa J, Kaku Y, Watarai T, Tanaka T, Hatsuda N, Ando T. Pure vasogenic edema caused by cerebral hyperperfusion after superficial temporal artery to middle cerebral artery anastomosis—case report. Neurol Med Chir (Tokyo). 2010; 50(3):250–253

[19] Kurashvili P, Olson D. Temperature management and nursing care of the patient with acute ischemic stroke. Stroke. 2015; 46(9):e205–e207

[20] National Stroke Association. http://www.stroke.org. Accessed June 29, 2017.

[21] North American Symptomatic Carotid Endarterectomy Trial Collaborators. Beneficial effect of carotid endarterectomy in symptomatic patients with high-grade carotid stenosis. N Engl J Med. 1991; 325(7):445–453

[22] Passacantilli E, Zabramski JM, Lanzino G, Spetzler RF. Cavernous malformations: genetics, molecular biology, and familial forms. Operative Techniques in Neurosurgery. 2002; 5(3):145–149

[23] Raaymakers TW, Rinkel GJ, Limburg M, Algra A. Mortality and morbidity of surgery for unruptured intracranial aneurysms: a meta-analysis. Stroke. 1998; 29(8):1531–1538

[24] Ryan D. Cavernous malformations. J Neurosci Nurs. 2010; 42(5):294–299

[25] Schievink WI. Genetics of Intracranial Aneurysms. In: Winn HR, ed. Youmans Neurological Surgery. 5th ed. Philadelphia, PA: WB Saunders; 2004

[26] Society of Neurointerventional Surgery. Brain Aneurysms. http://www.brainaneurysm.com. Accessed June 29, 2017

[27] Söderman M, Andersson T, Karlsson B, Wallace MC, Edner G. Management of patients with brain arteriovenous malformations. Eur J Radiol. 2003; 46(3):195–205

[28] Spetzler RF, Martin NA. A proposed grading system for arteriovenous malformations. J Neurosurg. 1986; 65(4):476–483

[29] Vajkoczy P. Moyamoya disease: collateralization is everything. Cerebrovasc Dis. 2009; 28(3):258

[30] Zabramski JM, Han PP. Epidemiology and natural history of cavernous malformations. In: Winn HR, ed. Youmans Neurological Surgery. 5th ed. Philadelphia: WB Saunders; 2004

[31] Zabramski JM, Henn JS, Coons S. Pathology of cerebral vascular malformations. Neurosurg Clin N Am. 1999; 10(3):395–410

[32] Zabramski JM, Wascher TM, Spetzler RF, et al. The natural history of familial cavernous malformations: results of an ongoing study. J Neurosurg. 1994; 80(3):422–432

9 Traumatic Brain Injury

Denita Ryan

Abstract

Traumatic brain injury (TBI) is a term that encompasses a wide variety of diagnoses, ranging from mild concussions to severe brain injury such as a hematoma or diffuse axonal injury. Severe brain injury can have devastating effects on the patient, and any TBI has the potential to be life-changing, with severe personal, physical, and socioeconomic consequences. The signs and symptoms of traumatic injury may be subtle or immediately recognizable. No matter the presentation, all neuroscience nurses must be familiar with the types of TBI and know the appropriate interventions and treatments.

Keywords: concussion, diffuse axonal injury, epidural hematoma, herniation syndromes, intracerebral hematoma, subdural hematoma

9.1 Traumatic Brain Injury

Injury to the brain from an external force that results in altered brain function has been a major health problem for centuries, indicated by archeological evidence that demonstrates clubbing injuries occurring 1 million years ago. Brain injuries have long been considered fatal. As recently as the 1970s, approximately 90% of patients suffering brain trauma died from their injuries. Today, that rate is less than 20%. Although outcomes are better today, patients with traumatic brian injury (TBI) still face a significant risk of long-term disability or death.

Acute head injury occurs in varying degrees of severity. Severity can range from a relatively simple scalp laceration requiring little or no treatment to a devastating TBI with severe impairment, prolonged hospitalization, and permanent disability or death.

9.1.1 Epidemiology

The U.S. Centers for Disease Control and Prevention (CDC) estimate that each year approximately 275,000 patients with TBI are admitted to hospitals in the United States and 52,000 persons die due to brain injury. In 2017, the CDC reported that approximately 282,000 people were diagnosed with TBI in 2013. Of these, nearly 50,000 died.

Causes of Traumatic Brain Injury

Although there are thousands of possible causes for TBI, the more common ones vary based on sex, age, and locale.

- Men are three times more likely than women to sustain a TBI
- American Indian/Alaska natives have the highest overall rate of TBI of any racial group; African-Americans have the second-highest rate
- The incidence of penetrating injuries such as gunshot wounds is higher in the United States than in any other developed country in the world
- Military personnel are more likely to suffer TBI from explosive blasts than regular civilians
- Motor vehicle accidents were the leading cause of death in persons 5 to 24 years old
- Rates of TBI-related death are highest in the elderly (> 75 years), with falls accounting for most deaths

Costs of Traumatic Brain Injury

The actual cost of TBI is incalculable. The direct and indirect costs of treatment and rehabilitation of patients who have sustained TBI in the United States have been estimated at $48.3 billion annually. However, the cost in suffering of patients, their families, and the community is immeasurable (Box 9.1 Risk Factors for TBI).

Box 9.1 Risk Factors for TBI

- Age 18 to 25 years or ≥70 years
- Male sex (1.5:1)
- Use of alcohol or drugs
- Active-duty military status
- Lack or insufficient use of restraint or safety measures (e.g., helmet or seat belt)
- Participation in certain sports (e.g., football)

9.2 Types of Traumatic Brain Injury

Traumatic brain injuries occur as either closed or open injuries. Closed injuries are more common. They frequently are caused by acceleration–deceleration incidents, which cause the brain to strike against one side of the skull, and then rebound to strike the opposite side of the skull. These injuries are also referred to as *coup-contrecoup* injuries (▶ Fig. 9.1; Video 9.1). Closed head injuries may result in hematomas, contusions, concussions, or diffuse axonal injuries.

Open injuries are those in which the cranial vault is breached, with injury to the brain itself. These injuries are usually seen as skull fractures caused by falls or motor vehicle accidents or as penetrating injuries such as gunshot wounds.

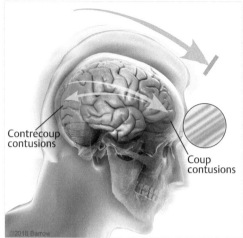

Fig. 9.1 Coup-contrecoup injury.

Contrecoup contusions

Coup contusions

It is common for a patient with TBI to have more than one type of head injury, and often several types, both open and closed (Box 9.2 Mechanisms of TBI).

Box 9.2 Mechanisms of Traumatic Brain Injury

- Acceleration–deceleration injuries
  - Motor vehicle accidents
  - Shaken baby syndrome
  - Falls
- Direct blow to the head
  - Falls
  - Sports injuries
  - Physical assaults
  - Debris falling from overhead
- Penetrating injuries
  - Gunshot wounds
  - Knives/impalement

May be combination of mechanisms.

9.2.1 Superficial Injuries

Patients with TBI often have superficial injuries to the scalp that also require medical attention. Superficial injuries are not brain injuries; however, they

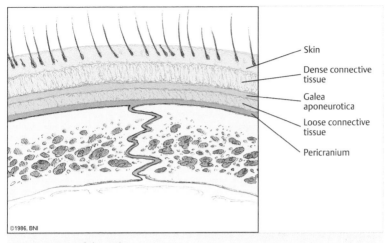

Fig. 9.2 Layers of the scalp.

commonly occur in conjunction with TBI (Box 9.3 Clinical Alert: Scalp Lacerations).
- The scalp consists of five layers that cover the skull (▶ Fig. 9.2)
- The subgaleal space is a common space for blood to collect, forming a "goose egg."
- The scalp is extremely vascular, making exsanguination (i.e., extensive blood loss) possible
- Treatment of scalp lacerations depends on the extent of injury
- Scalp lacerations may indicate the presence of a skull fracture beneath the scalp

---

Box 9.3 Clinical Alert: Scalp Lacerations

The presence of a scalp laceration may indicate the following:
- Extensive blood loss, possibly exsanguination
- Presence of a skull fracture under the laceration
- Potential for infection

9.2.2 Skull Fractures

The skull is the bony structure housing the brain.
- Composed of frontal, temporal, parietal, and occipital bones
- Includes multiple facial bones

- The floor of the skull is called the *skull base* and is rough and uneven
- Asymmetrical
- Variable thickness

Types of Skull Fractures

Fractures of the skull are categorized by type of break
- Linear
- Comminuted
- Basal
- Depressed

Linear Skull Fracture

- Simple break with no bone displacement (▶ Fig. 9.3)
- Most common in a low-velocity-impact accident

Comminuted Skull Fracture

- Fragmented interruption of the skull (▶ Fig. 9.4)
- Caused by multiple linear fractures

Basal Skull Fracture

- Linear fracture of the skull base (▶ Fig. 9.5)
- When fractured, the rough skull base may tear the dura, resulting in a cerebrospinal fluid (CSF) leak (Box 9.4 Causes and Signs of Cerebrospinal Fluid Leaks)

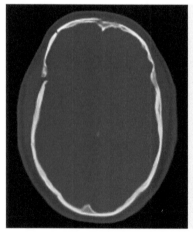

Fig. 9.3 Linear skull fracture.

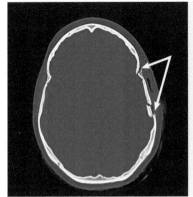

Fig. 9.4 CT scan using bone window of a comminuted skull fracture (arrows).

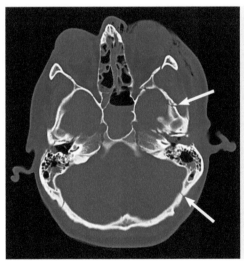

Fig. 9.5 CT scan using bone window of a patient with extensive basal skull fractures (arrows).

- Watch for characteristic signs of basal skull fracture; see also Chapter 2: Assessment
  - Battle's sign (ecchymosis over mastoid bone)
  - Raccoon eyes (periorbital ecchymosis)

Box 9.4 Causes and Signs of Cerebrospinal Fluid Leaks

- CSF leaks may occur because of the following causes:
  - Certain surgical approaches (e.g., retrosigmoid, transsphenoidal), see also Chapter 15: Neurosurgical Interventions
  - Basal skull fractures
- Signs of CSF leaks
  - Rhinorrhea
    - Clear liquid dripping from the nose
    - Awareness of fluid dripping down back of the throat
    - Metallic taste in the back of the throat
  - Otorrhea
    - Clear liquid discharge from ear
  - Halo sign
    - Stain on bed linens or clothes from the wound, nose, or ears
    - Usually clear with yellow ring (halo)
  - Reservoir sign
    - Dripping of fluid from the nose upon leaning forward

Depressed Skull Fracture

- Displacement of comminuted fracture (▶ Fig. 9.6)
- Usually seen in conjunction with other injuries, such as contusions or lacerations

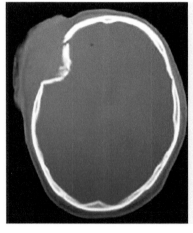

Fig. 9.6 Depressed skull fracture.

- Degree of neurologic impairment depends on the location and severity of the injury to the brain

Clinical Manifestations of Skull Fractures

Skull fractures alone do not cause neurologic symptoms.
- Often occur in conjunction with other types of brain injuries
  - Hematomas
  - Contusions
  - Penetrating wounds (e.g., gunshot wounds; ▶ Fig. 9.7)
- Clinical manifestations are related to TBI associated with the skull fracture

9.2.3 Hematomas

A hematoma is a localized collection of blood that is often clotted. Intracranial hematomas are defined by their location (▶ Fig. 9.8 and ▶ Table 9.1)
- Epidural
- Subdural
- Intraparenchymal

Epidural Hematoma

- Bleeding into the space between the skull and the dura (▶ Fig. 9.9)
- Usually caused by laceration of an artery or vein
  - About 85% of epidural hematomas (EDHs) are caused by arterial bleeding

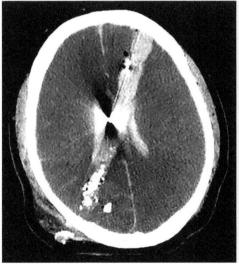

Fig. 9.7 Gunshot wound.

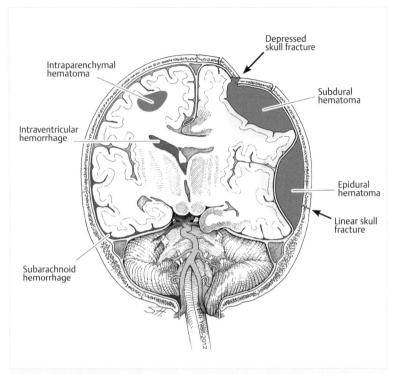

Fig. 9.8 Locations of hematomas.

Table 9.1 Characteristics of hematomas

Type of hematoma	Onset of symptoms	Appearance on CT
EDH	Immediate, with initial loss of consciousness, followed by lucid interval, then neurologic decline	Hyperdense, elliptical
IPH	Immediate	Hyperdense, frequently in frontal or temporal lobes
Acute SDH	Within 48 h after injury	Hyperdense
Subacute SDH	48 h to 3 wk after injury	Isodense
Chronic SDH	3 wk to several months after injury	Hypodense

Abbreviations: CT, computed tomography; EDH, epidural hematoma; IPH, intraparenchymal hemorrhage; SDH, subdural hematoma.

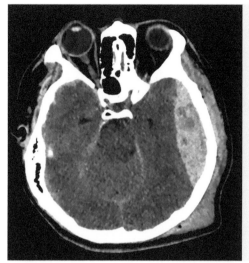

Fig. 9.9 Epidural hematoma.

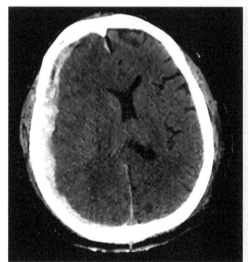

Fig. 9.10 Subdural hematoma.

Subdural Hematoma

- Bleeding between the dura and arachnoid layers of the meninges
  (▶ Fig. 9.10)
- Usually caused by tearing of the bridging veins on the surface of the brain

- Patients can have multiple episodes of bleeding (e.g., acute and chronic subdural hematoma [SDH])
- Divided into categories based on the amount of time between the original injury and the presentation of signs and symptoms
  - Acute
    - Symptoms present within 48 hours after injury
  - Subacute
    - Symptoms present from 48 hours to 3 weeks after injury
  - Chronic SDH
    - Symptoms present 3 weeks or longer after injury
    - Most common in the elderly
    - Composed of a hematoma with the consistency of motor oil.

Intraparenchymal Hematoma

- Intraparenchymal hematoma (IPH) is also referred to as *intracerebral hematoma*
- Hemorrhage causes blood clot within brain tissue
- Subarachnoid or intraventricular hemorrhages are also included in this category
- Vessel laceration caused by severe shearing forces of brain movement during acceleration–deceleration events
- Occurs in TBI but is more commonly caused by hypertension. Figure 8.18 in Chapter 8 demonstrates intraparenchymal hemorrhage, also known as hemorrhagic stroke

Clinical Manifestations of Hematomas

The classic clinical presentation of EDH is an immediate period of unconsciousness, followed by a lucid interval before neurologic decline. A growing hematoma rapidly increases intracranial pressure (ICP) and exerts pressure on surrounding structures in the brain, a phenomenon also known as *mass effect*; see also Chapter 3: Principles of Intracranial Pressure. Although symptoms depend on the location of the injury, some common manifestations of EDH may include the following:

- Enlargement of the pupil on the ipsilateral side
- Motor weakness
- Seizures
- Increasing headache

9.2.4 Contusion

Brain contusions are bruising of the brain.
- May occur with other types of brain injury, such as skull fractures or hematomas
- Result from blunt trauma, acceleration–deceleration injuries, or penetrating injuries

Coup-Contrecoup Contusions

Coup refers to a contusion directly over the brain at the point of impact; *contrecoup* refers to a contusion on the opposite side, at the point where the brain rebounds against the skull.

- Result from the brain moving about inside the skull
- Result from various types of impact, including the following:
  - Acceleration–deceleration injuries
  - Shaken baby syndrome
  - Falls

Clinical Manifestations of Contusions

Symptoms depend on the location and severity of the brain injury and the associated cerebral edema; see also Chapter 2: Assessment. Symptoms include the following:

- Cognitive deficits
- Motor and/or sensory deficits
- Headaches
- Seizures

9.2.5 Concussion

Concussion is a recognized collection of neurologic and cognitive symptoms that result from mild head injury. It is usually caused by blunt trauma to the head. Concussion can be caused by

- Sports injuries
- Motor vehicle accidents
- Falls
- Physical assaults

Clinical Manifestations of Concussion

- Confusion
- Headache
- Cognitive impairment (e.g., memory loss)
- Usually a nonfocal (i.e., diffuse) injury
- Patients may lose consciousness
  - Extended period of loss of consciousness warrants hospital admission for further testing to rule out a more serious TBI

Second Impact Syndrome

Second impact syndrome is a rare but devastating outcome of a second concussion that occurs before the brain can heal from a prior concussion.

- Caused by the loss of autoregulation of the brain's blood supply due to the first injury; see also Chapter 3: Principles of Intracranial Pressure

- Can result in cerebral edema and death
- Associated with high morbidity and death
- Patients who continue to participate in risky behavior or activities after concussion are considered to be at high risk for second impact syndrome (Box 9.5 American Association of Neurology Position on Sports Concussions)

Box 9.5 American Association of Neurology Position on Sports Concussions

Because of the gravity of second impact syndrome, the American Association of Neurology has issued a position statement on athletes that are returning to participation in high-risk activities.

- A possible concussion mandates the immediate cessation of participation in sports activity
- Any sign of concussion must be evaluated by a health care provider with specific training in the recognition of concussion
- A return to sports activities requires clearance by a medical professional

---

Postconcussion Syndrome

- Follows concussion
- Is characterized by one or more symptoms (Box 9.6 Symptoms of Postconcussion Syndrome)
- May take months to completely resolve
- Treatment is multilevel
  - Symptom support
  - Counseling
  - Cognitive testing
  - Education for the patient and family

Box 9.6 Symptoms of Postconcussion Syndrome

- Headache
- Dizziness or various types of vertigo
- Blurred vision
- Hearing loss or tinnitus (e.g., ringing or buzzing in ears)
- Anxiety
- Depression
- Decrease in or loss of appetite
- Alteration in sleep patterns
- Personality changes
- Light or noise sensitivity
- Cognitive decline

9.2.6 Diffuse Axonal Injury

Damage to the white matter of the brain caused by the tearing of small blood vessels and axons is called *diffuse axonal injury* or *shearing injury.*

Clinical Manifestations of Diffuse Axonal Injury

- Symptoms depend on the degree and location of the injury
- Damage ranges from mild cognitive loss to severe neurologic devastation and death

9.3 Diagnosis of Traumatic Brain Injury

Traumatic brain injury is diagnosed by obtaining the patient's medical history and by using the appropriate medical tests, usually diagnostic imaging (▶ Table 9.2).

9.3.1 Medical History

- Includes the suspected mechanism of injury (e.g., in the case of motor vehicle accident, documents use of seat belts, details of accident such as rollover or head-on collision, and whether it necessitated extraction from the vehicle by emergency personnel)
- Documents the time the injury occurred in relation to the present time
- Documents the patient's symptoms, including their duration

9.3.2 Imaging Studies

- Plain skull radiographs to diagnose fractures
- Computed tomography (CT) imaging to rule out or document underlying brain trauma
  - Hematomas
  - Hydrocephalus
  - Contusions
  - Edema
- Magnetic resonance imaging (MRI)
  - Diffuse axonal injury (not seen on CT)

9.3.3 Treatment of Traumatic Brain Injury

Treatment depends on the type, location, and severity of the TBI. Such treatment can be conservative or surgical, or it can be limited to end-of-life care.

Medical or Conservative Treatment

Linear fractures usually do not require intervention; however, the possibility of infection should be addressed. No specific treatment for concussion exists other than management of symptoms.

Table 9.2 Diagnostic tests for traumatic brain injury

Test	Expected findings	Rationale
Diagnostic imaging		
Plain films	Fractures (e.g., skull, spine, extremities, ribs)	Fractures are seen best in plain radiographs
CT	Hematomas, contusions, hydrocephalus Test is time-sensitive, as the presence of blood changes characteristics over time	CT is the best method to examine patients for the presence of blood, edema, and CSF
MRI	DAI	MRI will demonstrate small lesions not visible on CT imaging
Electroencephalography	Seizure activity	Commonly used in head trauma, due to altered electrical activity in brain
Laboratory tests		
Serum electrolytes	Abnormalities in sodium: either hyponatremia or hypernatremia	Hyponatremia is a risk factor for increased cerebral edema
	Blood glucose may be elevated	Hypernatremia may indicate dehydration, associated with hypotension
Complete blood cell count	Elevated white blood cell count	Indicates infection
	Possible decrease in hematocrit	Indicates excessive blood loss due to trauma, especially scalp trauma
Blood alcohol level, drug screen	Presence of alcohol or drugs in blood or urine	Presence of drugs or alcohol may alter neurologic examination
ABGs	Presence of hypoxia or hypercapnia	Depressed neurologic state may also indicate depressed respiratory drive Decreased levels of oxygen and increased levels of CO_2 are concerning for increasing ICP

Abbreviations: ABGs, arterial blood gases; CSF, cerebrospinal fluid; CT, computed tomography; DAI, diffuse axonal injury; ICP, intracranial pressure; MRI, magnetic resonance imaging.

For prolonged cognitive impairment, cognitive testing with possible neuro-psychological evaluation may be warranted. Even a patient with mild TBI may experience neurologic or cognitive sequelae and should be monitored closely (Box 9.7 Evidence-Based Practice: Mild TBI).

- Possible infection should be addressed in the case of a contaminated wound
- Observation may be sufficient for small hematomas without neurologic deficits
- Patients should be assessed individually and observed closely to avoid repeated injury
- Serial CT scans are used to monitor edema and check for hematomas or contusions.
  - "Blossoming," or the expansion of a contusion, may occur at about 3 days, with possible neurologic compromise
- Initial admission to intensive care unit for close monitoring and observation
- Antiepileptic drugs are usually not indicated unless seizures occur (Box 9.8 Clinical Alert: Antiepileptic Drugs and TBI)
- Steroids are not indicated
- Therapies are variable and often include more than one type; see also Chapter 17: Rehabilitation
  - Physical
  - Occupational
  - Cognitive therapy

Box 9.7 Evidenced-Based Practice: Mild Traumatic Brain Injury

- Mild TBI accounts for about 75% of the cases of diagnosed TBI
- Because symptoms are mild, they may go unnoticed. Examples include the following:
  - Memory problems
  - Concentration
  - Personality changes
  - Other cognitive disturbances
  - Headache
- Management of mild TBI means managing symptoms
- Prolonged symptoms and deficits in patients with mild TBI may be managed more effectively with early screening and education for patients and families

---

Box 9.8 Clinical Alert: Antiepileptic Drugs and Traumatic Brain Injury

- Unless the patient has had a seizure, antiepileptic drugs for patients with TBI are controversial
- If the potential risk of seizures is deemed significant, use of antiepileptic drugs is usually limited to 7 days, at which time they may be discontinued

Surgical

Patients with more severe TBIs may require surgery to debride the wound, repair the skull fracture, or relieve ICP. Such surgeries may include the following:

- Wound debridement
  - Comminuted or depressed skull fractures due to wound contamination
  - Gunshot wounds or any penetrating wounds
- Craniotomy
  - Elevation of depressed skull fracture
  - Evacuation of hematoma (e.g., SDH, EDH, IPH)
  - Subdural drain (i.e., burr holes)
- External ventricular drain
  - ICP monitoring
  - Hydrocephalus
- Craniectomy (or hemicraniectomy)
  - Decompresses wound and relieves pressure
  - Bone flap is completely removed
- Shunt
  - Used to drain CSF to relieve hydrocephalus

End-of-Life Care

Too often, TBI results in irreparable and irreversible damage. Extremely difficult decisions must be made by the patient's family or medical power of attorney with the assistance and support of health care professionals.

- The patient's quality of life must be considered
- Advance directives should be discussed
- If appropriate, the possibility of organ donation should be discussed with the family, including referral to a local organ donation organization
- Brain death determination; see also Chapter 2: Assessment

9.4 Specific Conditions and Terms Associated with Traumatic Brain Injury

9.4.1 Primary/Secondary Injury

The TBI resulting from a precipitating event is called the *primary injury*. Its sequelae (i.e., the body's response to the primary injury) are called *secondary injuries*.

Primary Injury

- Initial mechanical TBI
- Concussion, contusion, hematoma, or diffuse axonal injury

Secondary Injury

Management of patients with TBI is aimed at preventing secondary injury.
- Results from a chain of events that eventually lead to cerebral ischemia
- May be individual or multiple events, including the following:
  - Respiratory insufficiency
  - Hypoxia
  - Hypotension
  - Metabolic dysfunction (e.g., hyperglycemia or hyponatremia)
  - Sepsis
  - Increased ICP
  - Seizures
  - Hydrocephalus

9.4.2 Herniation Syndromes

Herniation syndromes are a type of secondary injury; see Chapter 2: Assessment and Chapter 3: Principles of Intracranial Pressure. A brain herniation occurs when the contents of the skull (brain, CSF, blood vessels) are pressed away from their usual position by increased Intracranial Pressure
- Result most often from brain swelling after TBI, stroke, or brain tumor
- Can have devastating neurologic consequences

9.5 Nursing Management for Patients with Traumatic Brain Injury

Neurologic assessment should be the primary concern of nurses caring for patients with TBI. Neurologic assessments are described in detail in Chapter 2: Assessment, but assessment for patients with suspected or confirmed TBI must include the components below. Any changes in the findings of a neurologic assessment must be communicated to the health care team so that appropriate management strategies can be implemented (▶ Table 9.3).

A nurse caring for a patient with TBI has the critical task of managing the patient's ICP. This is discussed in greater detail in Chapter 3: Principles of Intracranial Pressure. Patients with TBI often also have other injuries, so all systems must be examined for evidence of other injuries—not just neurologic issues (Box 9.9 Examples of Injuries Associated with TBI).

This chapter is meant to be a basic reference for individuals caring for neurologic patients with TBI. For further information, references are included at the end of this chapter, and the reader is encouraged to consult them to learn more about subjects of interest. A comprehensive nursing management table is provided in **Appendix A8: Nursing Management of Patients with Traumatic Brain Injury.**

Table 9.3 Traumatic brain injury: what to watch for

Problem	Indication	Nursing action	Rationale
Decline in neurologic status, with potential for secondary injury	Increased ICP Cerebral edema Hemorrhage	CT of head to rule out hemorrhage, increased edema, actual or pending herniation, hydrocephalus	Any type of TBI puts patient at risk for secondary injury with increased cerebral edema, increased ICP, decreased neurologic examination Life-threatening causes such as increased cerebral edema and herniation must be ruled out first, usually with CT scan
		Look for other causes for decreased LOC, such as Hypoxia Anemia Infection/fever Seizure (including nonconvulsive status epilepticus); see Chapter 6: Seizures Hyponatremia See Chapter 3: Principles of Intracranial Pressure	Many nonneurologic conditions may cause decreased LOC
Respiratory distress	Respiratory failure Atelectasis Pneumonia	Perform respiratory assessment, including respiratory rate and rhythm, oxygen saturation rate, ABG, auscultation of lungs	Respiratory failure is a risk for patients with decreased LOC due to risk of aspiration, pneumonia, and/or inability to protect airway
		Supplementary oxygen if needed	Patients who are intubated and on mechanical ventilation are at risk for ventilator-associated pneumonia
Rhinorrhea Otorrhea "Halo" sign on bed linens	CSF leak due to basal skull fracture	Place patient in bed with head of bed elevated 45° Report if new finding	CSF leak puts patient at risk for meningitis

Abbreviations: ABG, arterial blood gas; CSF, cerebrospinal fluid; CT, computed tomography; ICP, intracranial pressure; LOC, level of consciousness; TBI, traumatic brain injury.

Box 9.9 Examples of Injuries Associated with Traumatic Brain Injury

- Facial injury or fracture
- Vertebral injury or fracture
- Spinal cord injury
- Rib fracture with or without flail chest
- Pneumothorax
- Hemothorax
- Ruptured spleen
- Retroperitoneal hemorrhage
- Kidney contusion or laceration
- Musculoskeletal injury or bone fracture

9.5.1 Neurologic Assessment

- Assess level of consciousness (LOC); see also Chapter 2: Assessment
- Test cognition, motor, sensory, and cranial nerve function
- Perform neuropsychological assessment

9.5.2 Respiratory Assessment

- Respiratory failure is common in patients with decreased LOC
- Protect airway
- Monitor arterial blood gases (ABGs)

9.5.3 Cardiovascular Assessment

- Perform hemodynamic monitoring
- Monitor electrocardiogram
- Observe patient for signs of anemia, which may occur after blood loss

9.5.4 Musculoskeletal Assessment

- Check for fractures elsewhere in the body (common in patients with TBI)

9.5.5 Gastrointestinal Assessment

- Check for gastrointestinal bleeding
- Check for gastrointestinal distress possibly due to increased stress

9.5.6 Endocrine Assessment

- Monitor glucose level
- Watch for hyperglycemia and treat as needed
- Monitor serum sodium; see Chapter 5: Electrolyte Disturbances
- Watch for hyponatremia and treat as needed

9.5.7 Nutrition Assessment

- Start nutrition as soon as possible

9.5.8 Coagulopathy Assessment

- Monitor for coagulopathy
- Monitor for deep vein thrombosis
- Administer enoxaparin, unless contraindicated
- Institute prophylactic treatment for deep vein thrombosis
- Mobilize the patient as soon as possible, unless contraindicated

9.5.9 Patient and Family Teaching

- Provide family support and education
- Provide and review discharge instructions; see **Appendix B10: Sample Discharge Instructions After Concussion (or Other Closed Head Injury) and Appendix B11: Sample Discharge Instructions After Subdural Hematoma**

9.5.10 Collaborative Management

The health care team for patients with TBI consists of practitioners in numerous specialties.
- Nursing
- Neurosurgery
- Neurology for seizure management
- Pulmonology and critical care intensivists
- Internal medicine
- Cardiology, if warranted
- Endocrinology for management of diabetes mellitus or sodium abnormalities
- Therapies, including the following:
  - Physical therapy
  - Occupational therapy
  - Speech therapy
- Rehabilitation specialists or physiatrists

- Neuropsychology for cognitive monitoring
- Clergy
- Palliative care workers or hospice workers
- Social workers or case management personnel.

Video

Video 9.1 Coup-contrecoup injury.

Suggested Reading

[1] American Association of Neuroscience Nurses. Care of the Patient with Mild Traumatic Brain Injury. AANN and ARN Clinical Practice Guideline Series. Chicago, IL: American Association of Neuroscience Nurses; 2011

[2] Bay E, McLean SA. Mild traumatic brain injury: an update for advanced practice nurses. J Neurosci Nurs. 2007; 39(1):43–51

[3] Bay EH, Chartier KS. Chronic morbidities after traumatic brain injury: an update for the advanced practice nurse. J Neurosci Nurs. 2014; 46(3):142–152

[4] Burnett DM, Kolakowsky-Hayner SA, Slater D, et al. Ethnographic analysis of traumatic brain injury patients in the national Model Systems database. Arch Phys Med Rehabil. 2003; 84(2):263–267

[5] Cantu RC. Second impact syndrome: immediate management. Phys Sportsmed. 1992; 20:55–66

[6] Centers for Disease Control and Prevention. Brain injuries and mass trauma events. 2015; http://www.cdc.gov/masstrauma/factsheets/public/braininjuries_public.pdf. Accessed 01/19/2016

[7] Centers for Disease Control and Prevention. Rates of TBI-Related Emergency Department Visits, Hospitalizations, and Deaths—United States, 2001–2010. 2016; http://www.cdc.gov/traumaticbraininjury/data/rates.html. Accessed June 21, 2017

[8] Centers for Disease Control and Prevention. http://www.cdc.gov. Accessed August 3, 2017

[9] Evans RW, ed. Neurology and Trauma. 2nd ed. New York, NY: Oxford University Press; 2006

[10] Finkelstein E, Corso P, Miller T. The incidence and economic burden of injuries in the United States. New York, NY: Oxford University Press; 2006

[11] Gamble KH. A new game plan for concussion: as new research on the dangers of concussions is uncovered, treatment on sports sidelines is changing—from the little leagues to the professional level. Neurol Now. 2011; 7(1):28–31, 35

[12] Greenberg MS. Handbook of Neurosurgery. 8th ed. New York, NY: Thieme Medical Publishers, 2016

[13] Hwang DY, Yagoda D, Perrey HM, et al. Assessment of satisfaction with care among family members of survivors in a neuroscience intensive care unit. J Neurosci Nurs. 2014; 46(2):106–116

[14] Meier C. Airway management in patients with brain injury. Emerg Nurse. 2013; 21(8):18–23

[15] Rutland-Brown W, Langlois JA, Thomas KE, Xi YL. Incidence of traumatic brain injury in the United States, 2003. J Head Trauma Rehabil. 2006; 21(6):544–548

[16] Senelick RC. Living with Brain Injury: A Guide for Families. 3rd ed. Birmingham, AL: HealthSouth Press; 2012

10 Infectious Diseases

Denita Ryan

Abstract

Infectious diseases can occur anywhere within the central nervous system (CNS). They may be caused by bacteria, virus, fungus, or parasites and may be introduced into the body by various methods, including injury, surgery, insects, or other infections. CNS infections may result in mild symptoms or critical illness. The appropriate treatment varies by the type and location of the infection, and it is further subject to other patient comorbidities. Early recognition and intervention are critical in treating patients with infectious diseases of the CNS.

Keywords: abscess, encephalitis, meningitis, neurocysticercosis, prion disease, shunt infection

10.1 Infectious Diseases

The central nervous system (CNS) is vulnerable to many infectious diseases. Meningitis, encephalitis, and abscesses are all examples of infections of the CNS that can be caused by various bacterial, viral, or fungal pathogens. Infectious diseases may be community-acquired or nosocomial.

Nosocomial infections are infections acquired during hospitalization. Common examples include pneumonia, urinary tract infections, or postoperative wound infections. Most nosocomial infections occur in critical care units.

Although infections of the CNS can occur in patients who have had neurosurgical procedures, most do not warrant neurosurgical treatment. Instead, these infections are treated by infectious disease specialists.

10.2 Meningitis

Meningitis is inflammation of the meninges (▶ Fig. 10.1). It can be caused by bacteria, a virus, or fungus. Bacterial or viral meningitis are the most common types.

10.2.1 Bacterial

- Caused by a bacterial pathogen (Box 10.1 Common Bacterial Pathogens)
- Commonly affects very young or very old individuals
- Morbidity is variable and dependent on the specific pathogen

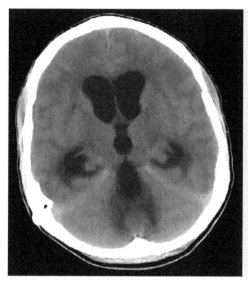

Fig. 10.1 Meningitis.

- Diabetic patients are more susceptible to bacterial meningitis
- Prognosis is good if treated, poor if untreated (Box 10.2 Mortality Rate of Bacterial Meningitis)

Box 10.1 Common Bacterial Pathogens

- Community-acquired
  - *Streptococcus pneumoniae*
  - *Neisseria meningitidis*
  - *Haemophilus influenzae*
  - *Listeria monocytogenes*
- Nosocomial
  - *Staphylococcus aureus*
  - *Pseudomonas aeruginosa*
  - *Staphylococcus* species
  - Other gram-negative bacteria

Box 10.2 Mortality Rate of Bacterial Meningitis

- More than 70% of persons who contract bacterial meningitis will die if the disease is not treated

10.2.2 Viral

- Caused by a viral pathogen (Box 10.3 Common Viral Pathogens)
- Can affect patients of any age
- Incidence and type influenced by geographic region
- May occur as a single isolated case or can be epidemic
- The virus that causes acquired immune deficiency syndrome (AIDS) interferes with the immune system; resulting infections may affect many organ systems, including the central nervous system (Box 10.4 Focus on: Central Nervous System Manifestations of AIDS)

Box 10.3 Common Viral Pathogens

- Herpes simplex 1 and 2 (HSV-1 and HSV-2), also called human herpesvirus 1 and 2
  - Common cold sore
  - Genital herpes
- Herpes zoster, also called human herpesvirus 3 (HHV-3)
  - Shingles
- Arbovirus (arthropod-borne)
  - West Nile virus
  - Zika virus
- Enterovirus
  - Coxsackievirus
  - Echovirus
  - Poliomyelitis
- Postviral
  - Measles
  - Mumps
  - Chickenpox

Box 10.4 Focus on: Central Nervous System Manifestations of AIDS

- About 40 to 60% of all patients with AIDS will develop neurologic symptoms
- Most common conditions include the following:
  - Toxoplasmosis
  - Primary CNS lymphoma
  - Cryptococcal abscess
  - Progressive multifocal leukoencephalopathy
  - Neurosyphilis

- Most common CNS effects of HIV infections include the following:
  - AIDS encephalopathy
  - AIDS dementia
  - Cranial neuropathies
  - Meningitis (aseptic)

10.2.3 Fungal

- Caused by a fungal pathogen
- Most common examples are *Cryptococcus* and *Coccidioides* (regional)

10.2.4 Epidemiology of Meningitis

- Involves inflammation of the meninges, the subarachnoid space, and the cerebrospinal fluid (CSF)
- Ventriculitis is an infection involving the ventricular system
- Bacteria enter the meninges by various methods. The bacteria that cause meningitis commonly travel through the CSF after trauma, after a surgical procedure, or after a lumbar puncture. However, bacteria may also reach the meninges via the following:
  - Blood (bacteremia)
  - Colonization of the mucosa with passage (e.g., sinus) to the submucosa
  - Contiguous spread
  - Dental procedures
  - Endocarditis

10.2.5 Clinical Manifestations

- Meningismus, also called meningism, is the clinical manifestation of meningeal irritation. It involves the following:
  - Nuchal rigidity (stiff neck)
  - Kernig's sign; see Chapter 2: Assessment
  - Brudzinski's sign; see Chapter 2: Assessment
- Headache
- Fever
- Altered level of consciousness (LOC)
- Seizure
- Rash may be present in meningococcal meningitis
- Chemical meningitis is inflammation of the meninges not caused by bacteria (Box 10.5 Chemical Meningitis)

Box 10.5 Chemical Meningitis

- Chemical meningitis, also called *aseptic meningitis*, is an inflammation of the meninges.
  - Not caused by infection
  - Commonly occurs after subarachnoid hemorrhage (blood in the subarachnoid space acts as the irritant)
- Clinical manifestations of chemical meningitis include the following:
  - Headaches (often severe)
  - Nausea and vomiting
  - Meningeal signs (e.g., stiff neck, photophobia, low back pain)
  - Fever is not a clinical manifestation of chemical meningitis
- Treatment options include the following:
  - Time
  - Support of symptoms (i.e., pain relief, antiemetics)
  - Dexamethasone is usually helpful

10.2.6 Diagnosis

After a complete history is obtained and a physical assessment is performed, various laboratory studies are carried out before meningitis can be diagnosed.

Laboratory Studies

- Lumbar puncture (LP) with CSF studies, including culture (▶ Table 10.1)
- Serum C-reactive protein (CRP) has high negative predictive value for bacterial meningitis
- Complete blood count (CBC) and erythrocyte sedimentation rate (ESR)
- Polymerase chain reaction (PCR) is highly predictive of enteroviral meningitis
- Blood cultures
- Procalcitonin (Box 10.6 Procalcitonin and ▶ Table 10.2)

Box 10.6 Procalcitonin

- Elevated procalcitonin is an early indication of inflammatory response and is highly suggestive of infection, especially in postoperative wounds
- High correlation between level of procalcitonin and poor prognosis
- Level of procalcitonin may increase within 3 to 6 hours of stimulation, and this level is detectable in blood

Table 10.1 Examination of cerebrospinal fluid in infections of the central nervous system

Condition	Opening pressure (cm H_2O)	Appearance	Cells (cells/µL)	Protein (mg/dL)	Glucose	Cultures
Normal	8–18	Clear	0–5	<45	60% of blood glucose level	No organisms
Bacterial meningitis	Increased	Clear or cloudy	>100	Increased (>50)	Decreased (<50% blood glucose)	Bacterial pathogens
Viral meningitis	May be normal or increased	Clear or cloudy	10–1000	Slightly increased (>50)	Normal or slightly decreased	Viral pathogens

Table 10.2 Possible causes of elevated procalcitonin levels in blood

Level (ng/mL)	Possible cause
< 0.05	Normal Local inflammatory possible; systemic disease unlikely
≥ 0.05 to < 2	Systemic inflammatory response present due to infection
≥ 2 to < 10	Sepsis likely
> 10	Severe sepsis or septic shock Organ dysfunction High risk of death

10.2.7 Treatment

Medical

- Infectious disease consultation
- Antibiotics for bacterial meningitis (Box 10.7 Starting Antibiotics), antiviral medication for viral meningitis, and antifungal medication for fungal meningitis
- Dexamethasone has been shown to decrease mortality when administered early in the disease course (Box 10.8 Vasogenic Edema)
- Relief of symptoms such as pain or fever
- Respiratory and circulatory support may be necessary in extreme cases
- Antiepileptic drugs (AEDs) for seizures (Box 10.9 Antiepileptic Drugs and Antibiotics)

- Except in cases of meningococcal meningitis, isolation is not necessary (universal precautions suffice)
- Treatment guidelines are outlined by the Infectious Diseases Society of America

---

Box 10.7 Starting Antibiotics

- Early treatment is imperative to ensure a good outcome
- As soon as bacterial meningitis is suspected, collect the appropriate specimens and send them immediately for culture and sensitivity analysis; then begin appropriate antibiotics
- Do not allow ancillary tests to delay initiation of antibiotics

---

Box 10.8 Vasogenic Edema

- Vasogenic edema is often seen with meningitis or encephalitis
- Associated with increased intracranial pressure (ICP)
- Dexamethasone is associated with improved outcome.

Box 10.9 Antiepileptic Drugs and Antibiotics

- Some antibiotics (e.g., phenytoin) interfere with the absorption or metabolism of some AEDs
- Patients with CNS infections are susceptible to seizure activity, so be sure to monitor blood levels of AED if appropriate

---

Surgical

- External ventricular drain (EVD) may be needed for patients with ventriculitis
  - Management of increased intracranial pressure (ICP). See also Chapter 3: Principles of Intracranial Pressure
  - Route for intrathecal antibiotics

10.3 Shunt Infections

10.3.1 Epidemiology

- Infection rate is approximately 6%
- May present within 2 weeks of shunt placement
- Late presentation (i.e., presentation > 6 months after shunt placement) is not uncommon
- *Staphylococcus* is the most likely infectious agent

10.3.2 Clinical Manifestations

- General malaise
- Fever
- Nausea and vomiting
- Abdominal pain (if shunt is ventriculoperitoneal)
- May present as shunt failure

10.3.3 Diagnosis

- Positive CSF cultures from shunt tap or EVD

10.3.4 Treatment

- Removal of all components of the infected shunt plus intravenous (IV) antimicrobial therapy as appropriate
- Shunt should be replaced only after CSF cultures remain negative for a determined length of time
- If shunt cannot be removed, antibiotics should be pumped into the ventricle through a shunt reservoir or via EVD

Intraventricular (Intrathecal) Antibiotics

- Potentially toxic
- No specific antibiotic has been approved by the Food and Drug Administration
- Should only be used in situations in which conventional IV therapy has not been effective

10.4 Encephalitis

Encephalitis is an inflammation of brain tissue. It has been known to mimic the characteristics of brain lesions and is often seen in conjunction with meningitis.

- Cause may be bacterial, viral (most common), fungal, or parasitic
- Specific pathogen is highly influenced by geographic location
- Viral form is the most common type found in the United States (herpes simplex)
- Viral pathogens are the same as for meningitis
- Postviral diseases such as measles, mumps, and chickenpox can also cause encephalitis.
  - Acute disseminated encephalomyelitis is an example of postinfectious or postimmunization encephalitis

10.4.1 Clinical Manifestations

Symptoms depend on the type of virus but are usually the same as the symptoms for meningitis. Symptoms of encephalitis, however, are usually more pronounced than symptoms for meningitis. LOC is especially affected.

- Alterations in LOC/sensorium
- Severe headache
- Fever
- Nausea and vomiting
- Focal deficits, such as motor weakness, may occur
- Seizures
- Signs of increased ICP
- Hydrocephalus

10.4.2 Diagnosis

Laboratory Studies

- LP with CSF studies, including cultures
- Blood cultures
- CBC, CRP, ESR, PCR

Imaging Studies

- Magnetic resonance imaging (MRI) may show abnormalities (e.g., small hemorrhages) (▶ Table 10.3)

10.4.3 Treatment

Medical

- Antiviral medications
- Dexamethasone
- Improve symptoms (e.g., pain, fever, seizure)
- Treatment guidelines are outlined by the Infectious Diseases Society of America

Surgical

- Brain tissue affected by encephalitis rarely requires biopsy
- Shunts are often placed in this population due to the common occurrence of hydrocephalus

Table 10.3 Diagnostic tests for patients with infections of the central nervous system

Test	Indication	Nursing implication
CBC	WBC increase indicates body's response to infection	Watch for signs and symptoms of infection
ESR	Inflammation	Watch for infection
CRP	Presence of inflammation, especially postoperative infection, somewhere in the body	Watch for infection
Electrolyte panel	Hyponatremia, especially in the setting of cerebral edema	Monitor laboratory values for hyponatremia Administer salt supplements if indicated Maintain strict intake and output, and restrict fluids if indicated
	Hyperglycemia may result after dexamethasone is administered	Monitor glucose levels Administer insulin if indicated Report if hyperglycemia is a new finding
LP	Measurement of opening pressure is contraindicated in patients with suspected abscess	Assist with proper positioning of patient
	CSF examination, including culture	Assist in maintaining sterile procedure
Blood culture	Indicates presence of bacterial or fungal pathogens in blood (bacteremia or fungemia)	Administer antibiotics as ordered May need PICC when long-term antibiotics are indicated Often seen in conjunction with CSF infections, such as meningitis or ventriculitis
MRI	Lesions such as neurocysticercosis, cerebral abscess, or hemorrhagic areas resulting from encephalitis Rule out other lesions as cause of neurologic symptoms	
EEG	Identifies seizure activity	Administer AEDs as ordered Follow seizure safety protocols; see also Chapter 6: Seizures

Abbreviations: AEDs, antiepileptic drugs; CBC, complete blood count; CRP, C-reactive protein; CSF, cerebrospinal fluid; EEG, electroencephalogram; ESR, erythrocyte sedimentation rate; LP, lumbar puncture; MRI, magnetic resonance imaging; PICC, peripherally inserted central catheter; WBC, white blood cell count.

10.5 Abscess

A brain abscess is a localized infection that has migrated to the brain from another part of the body.

- Usually bacterial
- Most common causes include the following:
  - Infection in the sinus, inner ear, or mouth
  - Dental procedures
  - Trauma, such as a penetrating head wound
  - Neurosurgical procedure
  - Endocarditis (Box 10.10 Brain Abscess in Intravenous Drug Users)

> ### Box 10.10 Brain Abscess in Intravenous Drug Users
>
> - Brain abscesses in IV drug users carry especially high rates of morbidity and mortality

10.5.1 Clinical Manifestations

- Depend on site and size of abscess
- Headache
- Nausea and vomiting
- Altered LOC
- Focal neurologic signs, such as motor weakness and speech difficulty
- Seizures
- Brain abscesses may cause mass effect

10.5.2 Diagnosis

History

- Medical
- Surgical
- Dental
- Travel history

Imaging Studies

- Computed tomography (CT)
- MRI
- Echocardiogram, if endocarditis is suspected (Box 10.11 Clinical Alert: Contraindicated Diagnostic Tests)

- Lumbar puncture is absolutely contraindicated if brain abscess is suspected; an abscess is a space-occupying lesion and is therefore capable of causing brain herniation in some cases

10.5.3 Treatment

Medical

- Antibiotics
- Steroids
- Management of pain and fever
- Management of ICP if warranted; see also Chapter 3: Principles of Intracranial Pressure

Surgical

- Drainage of the abscess (if possible)
- Craniotomy
- Management of ICP if warranted

10.6 Parasites

10.6.1 Cysticercosis

Cysticercosis is a parasitic disease found in various geographic regions of the world, including certain areas of the United States. When it affects the CNS, it is called *neurocysticercosis* (▶ Fig. 10.2). It is sometimes referred to as *brain worms.*

- Caused by the cysticerci (i.e., larvae) of *Taenia solium*, a tapeworm commonly found in pigs
- Tapeworm eggs are ingested via infected water or food (fecal–oral transmission) and then hatch in the gastrointestinal tract
- Once hatched, the tapeworms enter the bloodstream and infect CNS tissue, such as brain parenchyma

Clinical Manifestations

- Host is usually asymptomatic while parasite is alive
- Host immune system activates an adaptive response when parasite dies within its fluid-filled cyst
- Host develops symptoms (e.g., seizures, hydrocephalus, or mental status changes) as the cyst becomes calcified

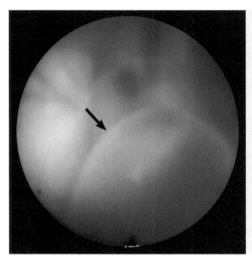

Fig. 10.2 Neurocysticercosis (arrow).

- Symptoms depend on the location of the cyst within the brain
- Lesions often cause vasogenic edema

Diagnosis

History

- Include travel history (Box 10.12 Neurocysticercosis)

Box 10.12 Neurocysticercosis

- In the United States, neurocysticercosis is more common in areas with large immigrant populations, especially where immigrants have arrived from third world countries
- It is imperative to obtain a travel history for any patient suspected of a parasitic disease
- Parasitic disease should be suspected in patients who have traveled outside the United States, especially to Mexico and Central or South America

Imaging Studies

- MRI
- CT (▶ Fig. 10.3).

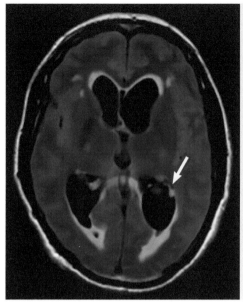

Fig. 10.3 Computed tomography scan of a patient with neurocysticercosis (arrow).

Treatment

Medical

- Antiparasitic, such as albendazole
- Symptom support, such as AEDs for seizures

Surgical

- Craniotomy for resection of the neurocysticercosis lesions

10.7 Prion Diseases

It is also known as *transmissible spongiform encephalopathies*; human prion diseases are fatal neurodegenerative diseases that affect both humans and animals.
- Distinguished by the presence of an abnormal, mutant form of cellular protein
- Mechanism of infection is as yet unknown
- Usually occur sporadically, but about 10% are hereditary
- Caused by ingesting animal tissue infected with prions
- Most common prion disease is Creutzfeldt-Jakob disease (CJD)

10.7.1 Creutzfeldt-Jakob Disease

Clinical Manifestations

- Myoclonus is a hallmark sign of CJD
- Personality changes
- Memory loss
- Gait ataxia
- Hallucinations
- Rapidly progressive dementia

Diagnosis

- The only way to achieve a definitive diagnosis of CJD is through pathologic analysis of brain tissue at biopsy or autopsy (Box 10.13 Prion Disease)

Box 10.13 Prion Disease

- Prion diseases such as CJD are transmissible but are not infectious
- Because prions are transmissible and not easily destroyed, diagnostic biopsies are controversial
- CJD is often diagnosed by history and physical examination; however, definitive diagnosis is possible only by examination of brain tissue at biopsy or autopsy

Treatment

- There is no treatment or cure for CJD
- Treatment is aimed at diminishing severity of symptoms
- Death is inevitable, usually within a year

10.8 Other Infections

10.8.1 Osteomyelitis

- Osteomyelitis is infection of the bone (▶ Fig. 10.4)
- It may occur in the skull, or in the spine (end plate or vertebral body)
- Diskitis and osteomyelitis often occur together
- Diskitis is inflammation of or infection in the vertebral disk space (▶ Fig. 10.5)
- Lumbar spine is the most common site for spinal osteomyelitis.

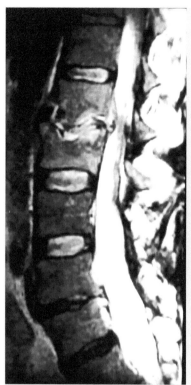

Fig. 10.4 Osteomyelitis.

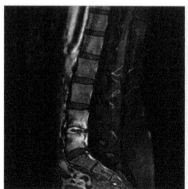

Fig. 10.5 Diskitis.

Etiology

- May occur after surgery
- May result from wound infection or from infection in another area of the body and spread via blood
- In cases of bacterial osteomyelitis, *Staphylococcus aureus* is the most common infecting agent (Box 10.14 Risk Factors for Osteomyelitis)

Box 10.14 Risk Factors for Osteomyelitis

- Advanced age
- IV drug abuse
- Diabetes
- Hemodialysis

Clinical Manifestations

- Local pain that worsens with movement
- Radicular pain
- Neck or back spasm
- Limited range of movement, intolerance of physical activity
- Some patients experience fever and chills

10.8.2 Spinal Epidural Abscess

- Often associated with diskitis and/or osteomyelitis
- Epidural abscess most common in the thoracic spine
- Classified as either acute or chronic
  - Acute
    - Clinical manifestations arise less than 16 days after exposure
    - Sepsis and pus in epidural space are common presentations
  - Chronic
    - Abscess can be present for months before becoming symptomatic
- Associated with weakened immune system
- Associated with diabetes mellitus, chronic renal failure, IV drug use, and alcoholism

Clinical Manifestations

- Severe back pain
- Fever and chills
- Encephalopathy
- Meningism
- Muscle weakness

Causes

- Spread via blood (most common)
- Skin infection
- IV drug use
- Bacterial endocarditis
- Urinary tract infection
- Respiratory infection
- Dental abscess
- Postoperative infection (from spinal procedures)
- Back trauma
- Direct extension from surrounding tissue (decubitus ulcer; neck, back, or abdominal wound)

Causative Agents

- *Staphylococcus aureus* is most common
- Chronic infections (e.g., tuberculosis; fungal or parasitic infection)
- Multiorganism infection

Treatment of Spinal Infections

- About 90% of cases can be treated with antibiotics and immobilization (back braces)
- Surgery is occasionally required to stabilize the spine

10.9 Nursing Management for Patients with Infectious Diseases

This chapter is intended to be a source of information for individuals caring for neurologic patients with infectious diseases of the CNS. The reader is encouraged to refer to the references listed at the end of this chapter to follow up on subjects of interest (▶ Table 10.4, ▶ Table 10.5, **and Appendix A9: Nursing Management of Patients with Infection of the Central Nervous System**).

10.9.1 Neurologic Assessment

- Evaluate LOC; see also Chapter 2: Assessment
- Be vigilant for signs of increased ICP; see also Chapter 3: Principles of Intracranial Pressure
- Assess motor, sensory, and cranial nerve function
- Observe for signs of meningism (e.g., nuchal rigidity, Kernig's sign, Brudzinski's sign)

Table 10.4 Pharmacology for patients with infections of the central nervous system

Drug	Category	Indication	Nursing implication
Phenytoin (Dilantin) or other AED; see also Chapter 6: Seizures	Antiepileptic drug	Seizures	Monitor drug levels Be aware of the potential effects of antibiotics and on phenytoin or other AEDs AEDs have many side effects
Dexamethasone (Decadron)	Corticosteroid	Reduce vasogenic edema	Increases WBC Increases glucose level May suppress wound healing May cause psychosis
Morphine Oxycodone Hydromorphone Hydrocodone Fentanyl citrate	Narcotic	Pain relief	May depress respiration rate May mask neurologic status May cause delirium or confusion, especially in the elderly
Acetaminophen Ibuprofen	Antipyretic	Fever reduction Mild pain relief	Use cautiously in patients with liver disease; monitor daily maximum dose May cause gastric irritation
Albendazole	Antiparasitic	Effective against neurocysticercosis	
Acyclovir (Zovirax)	Antiviral	Effective against herpes virus	Monitor renal function
Antibiotics[a]	Antibacterial		Be aware of potential interaction with other medications, especially AEDs Be aware of potential drug allergies Some antibiotics are extremely costly and are not available on all insurance plans

Abbreviations: AED, antiepileptic drug; WBC, white blood cell count.
[a]Antibiotics are evolving constantly, so the number of new, more effective drugs is ever-increasing. Specific antibiotics are therefore not addressed in this table.

10.9.2 Respiratory Assessment

- Perform airway assessment
- Document and monitor respiratory rate and rhythm
- Assess arterial blood gases (O_2 saturation monitor if appropriate)

Table 10.5 Infections of the central nervous system: what to watch for

Problem	Indication	Nursing action	Rationale
Decline in neurologic assessment	Increased ICP due to infection	See Chapter 3: Principles of Intracranial Pressure	
Meningism/ fever	Meningitis	Perform complete neurologic assessment Monitor vital signs, including current temperature Prepare for LP Report new findings	Early diagnosis is a positive indicator for good neurologic outcome Diagnosis is made by laboratory tests of CSF

Abbreviations: CSF, cerebrospinal fluid; ICP, intracranial pressure; LP, lumbar puncture.

10.9.3 Cardiovascular Assessment

• Perform hemodynamic monitoring, if appropriate
• Monitor electrocardiogram for cardiac arrhythmia

10.9.4 Fluid and Electrolyte Assessment

• Monitor serum sodium level and watch for hyponatremia. Report new findings. See also Chapter 5: Electrolyte Disturbances
• Check glucose levels, especially in patients on steroids. Administer insulin as directed

10.9.5 Fever Management

• Monitor vital signs for increased temperature and for signs of sepsis
• Administer antipyretic medication as indicated
• Obtain cultures (e.g., from blood, sputum, CSF, or wound) as indicated
• Administer antibiotics as directed

10.9.6 Pain Management

• Give narcotics as ordered
• Be mindful of the effectiveness of environmental changes, such as keeping the patient's room dark and quiet, if warranted
• Provide ice bags for comfort as needed

10.9.7 Seizure Assessment

- Medications, including drug interactions and levels, if indicated
- Patient safety; see also Chapter 6: Seizures

10.9.8 Immobility

- Administer enoxaparin sodium (Lovenox) unless contraindicated
- Use sequential compression devices
- Encourage early ambulation and emphasize the importance of mobility
- Watch for signs and symptoms of deep vein thrombosis

10.9.9 Patient and Family Teaching

- Recommend home health care if necessary, especially for patients who require long-term IV antibiotics
- If the family opts to administer IVs at home without professional assistance, be sure to offer comprehensive instruction on techniques for administering IV antibiotics

10.9.10 Collaborative Management

Patients with infectious disease of the CNS often require support from experts in other specialties, especially infectious diseases. Other groups with whom collaboration is common may include the following:

- Neurosurgery
- Neurology for seizure management
- Therapies
  - Physical
  - Occupational
  - Speech (for cognition)
- Rehabilitation
- Clergy, chaplain, or spiritual support
- Palliative care

Suggested Reading

[1] Gambetti P, Parchi P, Chen SG. Hereditary Creutzfeldt-Jakob disease and fatal familial insomnia. Clin Lab Med. 2003; 23(1):43–64

[2] Greenberg BM. Central nervous system infections in the intensive care unit. Semin Neurol. 2008; 28(5):682–689

[3] Greenberg MS. Handbook of Neurosurgery. 8th ed. New York, NY: Thieme Medical Publishers, 2016

[4] Hill M, Baker G, Carter D, et al. A multidisciplinary approach to end external ventricular drain infections in the neurocritical care unit. J Neurosci Nurs. 2012; 44(4):188–193

[5] Johnson KG. Spinal epidural abscess. Crit Care Nurs Clin North Am. 2013; 25(3):389–397

[6] Meiner Z, Gabizon R, Prusiner SB. Familial Creutzfeldt-Jakob disease. Codon 200 prion disease in Libyan Jews. Medicine (Baltimore). 1997; 76(4):227–237

[7] Simpson DM, Tagliati M. Neurologic manifestations of HIV infection. Ann Intern Med. 1994; 121 (10):769–785

[8] Slazinski T. Brain abscess. Crit Care Nurs Clin North Am. 2013; 25(3):381–388

[9] Smith DL, Levin SA, Laxminarayan R. Strategic interactions in multi-institutional epidemics of antibiotic resistance. Proc Natl Acad Sci U S A. 2005; 102(8):3153–3158

[10] Smith-Bathgate B. Creutzfeldt-Jakob disease: diagnosis and nursing care issues. Nurs Times. 2005; 101(20):52–53

[11] Tunkel AR, Glaser CA, Bloch KC, et al. Infectious Diseases Society of America. The management of encephalitis: clinical practice guidelines by the Infectious Diseases Society of America. Clin Infect Dis. 2008; 47(3):303–327

[12] Tunkel AR, Hartman BJ, Kaplan SL, et al. Practice guidelines for the management of bacterial meningitis. Clin Infect Dis. 2004; 39(9):1267–1284

[13] Tunkel AR, Pradhan SK. Central nervous system infections in injection drug users. Infect Dis Clin North Am. 2002; 16(3):589–605

[14] Tuppeny M. Viral meningitis and encephalitis. Crit Care Nurs Clin North Am. 2013; 25(3):363–380

[15] van de Beek D, Schmand B, de Gans J, et al. Cognitive impairment in adults with good recovery after bacterial meningitis. J Infect Dis. 2002; 186(7):1047–1052

[16] VanDemark M. Acute bacterial meningitis: current review and treatment update. Crit Care Nurs Clin North Am. 2013; 25(3):351–361

[17] Vandemark MV, Lovasik DA, Neatherlin JS, Omert T. Infectious and autoimmune processes. In: Bader MK, Littlejohns LR, eds. AANN Core Curriculum for Neuroscience Nursing. 4th ed. St. Louis, MO: W. B. Saunders; 2004

11 Spinal Disorders

Charlotte S. Myers and Simon Parkinson

Abstract

Spinal disorders are relatively common and include diagnoses such as disk herniation, stenosis, and spondylosis. These and other disorders of the spine may be found in the cervical, thoracic, and lumbar spine, causing a variety of symptoms, including pain and motor or sensory disturbances. Treatment may include observation, medical, or surgical intervention. Nurses should be knowledgeable on the many types of spinal disorders, as well as level of spinal involvement and associated symptoms.

Keywords: degenerative disk disease, disk herniation, myelopathy, radiculopathy, spinal stenosis, spondylolisthesis, spondylosis

11.1 Spinal Disorders

Spinal disorders may result from trauma, congenital factors, underlying diseases, or normal degenerative processes. Many painful acute and chronic conditions can be attributed to disorders of the spine. Although age-related degenerative changes are the most common cause, spinal disorders are not always the result of normal aging processes (Box 11.1 Causes of Spinal Disorders Other than Normal Aging).

This chapter will address common degenerative spinal disorders of each spinal region—cervical, thoracic, and lumbar. It will focus on clinical manifestations, treatment, and nursing care considerations for patients with these conditions.

Box 11.1 Causes of Spinal Disorders Other than Normal Aging

- Trauma
  - Fracture
  - Hematoma
  - Ligamentous strain
  - Dislocation
- Tumors
  - Schwannoma
  - Ependymoma
  - Metastatic
- Vascular
  - Arteriovenous malformation
  - Cavernous malformation
  - Infarction

- Infection
  - Osteomyelitis
  - Epidural abscess
- Systemic diseases
  - Rheumatoid arthritis
  - Ankylosing spondylitis

11.2 Specific Types of Spinal Disorders

11.2.1 Degenerative Disk Disease

Degenerative disk disease (DDD) is part of the natural aging process (Box 11.2 Degenerative Disk Disease) that is thought to begin during the third decade of life. DDD can result in loss of disk height, development of tears or fissures of the annulus fibrosis, formation of bone spurs, compression of nerve roots and facet joints, and vertebral end plate changes. It is the likely precursor to other spinal disorders, including the following:

- Disk herniation
- Spondylosis (i.e., degenerative changes due to osteoarthritis)
- Spondylolisthesis (i.e., forward displacement of one vertebra over another)
- Spinal stenosis (i.e., narrowing of the spinal canal)

DDD results from the loss of normal elasticity and flexibility of the vertebral disk, but it may be accelerated or exacerbated by several factors as follows:

- Smoking
- Sedentary lifestyle
- Obesity
- Repetitive injuries
- Congenital abnormalities

Box 11.2 Degenerative Disk Disease

- Degenerative disk disease is a part of normal aging
- Not everyone with degenerative spinal changes develops pain or neurologic impairments
- Many people without symptoms have incidental magnetic resonance imaging findings of abnormalities (e.g., disk herniation, degenerative changes, spinal stenosis)

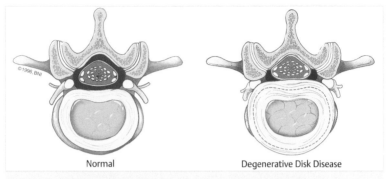

Normal   Degenerative Disk Disease

Fig. 11.1 Normal vertebral disk versus disk with degenerative disk disease.

Etiology of Degenerative Disk Disease

- The annulus fibrosis becomes less supple with age and is more easily torn (▶ Fig. 11.1)
- The nucleus pulposus starts to dry out and shrink, resulting in loss of disk height
- The entire spine becomes less flexible because of deteriorated disks

Epidemiology of Degenerative Disk Disease

- Affects about 20% of the U.S. population
- Slightly more prevalent among women
- Most common among those aged 45 to 75 years
- Causes loss of mobility and significant physical disability

11.2.2 Spondylosis

Spondylosis is a term that refers to osteoarthritis of the spine, but it is often used to describe any manner of spinal degeneration. It leads to the formation of bone spurs, or osteophytes, where the vertebral body and disk connect to the end plate (▶ Fig. 11.2). It can occur at any level of the spine and is categorized according to the affected level (i.e., cervical, thoracic, or lumbar).

Etiology of Spondylosis

- Results from degenerative changes in intervertebral disks

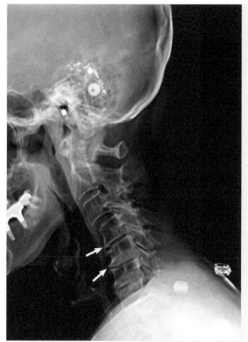

Fig. 11.2 Spondylosis, with arrows indicating osteophytes of the lower cervical spine.

- Disks become stiff, subjecting the bony end plates to increased load bearing and dynamic stress, causing thickening and sclerosis, which over time leads to the formation of osteophytes.
  - Osteophytes affect other structures around the vertebrae, such as the surrounding ligaments (e.g., anterior longitudinal ligaments, posterior longitudinal ligaments, and ligamenta flava), disks, facet joints, and laminae
  - Osteophytes can occur anteriorly or posteriorly
  - Anterior osteophytes rarely produce symptoms
  - Posterior osteophytes can result in stenosis of the spinal canal or neural foraminal stenosis

Epidemiology of Spondylosis

- Between 27 and 37% of the population in the United States is thought to have asymptomatic lumbar spondylosis
- Affects between 50 and 75% of the U.S. population by age 50 years, 90% by age 60 years
- Roughly 74% of women and 84% of men have vertebral osteophytes (usually at T9-T10 or L3)
- About 28% of women and 30% of men between 55 and 64 years have osteophytes of the lumbar spine

11.2.3 Intervertebral Disk Herniation

Extruded disk material is referred to as *herniated nucleus pulposus* (Box 11.3 Terms for Herniated Disk). A herniated disk can result from trauma, although DDD is often a contributing factor.

Box 11.3 Terms for Herniated Disk

- Herniated intervertebral disk
- Herniated nucleus pulposus
- Prolapsed intervertebral disk
- Slipped disk
- Ruptured disk
- Sequestered disk

Etiology of Herniated Disk

- Disk extrusion can be a bulge or complete herniation through the annulus fibrosis
- Herniation may be lateral or central (▶ Fig. 11.3, ▶ Fig. 11.4), but central herniation is less common
- Disk herniation can result in disk fragmentation (i.e., pieces of disk material found outside the disk space, usually in the epidural space)
- Nerve root compression resulting from a herniated disk may cause radiculopathy (i.e., disease of the nerve root caused by compression or inflammation)

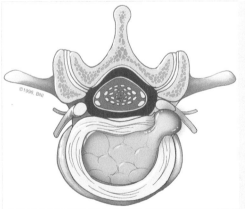

Fig. 11.3 Lateral disk herniation.

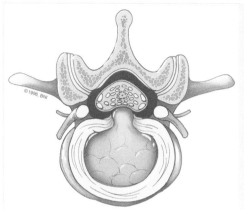

Fig. 11.4 Central disk herniation.

- Radiculopathy causes pain to radiate from a specific spinal segment to a distal site (i.e., to the arm or hand if a cervical nerve root is compressed; to the truncal region if thoracic nerve root is compressed; and to the buttocks, groin, or lower extremities if a lumbar nerve root is compressed)
- Radiculopathy is dermatome-specific to the spinal level and the side of disk herniation

Epidemiology of Disk Herniation

- Affects men more often than women
- Average age at onset is 30 to 50 years
- Occurs more often in the lumbar spine than in the cervical spine; it rarely occurs in the thoracic spine
- About 10% of patients experience herniation at multiple levels

11.2.4 Spondylolisthesis

The abnormal movement or slippage of one vertebral body onto another is called *spondylolisthesis* (▶ Fig. 11.5).

- Degree of displacement can be determined using the Meyerding Grading System (▶ Table 11.1). This scale measures the ratio of the overhanging portion of the vertebral body to the anteroposterior length of the inferior vertebral body. The grade of spondylolisthesis may help facilitate treatment decisions
- The most severe degree of spondylolisthesis is referred to as *spondyloptosis*. This rare condition is characterized by the complete anterior dislocation of the L5 vertebral body from the sacrum

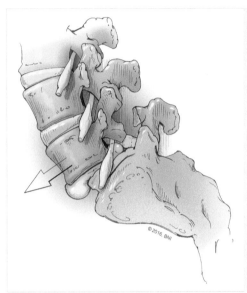

Fig. 11.5 Spondylolisthesis of L5 onto S1.

Table 11.1 Meyerding Grading System for spondylolisthesis

Grade	Degree of subluxation
Grade I	0–25%
Grade II	26–50%
Grade III	51–75%
Grade IV	76–99%
Grade V (spondyloptosis)	100%

Etiology of Spondylolisthesis

- May be congenital or developmental (i.e., present at birth or having developed during childhood)
- May be acquired from daily stress or from force exerted on the spine (e.g., resulting from arthritis, trauma, overuse, or as a complication of infection)

Epidemiology of Spondylolisthesis

- Can occur at any spinal level but is most common in the lower lumbar spine
- Affects approximately 5 to 6% of men and 2 to 3% of women
- Most common in individuals involved in physically demanding activities or sports (e.g., gymnasts, weightlifters, and football players)
  - Symptoms of spondylolisthesis are more common in men, as they are more likely to be involved in highly physical activities

11.2.5 Stenosis

Stenosis is narrowing of either the spinal canal or the neural foramen, leading to compression of the spinal cord or spinal nerve roots (▶ Fig. 11.6).

- Central canal stenosis is classified by the spinal level
- Foraminal stenosis can occur left, right, or bilaterally at any level and is classified accordingly
- Foraminal stenosis causes compression of individual spinal nerve roots as they exit the spinal canal through the neural foramen
- Neurologic symptoms are related to the affected spinal level
- Stenosis may be asymptomatic; if symptoms are present, they vary based on which structure is compressed
- Symptoms may involve radiculopathy or myelopathy (Box 11.4 Myelopathy vs. Radiculopathy)
  - Radiculopathy can occur at any level, usually from foraminal stenosis and resultant nerve root compression
  - Myelopathy results from severe central canal stenosis that compresses the spinal cord
- Severe central canal stenosis together with compression of multiple descending nerve roots in the lumbar spine is referred to as *cauda equina syndrome*, which is described in Section 11.5.2 of this chapter

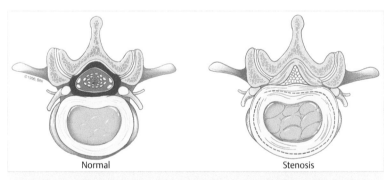

Fig. 11.6 Normal spinal canal versus spinal canal with central and neuroforaminal narrowing.

Box 11.4 Myelopathy versus Radiculopathy

- Myelopathy
  - Spinal cord compression
  - Subtle symptom onset with slow progression
  - Does not improve without decompressive surgery
  - Patients do not usually seek medical care early given that they do not have pain
  - Results in weakness, difficulties with ambulation may develop later
- Radiculopathy
  - Painful
  - Usually caused by herniated disks
  - Patients often do well with conservative treatment
  - Dermatome specific

Etiology of Stenosis

Stenosis is usually caused by a combination of congenital and acquired factors.
- Congenital
  - Spina bifida
  - Narrow spinal canal
- Acquired
  - Spinal trauma or fracture
  - DDD, thickened ligaments, and hypertrophied facets
  - Spondylosis
  - Spondylolisthesis or subluxation

Epidemiology of Stenosis

- More common in the lower lumbar spine than in the cervical spine
- Rarely occurs in the thoracic spine

11.3 Disorders of the Cervical Spine

11.3.1 Herniated Cervical Disk

- Affects men more often than women
- About 70% of cervical herniated disks occur at C5–C6 or C6–C7
- About 90% of patients are estimated to improve without surgery

Clinical Manifestations of Herniated Cervical Disk

- Symptoms are related to the following various factors:
  - The size of the herniation
  - The affected cervical spine level
  - The presence and degree of spinal cord compression
  - Symptoms can be of sudden onset with a known eliciting event or may develop slowly over time
- Examination findings indicative of cervical disk herniation may include the following:
  - Neck or arm radiculopathy relative to the affected cervical spine level (though central disk herniation may result in bilateral arm symptoms)
  - Arm muscle weakness with possible atrophy of associated arm muscles
  - Numbness or decreased sensation relative to the affected cervical spine level
  - Decreased range of motion of the neck, shoulders, and arms
  - Headache elicited by certain head movements (sometimes referred to as *cervicogenic headache*)

Cervical myelopathy may occur along with spinal cord compression, resulting in disturbance of motor or sensory function with or without pathologic change in the spinal cord (Box 11.5 Symptoms of Cervical Myelopathy).

Box 11.5 Symptoms of Cervical Myelopathy

- Neck stiffness
- Deep aching or pain in the neck
- Arm or shoulder pain (i.e., cervical radiculopathy)
- Stiffness or clumsiness while walking
- Heavy feeling in the legs
- Deterioration in fine motor skills (e.g., buttoning a shirt or writing)
- Intermittent electric-like shooting pains in the arms and legs, especially when the head is bent forward (this is known as *Lhermitte's sign*)

Treatment of Herniated Cervical Disk

- Conservative therapy
  - Bed rest; usually no more than 2 days
  - Analgesics (over-the-counter or prescription) and muscle relaxants should be administered sparingly (▶ Table 11.2). Pain relievers are available in oral, topical, or injectable forms
  - Topical pain medications are applied directly to the skin of the affected region to reduce pain resulting from arthritis or muscle soreness

Table 11.2 Pharmacology for management of spinal disorders

Drug	Category	Indication	Nursing implication
Ibuprofen (Motrin, Advil) Naproxen (Aleve, Naprosyn) Ketorolac (Toradol)	NSAIDs	Mild or moderate back or neck pain, tenderness, inflammation, and stiffness	May irritate the stomach Should be taken with food Use with caution in elderly patients and in those with renal disease or hypertension Has mild blood thinning effect Some IV preparations are available
Celecoxib (Celebrex)	COX-2 inhibitor (subclass of NSAIDs)	Arthritic pain Inflammation	Available by prescription Prolonged use should be avoided
Acetaminophen (Tylenol)	Analgesic	Mild to moderate pain	Take with food Watch for dosing limits
Methylprednisolone (Medrol)	Corticosteroid	Pain due to inflammation or irritation (i.e., radiculopathy)	May irritate the stomach Should be taken with food
Oxycodone with acetaminophen (Percocet) Hydrocodone with acetaminophen (Vicodin, Lortab)	Opioid analgesics	Moderate to severe pain; acute pain; postoperative pain	Sedating Respiratory depressant Constipating May cause urinary retention Habit-forming Not effective for neuropathic pain Additional preparations for sustained release and IV administration
Baclofen (Lioresal) Carisoprodol (Soma) Cyclobenzaprine (Flexeril)	Muscle relaxants	Muscle stiffness or spasm	Be aware of sedative side effects, especially when used with narcotics
Diazepam (Valium)	Benzodiazepine	Used for more severe spasm	Heaviest sedative; potential for drug dependence

Abbreviations: COX-2, cyclo-oxygenase 2; IV, intravenous; NSAIDs, nonsteroidal anti-inflammatory drugs.

- Topical remedies, such as Icy Hot, ArthriCare cream, Zostrix, Aspercreme, Bengay, and various store brands, are available over the counter
- A pain-relief patch such as Flector Patch is available with a prescription
  ○ Epidural steroid or analgesic injections
  ○ Physical therapy
  ○ Possible cervical traction
- Surgical therapy
  ○ Surgical therapy may be indicated when conservative therapy fails. This may be the case in patients with myelopathy and severe central stenosis or in patients with unmanageable pain. Possible surgical intervention may include the following:
    - Anterior cervical diskectomy and fusion
    - Anterior or posterior foraminotomy; see Chapter 15: Neurosurgical Interventions

11.3.2 Cervical Stenosis

Clinical Manifestations of Cervical Stenosis

- Symptoms are associated with the affected cervical level (▶ Fig. 11.7)

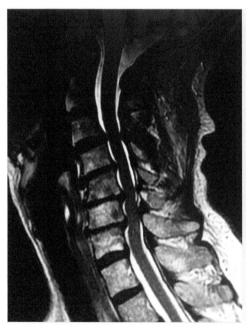

Fig. 11.7 Cervical stenosis resulting from multilevel degenerative disk disease.

- Symptoms are usually insidious and progressive, and they may include the following:
  - Neck and arm pain
  - Decreased motor function and dexterity
  - Altered sensory function
  - Spinal cord compression with severe stenosis
  - Difficulty walking
  - Spinal cord compression with no or little pain
  - May cause cervical myelopathy.

Treatment of Cervical Stenosis

- Surgical therapy; see also Chapter 15: Neurosurgical Interventions.
  - Decompressive laminectomy
  - Anterior cervical diskectomy

11.4 Disorders of the Thoracic Spine

Thoracic spinal disorders rarely occur without a precipitating traumatic event.
- DDD may predispose one to traumatic disk herniation
- Even a small thoracic herniation is associated with neurologic symptoms

11.4.1 Herniated Thoracic Disk

Epidemiology of Herniated Thoracic Disk

- More common in men than in women
- Thoracic disk herniations account for less than 1% of all herniated disks

Clinical Manifestations of Herniated Thoracic Disk

There is no characteristic presentation in a patient with a herniated thoracic disk (▶ Fig. 11.8). The condition is often misdiagnosed as angina, pleurisy, cholecystitis, arthritis, muscle strain, or fibromyalgia.
- Symptoms are variable and include the following:
  - Localized pain in the upper back or chest
  - Numbness, weakness, or spasticity
  - Radicular pain
  - Pain that often precedes neurologic symptoms
  - Myelopathy
  - Hyperactive reflexes such as clonus (e.g., rapidly alternating muscle contraction and relaxation in a continuous reflex tremor) and Babinski sign (e.g., plantar reflex with dorsiflexion of the big toe and fanning of the smaller toes elicited by stroking the bottom outer edge of the patient's foot)

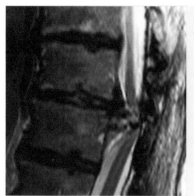

Fig. 11.8 Herniated thoracic disk compressing spinal cord.

Treatment of Herniated Thoracic Disk

Surgical therapy may be indicated in patients with unmanageable pain or with myelopathy. Several types of surgery may alleviate a herniated thoracic disk; see Chapter 15: Neurosurgical Interventions.

- Surgical therapy
  - Anterior
    - Thoracoscopic surgery
    - Thoracotomy for transthoracic diskectomy, with or without fusion
  - Posterior
    - Costotransversectomy
    - Transpedicular diskectomy and fusion, with or without anterior graft

11.5 Disorders of the Lumbar Spine

11.5.1 Herniated Lumbar Disk

- Common cause of low back pain (▶ Fig. 11.9)
- Frequently asymptomatic.

Epidemiology of Herniated Lumbar Disk

- Often occurs at multiple levels
- Most common at L4–L5 and L5–S1
- Herniation is usually posterolateral

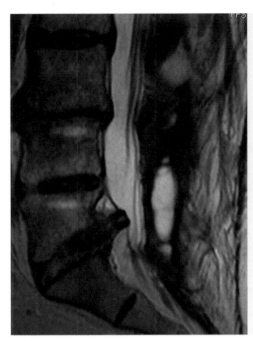

Fig. 11.9 Herniated lumbosacral disk.

Clinical Manifestations of Herniated Lumbar Disk

Patients with herniated lumbar disks may be asymptomatic or may have radiculopathy or, in severe cases, cauda equina syndrome. Symptoms of a herniated lumbar disk often include the following symptoms:

- Back pain
- Radiating leg pain
- Weakness or numbness in the associated dermatome
- Paresthesia
- Bladder or bowel dysfunction

Treatment of Herniated Lumbar Disk

- Conservative therapy
  - Same as for low back pain; see later
  - Epidural steroid injections (Box 11.6 Epidural Steroid Injections)
- Indications for surgery
  - Failure of conservative therapy after 1 to 2 months
  - Unmanageable pain

○ Progressive neurologic deterioration
  – New foot drop
  – Urinary retention
  – Cauda equina syndrome
• Surgical therapy; see Chapter 15: Neurosurgical Interventions.
  ○ Diskectomy
  ○ Microdiskectomy

Box 11.6 Epidural Steroid Injections

• Epidural steroid injections have been shown to provide short-term pain relief
• No demonstrated long-term benefit in treatment of chronic back pain

---

11.5.2 Cauda Equina Syndrome

The cauda equina consists of 10 spinal nerve pairs: 4 lumbar, 5 sacral, and 1 coccygeal (▶ Fig. 11.10). It is named for its horsetail appearance and is formed by the spinal nerve roots below the level of the spinal cord termination (i.e., the conus medullaris), which occurs around the L1–L2 vertebral level. Cauda equina syndrome is a group of symptoms caused by severe compression of the spinal nerves in the lumbosacral spine at the level of the cauda equina (▶ Fig. 11.11).

Etiology of Cauda Equina Syndrome

• Most common cause is a large central disk herniation at L4–L5 or L5–S1
• Trauma
• Hematoma
• Epidural abscess
• Tumor

Clinical Manifestations of Cauda Equina Syndrome

• Saddle anesthesia (i.e., loss of sensation or reduced sensation in the perineum and buttocks)
• Lower extremity motor or sensory changes
• Loss of bladder or bowel function
• New-onset cauda equina syndrome is a medical emergency (Box 11.7 Clinical Alert: Cauda Equina Syndrome Is a Medical Emergency)

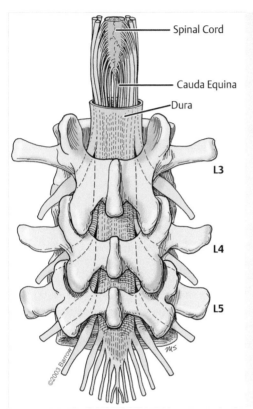

Spinal Cord

Cauda Equina

Dura

L3

L4

L5

Fig. 11.10 Cauda equina.

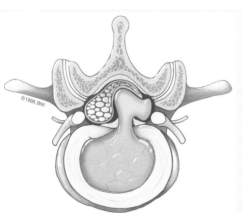

Fig. 11.11 Large centrally herniated disk causing cauda equina syndrome.

Treatment of Cauda Equina Syndrome

- Emergency surgical decompression to prevent symptoms from becoming permanent
- Bladder or bowel incontinence or paraplegia could result if it is left untreated

---

Box 11.7 Clinical Alert: Cauda Equina Syndrome Is a Medical Emergency

- Report any symptom of cauda equina syndrome immediately
  - New-onset saddle anesthesia
  - Weakness in both legs
  - Loss of sensation in lower extremities
  - Loss of bladder or bowel control
- Decompressive surgery within 48 hours of symptom onset significantly reduces the likelihood of long-term neurologic impairment

---

11.5.3 Lumbar Stenosis

Etiology of Lumbar Stenosis

- Congenital
- Trauma
- Acquired
- Spondylosis
- Spondylolisthesis

Clinical Manifestations of Lumbar Stenosis

- Low back pain
- Lower extremity weakness and sensory loss
- Leg fatigue
- Neurogenic claudication
  - Can be bilateral or unilateral
  - Pain, discomfort, or weakness in the buttocks, thighs, or calves
  - May be precipitated by prolonged standing or walking
  - Pain is classically relieved by a change in position or by bending forward; it is not simply relieved by rest (unlike vascular claudication, for which rest alone can relieve symptoms)
  - Patients with neurogenic claudication usually experience less difficulty with activities that allow bending or forward flexion (e.g., pushing a shopping cart, cycling, or climbing stairs)
  - In patients with severe neurogenic claudication, the pain associated with neurogenic claudication is ever-present instead of intermittent

Treatment of Lumbar Stenosis

- Conservative therapy: same as for low back pain (Box 11.8 Conservative Therapy for Spinal Stenosis)
- Surgical therapy; see also Chapter 15: Neurosurgical Interventions.
  - Decompressive laminectomy
  - Placement of interspinous process decompression device (e.g., X STOP [St. Francis Medical Technologies Inc./Medtronic plc] and Aspen MIS Fusion System [Lanx Inc./Biomet Inc./Zimmer Biomet Inc.])

Box 11.8 Conservative Therapy for Spinal Stenosis

- Diminishes symptoms in some patients with spinal stenosis
- Should be tried in all patients without significant neurologic deficits (e.g., lower extremity weakness, bladder or bowel dysfunction)
- Recurrence of neck, back, or radicular pain is often unavoidable with resumption of normal activity and may indicate the need for decompressive surgery

---

11.5.4 Low Back Pain

Low back pain is a common and challenging health concern among the general U.S. population. It is a major cause of disability and lost work time and is quite costly. As many as 80% of U.S. adults experience at least one episode of low back pain during their lifetime, and 5% experience chronic back pain. In the United States, back pain in workers has been estimated to cost employers $7.4 billion annually (Box 11.9 The Incidence and Cost of Low Back Pain).

- Affects men and women equally; it may be a dull ache, or it may be sharp and severe
- Often nonspecific
- Onset may be sudden, as when precipitated by trauma or by lifting a heavy object
- Pain may develop over time, as in patients with age-related degenerative spinal disorders
- A sedentary lifestyle may contribute to low back pain
- Often results in limitations of body positions and an inability to perform certain activities
- Usually acute in nature, lasting only a several days or weeks. Almost all patients (roughly 90%) recover within 4 to 6 weeks
- Often resolves on its own when patients seek conservative therapy and limit activities that may exacerbate the pain

○ Most acute low back pain results from a mechanical injury (i.e., an unusual movement or abnormal alignment of vertebrae, muscles, disks, or nerves).
  – Subacute low back pain is temporary, usually lasting between 4 and 12 weeks
  – Chronic back pain is pain that persists for 12 weeks or longer, even when the initial injury or cause has been treated

---

Box 11.9 The Incidence and Cost of Low Back Pain

- Up to 80% of people at some time in their life will experience neck or back pain
- About 20 to 40% of the population report having had back pain at some point
- Most common cause of job-related disability and a leading contributor to missed work days
- Back pain sufferers contribute more than $90 billion annually to health care expenses and account for 33 cents of every dollar spent on U.S. disability claims

---

Conservative Therapy for Low Back Pain

- Rest or reduced level of activity
  ○ Bed rest is usually no longer than 2 days
  ○ Restricting activities (e.g., avoiding bending, lifting, twisting)
- Pain medications (e.g., acetaminophen, nonsteroidal anti-inflammatory drugs [NSAIDs], and narcotics, used sparingly for severe, intractable pain not responsive to nonnarcotics)
- A short course of steroids may be helpful for radiculopathy
- Muscle relaxants
- Physical therapy
- Exercise: Stretching, strengthening, and low-impact aerobic exercise can help prevent low back pain, reduce flare-ups, and retain strength and flexibility
- Epidural injections
- Transcutaneous electrical nerve stimulation units
- Ultrasound treatment
- Massage
- Ergonomics: proper lifting techniques, supportive footwear, and avoidance of prolonged sitting or standing
- Education about lifestyle modification (e.g., weight loss, smoking cessation)
- Chiropractic manipulation (Box 11.10 Alternative Therapy: Acupuncture)

- Acupuncture may influence the electromagnetic field of the body, thereby altering the chemical neurotransmitters within the body
- Data are insufficient to judge the clinical efficacy of acupuncture for treatment of low back pain

11.6 Diagnosis of Spinal Disorders

11.6.1 Medical History

- Identify possible precipitating event
- Document preexisting known spinal disease
- Record current medications for an existing spinal disorder
- Document symptoms, including the following:
  - Onset of pain and sensory or motor changes
  - Location of pain, including radiation to arms or legs
  - Description of pain (e.g., dull, aching, deep, sharp, burning, throbbing, lancinating)
  - Description of numbness or tingling
  - Description of what exacerbates or improves symptoms (i.e., changing position, activity, heat, cold, rest)
  - Bladder and bowel dysfunction (i.e., neurogenic bladder, neurogenic bowel).
    - Urinary or bowel incontinence
    - Incomplete emptying or constipation
    - Increased frequency
  - Functional or lifestyle impairments

11.6.2 Medical Evaluation

The medical assessment of a patient with a spinal disorder involves physical, motor, and sensory assessment, with special attention paid to reflexes. See Chapter 2: Assessment for a detailed description of these evaluations.

- Physical evaluation
  - Muscle mass and symmetry
  - Normal or abnormal spine curvature
  - Localized regions of spinal pain or muscle spasm
  - Gait analysis to quantify weakness or spasticity in feet, legs, hips, and trunk
- Motor assessment
  - Assess for strength by specific muscle group
    - Muscle grading scale (▶ Table 11.3)

Table 11.3 Spinal nerve root motor assessment

Level	Affected muscles or motor groups	Muscle action
C4	Diaphragm	Respiratory inspiration
C5	Deltoid	Abduct arm
	Biceps	Elbow flexion
C6	Extensor carpi radialis	Wrist extension
C7	Triceps	Elbow extension
	Extensor digitorum	Finger extension
C8	Flexor digitorum profundus	Hand grip
	Intrinsic hand muscles	Abduct little finger
L2	Iliopsoas	Hip flexion
L3	Quadriceps	Knee extension
L4	Hamstrings (medial)	Ankle dorsiflexion
	Tibialis anterior	
L5	Posterior tibialis	Foot inversion
	Extensor hallucis longus	Extension of big toe
S1	Gastrocnemius	Ankle plantar flexion
S2	Bladder	Bladder tone
	Anal sphincter	Rectal tone

- Sensory assessment; dermatome sensory testing
- Reflexes
  - Presence of clonus
  - Hyperreflexia or areflexia
- Specific tests can be administered by the clinician to further assess the patient for common spine disorders (▶ Table 11.4)

11.6.3 Diagnostic Imaging

The most commonly used diagnostic imaging techniques to evaluate a patient with a suspected spinal disorder are radiography, computed tomography (CT), and magnetic resonance imaging (MRI) (▶ Table 11.5). See also Chapter 14: Neuroradiology and Neuroendovascular Interventions.

- Plain radiographs
  - Assess alignment and spacing between the occiput and vertebral bodies
  - Open-mouth view for visualization of C1–C2 joint
  - Swimmer's view for cervicothoracic junction
  - Flexion-extension view useful for identifying abnormal subluxation or movement suggestive of instability

Table 11.4 Specific tests for spinal disorders

Test	Indications	Testing method
Lasègue's sign (i.e., straight leg raise test)	Herniated lumbar disk	With the patient laying supine, lift the affected leg, keeping the knee straight. If the patient reports pain down the back of the leg when it is elevated to the 30- to 70-degree range, the test is positive (i.e., the nerve roots leading to the sciatic nerve may be compressed or irritated) If pain develops before an elevation of 30 degrees, the pain is likely not the result of a herniated disk If the test is performed on the unaffected leg (i.e., a contralateral straight leg raise test) and pain is reported in the affected leg, this serves as confirmation of the finding
Lhermitte's sign	Cervical cord compression Multiple sclerosis B_{12} deficiency Transverse myelitis	Gently flex the patient's head forward; test is positive if flexion produces shooting, electric-like shocks that travel from the head down the spine
Spurling's test	Cervical disk herniation with or without stenosis Cervical radiculopathy	Turn the patient's head to the affected side while extending and applying mild downward pressure to the top of the head A positive test is when the neck pain radiates in the direction of the corresponding dermatome
Hoffmann's sign (i.e., finger-flexor reflex)	Cervical myelopathy Spinal cord compression	Sharply flick or snap the patient's nail of the middle finger. The test is positive when the tip of the index finger, ring finger, and/or thumb suddenly flex in response

- CT
  - Best study for evaluating bony anatomy, spinal alignment, fractures, and dislocations
  - Useful for patients unable to undergo MRI due to the presence of a pacemaker or other metal implants or who have had previous spinal surgery
- MRI
  - Imaging of choice for evaluating disk disease, spinal cord and nerve root disorders, and most other spinal conditions
  - Performed without a contrast agent for evaluation of spinal disks, nerve roots, fractures, and degenerative disease
  - A contrast agent is used for evaluating spinal infections, spinal canal tumors, multiple sclerosis or other causes of myelitis, and syrinxes

Table 11.5 Diagnostic studies for spinal disorders

Type of test	Visualized structures	Nursing implication
Myelography (cervical, thoracic, or lumbar)	Size and location of disk herniation	Patient must be NPO Contrast agent is used[a] Patient may need to remain flat in bed for 2–6 h after the procedure
MRI	Highly specific for determining the level and degree of disk herniation, presence of tumors, hemorrhage, infection, and edema	Patient must be NPO if sedation is needed for claustrophobia or pain Contraindicated in patients with metallic implants (i.e., pacemakers or history of working with metal) Contrast agent may be used[a]
CT	Helpful in determining bony structures, including bone spurs, fragments, and bony alignment	Contrast agent may be used[a]
Plain films	Spinal fractures Bony alignment	

Abbreviations: CT, computed tomography; MRI, magnetic resonance imaging; NPO, nil per os (nothing by mouth).

[a]The use of contrast agents may cause allergic reactions, and caution must be used in patients with diabetes.

- Used to evaluate the following:
  - Ligaments
  - Herniated disks
  - Nerve roots
  - Cord compression
  - Cauda equina
  - Spinal canal

11.7 Other Spinal Disorders

11.7.1 Osteoporosis

Osteoporosis is a condition characterized by the thinning of bone. Bones naturally thin with age, and this process reduces the amount of weight they can support and external stresses that can be withstood. In the 2005 to 2008 National Health and Nutrition Examination Survey, the Centers for Disease Control and Prevention reported that 9% of adults 50 years and older had osteoporosis of the lumbar spine or the femoral neck. Of those 9%, roughly half had low bone mass at either the lumbar spine or femoral neck. The other half had normal bone mass at both sites.

Women are more likely than men to have low bone mass and osteoporosis, and the prevalence of these conditions is increased with age.

- Osteoporosis occurs most often in postmenopausal white women. Roughly 4 in 10 are likely to experience a hip, spine, or wrist fracture after age 50
- About 70% of women in the United States are osteoporotic by age 80

Treatment of Osteoporosis

- The best treatment is prevention
  - Calcium and vitamin D supplements
    - Adults younger than age 50 years should consume 1,000 mg/d of calcium and 400 to 800 IU/d of vitamin D; adults older than age 50 years should consume 1,200 mg/d of calcium and 800 to 1,000 IU/d of vitamin D
  - Good nutrition, including adequate amounts of dairy, protein, fruits, and vegetables
  - Normal body mass index of 20 to 25
  - Exercise. A well-rounded exercise program should include the following three elements:
    - Impact training (e.g., walking, running)
    - Strength training (e.g., weight lifting, resistance training)
    - Balance training (e.g., dancing, yoga)
  - Smoking cessation
  - Alcohol restriction (1 drink/d for women and 2 drinks/d for men)
- Medications to help slow bone loss and maintain bone mass
  - Bisphosphonates (alendronate [Fosamax], ibandronate [Boniva], risedronate [Actonel], zoledronic acid [Reclast])
  - Selective estrogen receptor modulators (e.g., raloxifene [Evista])
  - Calcitonin
  - Hormone replacement therapy (e.g., estrogen) should not be the first-choice treatment

11.7.2 Osteoporotic Vertebral Compression Fractures

Patients with osteoporosis are at risk of developing compression fractures of the thoracic or lumbar spine merely as a result of ordinary daily activities, without trauma (▶ Fig. 11.12). Accordingly, they are at significant risk for fracture in the setting of trauma. In fact, about 40% of white women and 13% of white men in the United States will experience at least one "fragility fracture" (i.e., a fracture resulting from a low-trauma event) after age 50 years. Osteoporotic vertebral compression fractures account for most vertebral fractures and are commonly caused by falls or motor vehicle accidents. This type of fracture is associated with increased risk of future vertebral and nonvertebral fractures. Related pain is expected to decrease with time as the fracture heals.

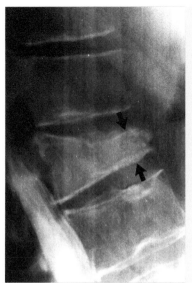

Fig. 11.12 Compression fracture.

Treatment of Osteoporotic Fractures

- Bracing with lumbosacral orthotic or thoracolumbosacral orthotic devices
- Pain control (acetaminophen, NSAIDs, muscle relaxants, narcotics)
- Heat therapy or cold therapy
- Physical therapy
- Early mobilization, with use of a brace or orthotic device
- Upright and supine thoracolumbar radiographs with the patient in a brace to determine the stability of the fractured spine
- Fractures can be expected to heal in 8 to 12 weeks
- Patients with one compression fracture are much more likely to develop another
- Vertebroplasty (i.e., percutaneous injection of medical-grade acrylic cement into the fractured vertebra) or kyphoplasty (i.e., repair of compressed vertebrae by percutaneous insertion of a balloon-type device to restore height, followed by injection of polymethacrylate cement) may be considered for refractory pain

11.7.3 Pathologic Spinal Fractures

Pathologic fractures occur in bone that has been weakened by an underlying preexisting disease or condition by long-term use of corticosteroids. These fractures may be precipitated by a minor traumatic event or by normal activity. A fractured, weakened vertebra is at risk for collapse (i.e., a compression fracture). This type of injury can occur at any spinal level, but it is most common in the thoracic and lumbar spine. Pain related to a pathologic spinal fracture may be acute and progressive, and may only be diminished once the underlying pathology is treated and resolved.

Disease Processes Leading to Pathologic Spinal Fractures

Pathologic spinal fractures may result in neurologic impairment with or without spinal cord injury. Various disease processes lead to pathologic spinal fractures, including the following:

- Metastatic lesions to the bone (most common); three out of four cases metastasize from breast cancer (▶ Fig. 11.13)
- Multiple myeloma
- Chordoma
- Metabolic-based bone disease (e.g., osteoporosis, osteomalacia, hyperparathyroidism, renal osteodystrophy)
- Bone tuberculosis
- Osteomyelitis (i.e., inflammation of bone from infection)
- Paget's disease of bone, known as *osteitis deformans*, marked by increased bone resorption that results in weakened bones
- Fibrous dysplasia of bone marked by thinning of the cortex and replacement of bone marrow with fibrous tissue containing bony, sharp, needle-like formations (i.e., spicules)

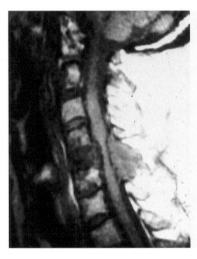

Fig. 11.13 Metastatic lesion leading to cervical vertebral fracture.

Treatment of Pathologic Spinal Fractures

- Treatment of the underlying disease is critical
- Needle biopsy is indicated if osteomyelitis or cancer of unknown primary origin is suspected
- Patients with fractures caused by osteomyelitis are not suitable for vertebroplasty or kyphoplasty
- Bracing, surgical intervention, or radiation therapy may be indicated, based on the primary process and whether the patient has compression of the spinal nerves
- Treatment of pain and muscle spasms

11.7.4 Rheumatoid Arthritis Associated with Cervical Spine Disease

Rheumatoid arthritis (RA) causes inflammation and destructive changes of the synovial joints of the cervical spine and the surrounding bone and cartilage.

- RA involvement in the cervical spine begins early in the course of the disease
- RA-related granulation tissue can cause spinal cord compression
- Enzymes produced by RA accelerate destruction of bone, ligaments, and tendons, causing more instability

Cervical Fractures Specific to Rheumatoid Arthritis

Atlantoaxial Instability (Anterior C1–C2 Subluxation or Instability)

- Caused by abnormal separation between the anterior arch of the atlas and the odontoid process of the axis
- Displacement of C1 on C2 is more pronounced with neck flexion and can cause spinal cord compression
- Secondary to loosening of the transverse ligament from RA-related inflammation of joints between C1 and the odontoid process

Vertical Atlantoaxial Instability (Atlantoaxial Impaction, Basilar Invagination, and Vertical Subluxation)

- Upward displacement of the odontoid process of C2 into the foramen magnum, with compression of the brainstem and vertebral artery
- Caused by inflammation and bony breakdown of C1 lateral masses
- Can cause quadriplegia
- Present in 3 to 4% of all patients with RA

Treatment of Rheumatoid Arthritis–Related Fractures

- Surgical stabilization of spine, with possible decompression; see Chapter 15: Neurosurgical Interventions
- Orthotic bracing; see Chapter 12: Traumatic Spine Injury
- Treatment of pain and muscle spasms
- Treatment of systemic disease
- Therapy and rehabilitation; see Chapter 17: Rehabilitation

11.7.5 Ankylosing Spondylitis

Ankylosing spondylitis is a rare rheumatological, inflammatory disorder of synovial joints and membranes that involves the spine and skeletal structures of the head and trunk (Box 111.11 Ankylosing Spondylitis).

- Onset occurs at age 25 to 35 years
- Causes inflammation and pain in joints of spine and pelvis
- Starts with inflammation, leading to bony erosion and ankylosis (i.e., immobilization and consolidation of a joint resulting in spine stiffness), with eventual fusing of involved joints and kyphotic deformities
- Spinal rigidity and comorbid osteoporosis increase the risk of vertebral fractures

Box 11.11 Ankylosing Spondylitis

- A blood test can determine the presence of the *HLA-B27* gene, which is found in about 90% of people with ankylosing spondylitis
- Only 10 to 15% of persons who inherit the *HLA-B27* gene will go on to develop ankylosing spondylitis
- Medications are being developed to inhibit certain immune-system cells, called *cytokines*, which appear to cause some of the symptoms of ankylosing spondylitis

Clinical Manifestations of Ankylosing Spondylitis

- Pain
- Stiffness, mostly in the morning
- Functional limitations
- May result in progressive kyphosis (i.e., abnormal outward curvature of spine, causing hunching of the back)
- May impede ability to stand upright

Diagnosis of Ankylosing Spondylitis

- Medical history
- Medical assessment
  - Limited range of motion

Imaging Studies

- Plain radiography best for visualizing fused joints

11.7.6 Failed Back Syndrome.

The persistence or worsening of pain and physical limitations after lumbar laminectomy or diskectomy is called *failed back syndrome*.
- Affects about 15% of patients after back surgery
- Possible causes
  - Misdiagnosis or inappropriate first surgery
  - Inadequate decompression from first surgery
  - Scar tissue
  - Recurrent disk herniation
  - Physically demanding job requirements or lifestyle
  - Smoking
  - Psychological factors
- May lead to permanent disability

Treatment of Failed Back Syndrome

- Repeat surgery, which is successful in about 50% of patients
- Pain management
- Physical therapy

11.7.7 Diskitis

Diskitis is an infection of the vertebral disk space.
- May lead to osteomyelitis or abscess
- Most common cause is prior spine surgery
- May occur as infection from another site in the body that travels to bone
- Diagnosed by image-guided needle biopsy to identify pathogen

Treatment of Diskitis

- Intravenous antibiotics, with infectious diseases consult
- Pain management, as diskitis causes severe pain and paraspinal muscle spasm

- Orthotic bracing may provide support
- Physical therapy
- Surgical debridement occasionally needed for refractory cases or for nerve compression; see Chapter 10: Infectious Diseases

11.7.8 Scoliosis

Scoliosis is characterized by abnormal sagittal, coronal, and/or axial curvature of the spine (► Fig. 11.14). It may be congenital or idiopathic, and can be degenerative.

Congenital Scoliosis

Congenital scoliosis is an abnormal condition present at birth, characterized by a lateral curvature of the spine. It is estimated to occur in only 1 in 10,000

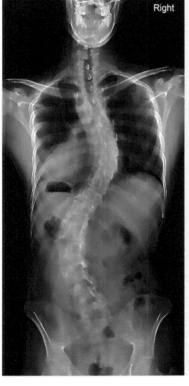

Right

Fig. 11.14 Scoliosis.

newborns, but it may not be diagnosed until adolescence. In patients with idiopathic scoliosis, the condition is often painless and may go unnoticed.

Idiopathic Scoliosis

Idiopathic scoliosis usually presents in children and adolescents. The precise etiology is unknown but has been the topic of much debate and investigation. It occurs more commonly in female patients.

Degenerative Scoliosis

Degenerative scoliosis, which usually affects the lumbar spine, occurs when the intervertebral disks deteriorate and the facet joints of the posterior spine become arthritic. The condition is characterized by lateral curvature of the lower back and loss of the lordotic curvature. Degenerative scoliosis usually affects older patients (individuals over 65 years of age) and worsens with age. As the spine degenerates and the facet joints become increasingly arthritic, the joints enlarge, which in turn narrows the spinal canal and results in spinal stenosis.

Diagnosis of Scoliosis

- Medical history
- Medical assessment
  - The physical examination should include the following:
    - The forward bending test, which makes any spinal deformity more noticeable. In this test, the patient is asked to lean or bend forward and their spine is examined
  - In patients with scoliosis, examination findings may include the following:
    - Tilted or uneven shoulders
    - Protrusion of one shoulder blade
    - Prominence of ribs on one side
    - An uneven waistline/one hip higher than the other
    - The appearance of leaning toward one side, or obvious abnormal spinal curvature
  - Patient may report weakness or numbness, which is indicative of nerve/ spinal cord compression
  - Patient may report back pain and/or muscle spasm
  - Patient may report new discomfort with the way clothing fits
  - In severe cases, patients may experience restriction of chest expansion
- Imaging studies
  - Plain radiographs: Full-length frontal and lateral views; right and lateral bending views; anteroposterior upright view
  - CT or MRI may also be indicated, depending on patient history and examination findings
- Rule out other potential causes of back pain

Clinical Manifestations of Scoliosis

Many persons with scoliosis have no back pain; in patients with pain, however, the pain is often chronic.
- If pain is present, it typically develops gradually
- Facet joints are exposed to the greatest pressure when standing
- Sitting or lying removes much of the stress from the joints
- Patients often feel worse in the morning

Treatment of Scoliosis

- Pain management
- Physical therapy
- Bracing or surgery (with possible extensive instrumentation) may be indicated

11.8 Nursing Management for Patients with Spinal Disorders

This chapter is intended as a basic reference for bedside care of neurologic patients with spine disorders. For further information, the reader should consult the references at the end of the chapter to learn more about subjects of interest (▶ Table 11.6 **and Appendix A10: Nursing Management of Patients with Spine Disorders**).

11.8.1 Neurologic Assessment

- Patient's medical history; refer to Chapter 2: Assessment
- Motor assessment
- Sensory assessment
- Assessment of reflexes
- Assessment of neck and back for spasms, tenderness, atrophy, and flexibility
- Gait analysis

11.8.2 Mobility Assessment

- Assess mobility and encourage early postoperative ambulation
- Watch for signs and symptoms of deep vein thrombosis (in the acute setting)
- Assist in repositioning the patient as needed (in the acute setting)

11.8.3 Integumentary Assessment

- Watch for signs and symptoms of skin breakdown due to immobility or orthosis
- Institute appropriate skin care and proper padding of orthotic devices

Table 11.6 Nursing management for patients with spinal disorders

Problem	Nursing action	Rationale
Neurologic Decreased motor or sensory function; gait abnormalities	Neurologic assessment, including motor and sensory assessment	Potential for worsening of function due to edema or hemorrhage
Urinary retention	Accurate intake and output Check postvoid residual urine volume Timed voiding (every 4–6 h) Notify medical team of any new symptoms of retention or incontinence	Urinary retention is a common complication of lumbar surgery or lumbar myelopathy Urinary retention also results from opioid use Urinary retention or incontinence could be a symptom of cauda equina syndrome
Pain	Administer analgesics and muscle relaxants as indicated by the patient's pain level and as ordered Assess patient's response to medications Use alternative methods of pain relief (e.g., ice, heat, massage, repositioning) when possible	Pain may cause the patient to refrain from activity
Patient and family education	Assess risk factors (e.g., smoking, excess weight, lack of exercise) Educate regarding proper body mechanics Educate regarding appropriate exercise program Recommend smoking cessation	Many spinal disorders (e.g., degenerative disk disease, disk herniation) are aggravated by poor body mechanics Smoking is detrimental to general health as well as to bone health and healing

11.8.4 Pain Management

- Narcotics, NSAIDs, or acetaminophen as ordered
- Steroids
- Antispasm medications
- Pregabalin (Lyrica) or gabapentin (Neurontin) for relief of neurogenic pain
- Cold or heat therapy as needed for comfort
- Massage

11.8.5 Patient Education and Family Support

- Patient and family education for mobility assistance (e.g., transfers, assistance with ambulation)

- Patient and family training for use of brace or assistive device if appropriate
- Patient and family education regarding use of narcotics if appropriate
- See **Appendix B** for appropriate sample discharge instructions, especially **Appendix B12: Sample Discharge Instructions After Anterior Cervical Diskectomy with Fusion and Plating; Appendix B13: Sample Discharge Instructions After Laminectomy; Appendix B14: Sample Discharge Instructions After Lumbar Diskectomy;** and **Appendix B15: Anterior Lumbar Spinal Fusion**

11.8.6 Collaborative Management

The management of patients with spinal disorders requires a team of specialists. Such specialties may include the following:
- Nursing
- Neurosurgery
- Internal medicine
- Neurology (for management of pain or conditions not requiring surgery)
- Specialists related to specific coexisting conditions (e.g., specialists in rheumatology, infectious diseases, chronic pain)
- Orthotists
- Physical, occupational, and rehabilitation therapy
  - Rehabilitation consult if appropriate
- Clergy members or other spiritual support if appropriate

Suggested Reading

[1] American Academy of Orthopaedic Surgeons. Congenital scoliosis. OrthoInfo 2010; http://orthoinfo.aaos.org/topic.cfm?topic=A00576. Accessed March 7, 2016

[2] American Academy of Pain Medicine. The cost of pain to business and society due to ineffective pain care. 2016; http://www.painmed.org/patientcenter/cost-of-pain-to-businesses/. Accessed March 7, 2016

[3] American Association of Neuroscience Nurses. Cervical Spine Surgery: A Guide to Preoperative and Postoperative Care. Glenview, IL: American Association of Neuroscience Nurses; 2007

[4] American Association of Neuroscience Nurses. Thoracolumbar Spine Surgery: A Guide to Preoperative and Postoperative Patient Care. Chicago, IL: American Association of Neuroscience Nurses; 2014

[5] Caridi JM, Pumberger M, Hughes AP. Cervical radiculopathy: a review. HSS J. 2011; 7(3):265–272

[6] Crow WT, Willis DR. Estimating cost of care for patients with acute low back pain: a retrospective review of patient records. J Am Osteopath Assoc. 2009; 109(4):229–233

[7] Dawodu ST. Cauda equina and conus medullaris syndromes. 2017; http://emedicine.medscape.com/article/1148690-overview. Accessed June 29, 2017

[8] Deyo RA, Tsui-Wu YJ. Descriptive epidemiology of low-back pain and its related medical care in the United States. Spine. 1987; 12(3):264–268

[9] DeWitt D. Medications for back pain and neck pain. 2016; http://www.spine-health.com/treatment/ pain-medication/medications-back-and-neck-pain. Accessed June 29, 2017

[10] Florence R, Allen S, Benedict L, et al. Diagnosis and Treatment of Osteoporosis. Bloomington, MN: Institute for Clinical Systems Improvement (ICSI); 2013

[11] Garfin SR. Rheumatoid arthritis of the cervical spine: overview of rheumatoid spondylitis. 2015; http://emedicine.medscape.com/article/1266195-overview. Accessed December 28, 2015

[12] International Osteoporosis Foundation. International Osteoporosis Foundation: Facts and Statistics. 2015; http://www.iofbonehealth.org/facts-statistics#category-23. Accessed 12/28/2015

[13] Jones J, Gaillard F. Spondylolisthesis grading system. 2016; http://radiopaedia.org/articles/spondylolisthesis-grading-system. Accessed March 7, 2016

[14] Kishner S. Degenerative disk disease. 2017; http://emedicine.medscape.com/article/1265453-overview#showall. Accessed June 29, 2017

[15] Lønne G, Johnsen LG, Rossvoll I, et al. Minimally invasive decompression versus x-stop in lumbar spinal stenosis: a randomized controlled multicenter study. Spine. 2015; 40(2):77–85

[16] Looker AC, Borrud LG, Dawson-Hughes B, Shepherd JA, Wright NC. Osteoporosis or low bone mass at the femur neck or lumbar spine in older adults: United States, 2005–2008. NCHS Data Brief. 2012(93):1–8

[17] Mayo Clinic Staff. Osteoporosis. 2016; http://www.mayoclinic.org/diseases-conditions/osteoporosis/home/ovc-20207808. Accessed July 19, 2017

[18] Mehlman CT, Talavera F, Shaffer WO, Goldstein JA. Idiopathic scoliosis. 2016; http://emedicine.medscape.com/article/1265794-overview#a4. Accessed February 29, 2016

[19] Patel RK. Lumbar degenerative disk disease. 2016; http://emedicine.medscape.com/article/309767-overview. Accessed June 29, 2017

[20] Prendergast V. Spine disorders. In: Bader MK, Littlejohns LR, eds. AANN Core Curriculum for Neuroscience Nursing. 5th ed. St. Louis, MO: Saunders; 2010

[21] Rajiah P. Idiopathic scoliosis imaging. 2015; http://emedicine.medscape.com/article/413157-overview. Accessed December 28, 2015

[22] Reed Group. Fracture, vertebra (pathological). MD Guidelines 2016; http://www.mdguidelines.com/fracture-vertebra-pathological. Accessed July 19, 2017

[23] Rodts M. Spondylolisthesis: back condition and treatment. 2017; http://www.spineuniverse.com/conditions/spondylolisthesis/spondylolisthesis-back-condition-treatment. Accessed June 29, 2017

[24] Rothschild BM. Lumbar spondylosis. 2016; http://misc.medscape.com/pi/iphone/medscapeapp/html/A249036-business.html. Accessed February 29, 2016

[25] Strayer AL, Hickey JV. Back pain and spinal disorders. In: Hickey JV, ed. The Clinical Practice of Neurological and Neurosurgical Nursing. 7th ed. Philadelphia, PA: Lippincott Williams & Wilkins, a Wolter Kluwer business; 2014

[26] Ullrich PF. Spondylosis: what it actually means. 2008; http://www.spine-health.com/conditions/lower-back-pain/spondylosis-what-it-actually-means. Accessed June 29, 2017

[27] Wheeler SG, Wipf JE, Staiger TO, Deyo RA, Jarvik JG. Evaluation of low back pain in adults. 2017; http://www.uptodate.com/contents/evaluation-of-low-back-pain-in-adults. Accessed June 29, 2017

12 Traumatic Spine Injury

Charlotte S. Myers and Laurie Baker

Abstract

Traumatic spine injuries occur in varying degrees of severity, ranging from mild cervical strain to complete spinal cord injury. Injuries to the spine may be caused by trauma, such as a car or diving accident, or a disease process, such as a tumor or abscess. Because spinal cord injuries may have devastating effects on the patient and family, a multidisciplinary team of health care providers (e.g., surgeons; nurses; occupational, speech, and physical therapists; medical staff; and case managers) is needed to ensure optimal recovery and rehabilitation.

Keywords: autonomic dysreflexia, cauda equina syndrome, central cord syndrome, spinal cord injury, spinal fractures, spinal shock

12.1 Traumatic Spine Injury

A traumatic spine injury involves damage to the spinal cord, spinal nerves, supporting ligaments, vertebral bodies, blood vessels, or a combination of these. Many cases of traumatic spine injury result in serious implications for patients, both initially and long term. Long-term outcomes are influenced by the type, level, and severity of the injury. Of all traumatic spine injuries, an injury to the spinal cord is the most calamitous.

12.2 Spinal Cord Injury

Spinal cord injury (SCI) is a devastating, life-changing event that may result from trauma, neoplasm, hemorrhage, infection, or a degenerative spine condition. Bony fracture or dislocation is frequently associated with SCI (Video 12.1). It results in major morbidity and is costly for the health care system (▶ Table 12.1). SCI does not take only a physical toll; it also results in significant psychological stress and can bring about major lifestyle changes. Injury to the spinal cord will alter the patient's independence, economic security, body image, lifestyle, and overall quality of life.

Patients with SCI pose a unique set of challenges for the bedside nurse. The many emotional and physiologic responses associated with this type of injury may affect different systems in the body. The ability to recover from SCI depends on a host of variables, including the level of injury; the patient's personal characteristics; the receipt of timely, evidenced-based medical care; and

Table 12.1 Costs of spinal cord injury: estimated average annual cost of health care and living expenses for a patient with spinal cord injury

Injury type	First year	Each subsequent year
C1–C4 injury	$1,044,197	$181,328
C5–C8 injury	$754,524	$111,237
Paraplegia	$508,904	$67,415
Incomplete motor	$340,787	$41,393

In 2013, the estimated annual indirect cost of SCI (i.e., loss of wages, employment benefits, and productivity) was $70,575

Abbreviation: SCI, spinal cord injury. Note: Data from the National Spinal Cord Injury Statistical Center, http://www.nscisc.uab.edu.

access to neurorehabilitation. Some patients may have no identifiable neurologic impairment, whereas, sadly, others experience severe and permanent disability.

12.2.1 Etiology of Spinal Cord Injury

Spinal cord injury can be caused by accidents, diseases, or developmental anomalies (Box 12.1 Etiology of Spinal Cord Injury). Following are some common causes
- Motor vehicle accidents
- Falls
- Acts of violence (e.g., gunshot wounds)
- Sports injuries
- Tumors
- Hemorrhage
- Infection

Box 12.1 Etiology of Spinal Cord Injury

- Etiology of SCI
  - Vehicle accidents: 38%
  - Falls: 30%
  - Violence: 14%
  - Sports-related injuries: 9%
  - Medical/surgical: 5%
  - Other: 4%
- Less than 10% of SCI result from medical causes (e.g., neoplasm or hemorrhage from a vascular abnormality)
- Since 2000, SCI categories at time of hospital discharge are as follows:

○ Incomplete tetraplegia: 45%
○ Complete tetraplegia: 14%
○ Incomplete paraplegia: 21%
○ Complete paraplegia: 20%

Data from the National Spinal Cord Injury Statistical Center, http://www.nscisc.uab.edu

Epidemiology of Spinal Cord Injury

- About 12,500 new cases of SCI occur annually in the United States alone (Box 12.2 Risk Factors for Spinal Cord Injury)
- In 2014, over 275,000 people in the United States had an SCI
- About 80% of patients with SCI are men
- Most are white, followed by African American, then Hispanic

Box 12.2 Risks Factors for Spinal Cord Injury

- Male sex (80% of people in the United States who sustain SCI are men)
- Age between 16 and 30 years
- Participation in certain sports, especially
  ○ Football, rugby, wrestling, gymnastics, horseback riding, diving, surfing, roller skating, in-line skating, ice hockey, downhill skiing, and snowboarding
- Underlying bone or joint disorder
  ○ A relatively minor accident can cause an SCI in someone who has arthritis or osteoporosis

12.2.2 Types of Spinal Cord Injury

Concussion

- Caused by a blow to the spinal column that jars or shakes the spinal cord
- Results in temporary loss of neurologic function; this impairment can last for just a few hours or many days

Contusion

- Bruising of the spinal cord caused by fracture, dislocation, or direct trauma
- Necrosis of spinal cord tissue may result from initial trauma or from later compression caused by bleeding or edema
- Resulting dysfunction depends on the severity of the contusion

Compression

- Caused by constriction or pressure on the spinal cord
- Pressure may be brief (e.g., hyperextension injury) or prolonged (e.g., mass effect from bone fragments, neoplasm, hemorrhage, or disk herniation)
- Compression may cause contusion, concussion, laceration, or transection of the spinal cord

Laceration

- Partial tear or cut into the spinal cord
- Deficits are permanent and irreversible

Transection

- Complete tear or cut through the spinal cord, severing it
- Permanent loss of neurologic function below the level of injury

Hemorrhage

- Bleeding within the spinal cord or its surrounding tissues
- Compression of the spinal cord, causing irritation to spinal nerves

Infarction

- Ischemia of the spinal cord due to interrupted blood flow
- Results from compression of the spinal cord or injury to the blood vessels that perfuse it

12.2.3 Mechanisms of Spinal Cord Injury

Hyperflexion

- Occurs when the head and neck are violently forced forward
- Deceleration injury. Occurs when a person in motion is abruptly stopped, as in a head-on motor vehicle collision or diving accident
- C5 and C6 typically experience the greatest amount of stress
- Compression fracture and wedge fractures are the most common fractures associated with hyperflexion (discussed in greater detail later)
- Neurologic deficits are expected only if the posterior ligament is torn and facets are dislocated (fracture or dislocation)

Hyperextension

- Occurs when the head and neck are suddenly forced backward
- Acceleration injury. Occurs when a person is suddenly pushed into motion from a stopped state, as in a rear-end motor vehicle collision or forward fall onto the face, with the chin forced backward (common in the elderly population)

- C4 and C5 experience the most stress
- Soft-tissue strain (i.e., whiplash) is common; contusion or ischemia of the spinal cord from stretching is less likely but possible
- Neurologic deficits may result if the spinal cord is damaged
- Plain radiographs are nondiagnostic because ligaments usually remain intact and neither fractures nor dislocations occur with this type of injury

Compression

- Injury results from axial loading, or force applied straight down on the vertebrae (▶ Fig. 12.1)
- Can result from a fall from a height, with the person landing on her feet or buttocks
- Compression injuries usually result in a burst fracture or wedge fracture in the thoracic or lumbar spine
- Usually no associated neurologic deficits

Rotation

- Occurs when there is extreme twisting of the head or neck
- Posterior ligaments may tear or rupture, resulting in dislocation of one or more facet joints
- No neurologic deficit is expected if only one facet joint is involved; however, neurologic deficit is expected if two or more facets are locked

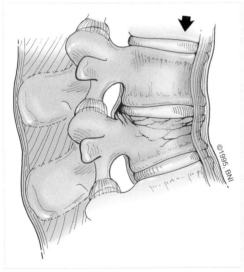

Fig. 12.1 Compression fracture.

Penetration

- Results when a foreign object (e.g., a bullet or knife) pierces the spinal column
- Damages soft tissue and may involve vertebrae or spinal cord transection
- Neurologic deficits are expected if the spinal cord is involved

12.2.4 Classification of Spinal Cord Injury

Complete Spinal Cord Injury

- Complete loss of voluntary motor and sensory functions below the level of injury
- Irreversible, permanent damage to the spinal cord
- Tetraplegia (also called quadriplegia) (▶ Fig. 12.2)
  - ○ Caused by injury to the cervical spinal cord
  - ○ Results in loss of motor and sensory function of both upper extremities, both lower extremities, and bladder and bowel function

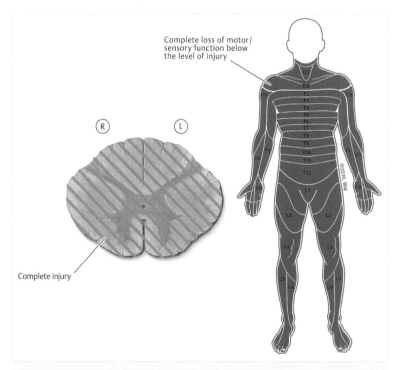

Fig. 12.2 Complete spinal cord injury at cervical spine level.

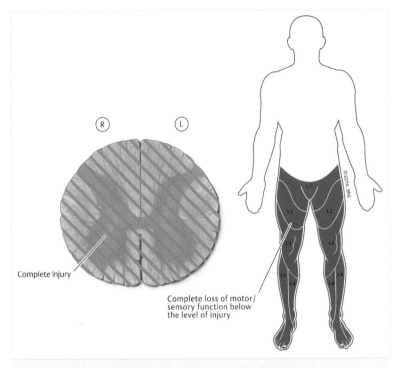

Fig. 12.3 Complete spinal cord injury at lumbar spine level.

- Paraplegia
  - ○ Results from injury to the thoracic or lumbar spinal cord
  - ○ Results in loss of motor and sensory function in both lower extremities and bladder/bowel function (▶ Fig. 12.3)

Incomplete Spinal Cord Injury

- Some sensory or motor function is preserved below the level of injury
- Spared spinal cord tracts allow some neurotransmission
- The SCI syndromes below are descriptive classifications of different types of incomplete SCI (▶ Table 12.2)
  - ○ Central cord syndrome
    - – Most common subset of incomplete SCI (▶ Fig. 12.4)
    - – Can occur at any age, but it is most common in older patients with cervical bony degeneration and cervical stenosis; see also Chapter 11: Spinal Disorders

Table 12.2 Spinal cord injury: clinical syndromes

Syndrome	Area of injury	Clinical symptoms	Prognosis
Central cord	Center of spinal cord	Upper extremity weakness	Variable
Anterior cord	Anterior spinal cord	Paralysis, loss of pain and temperature sensation below level of injury Vibration, light touch, and proprioception are preserved	Variable, but generally poor
Brown-Séquard	Transverse hemisection of spinal cord	Ipsilateral paralysis and loss of proprioception below level of injury Contralateral loss of pain and temperature sensation	Variable, but generally favorable
Cauda equina	Nerve roots below L1	Lower extremity weakness and/or sensory loss Loss of bowel/bladder/sexual function Saddle anesthesia Symptoms may vary depending on specific nerve roots involved	Can be excellent, early surgical intervention is critical
Conus medullaris	Conus medullaris	Lower extremity weakness and/or sensory loss Loss of bladder/sexual function	Variable with treatment

– Often caused by hyperextension injury, with damage to the center of the spinal cord where the nerve fibers that lead to the upper extremities are located
– Loss of motor and sensory function is more severe in the upper extremities than in the lower extremities (e.g., the patient can walk to the door, but cannot open it); bladder dysfunction may or may not result
– Function is usually restored in the lower extremities first, then bladder function is restored

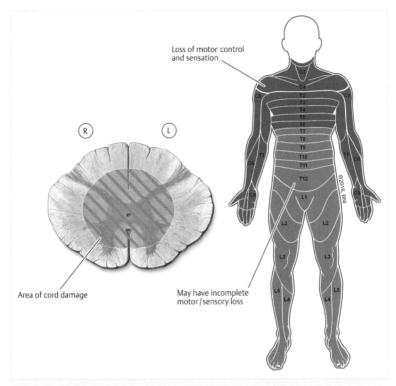

Loss of motor control and sensation

Area of cord damage

May have incomplete motor/sensory loss

©2016, BNI

Fig. 12.4 Central cord syndrome.

- Recovery of hand intrinsic function is variable and is often the last function to return
○ Anterior cord syndrome
   - Caused by direct injury to the anterior portion of the spinal cord or by disruption of the anterior spinal artery, anterior cord syndrome results in ischemia and infarction of the anterior two-thirds of the spinal cord (▶ Fig. 12.5)
   - Direct injury may result from an acute disk herniation or hyperextension injury with fracture dislocation of the vertebrae
   - Paralysis and loss of pain and temperature sensation are evident below the level of injury
   - Light touch, vibration, and proprioception are preserved, because these nerve tracts are located in the dorsal columns of the spinal cord, which are perfused by the posterior spinal arteries
   - Prognosis for recovery varies, but it is generally unfavorable

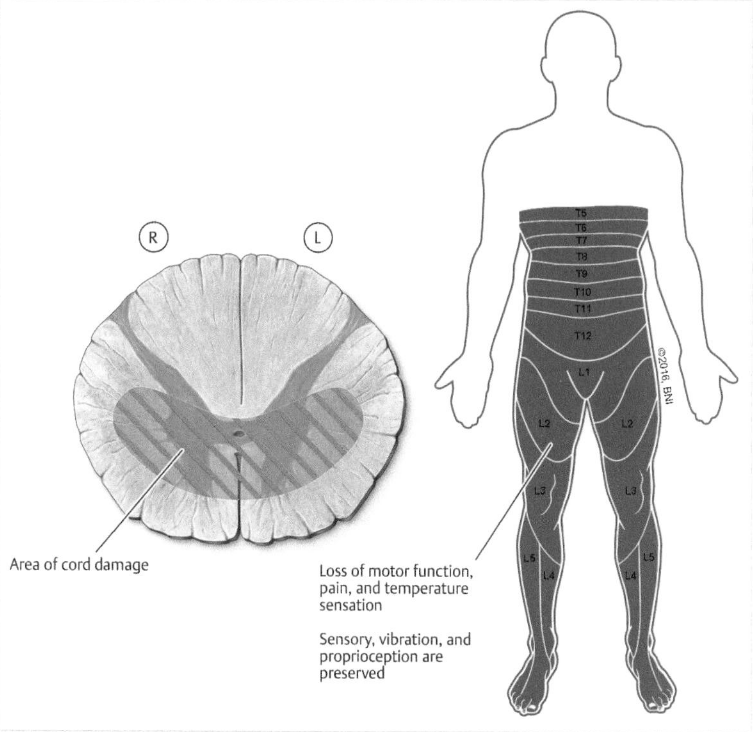
R
L
Area of cord damage
Loss of motor function, pain, and temperature sensation
Sensory, vibration, and proprioception are preserved
T5
T6
T7
T8
T9
T10
T11
T12
L1
L2
L2
L3
L3
L5
L4
L5
L4
©2016, BNI

Fig. 12.5 Anterior cord syndrome.

- Cauda equina syndrome
  - A neurosurgical emergency requiring urgent intervention, cauda equina syndrome is caused by compression of the lumbar nerve roots below L1 (Box 12.3 Clinical Alert: Cauda Equina Syndrome)
  - Most commonly occurs when large disk herniations at L4/L5 exert mass effect on the lumbar nerve roots descending through the spinal canal
  - Deficits vary depending on the specific nerve roots involved, but may include loss of motor and sensory functions of the pelvic organs (i.e., bladder, bowel, and sexual dysfunction) and the lower extremities
  - Recovery is variable, but early diagnosis and prompt surgical treatment are associated with improved outcomes
- Conus medullaris syndrome
  - Caused by pressure on the conus medullaris. Tumor growth, spinal trauma, infection or abscess, degenerative arthritis, or another element may be responsible for pressure exerted on the conus medullaris

– Symptoms include low back pain, numbness of the groin or inner thigh, numbness or weakness of the leg or foot, urinary incontinence, difficulty walking, and impotence

– Treatment depends on the underlying cause and may include corticosteroids to reduce swelling, decompressive surgery, or radiotherapy for spinal tumor

○ Brown-Séquard syndrome

– Accounts for less than 4% of all SCIs and rarely occurs alone

– Results from an inflammatory SCI or from a penetrating injury with transverse hemisection of the spinal cord (▶ Fig. 12.6)

– Paralysis and loss of proprioception occur on the side of injury (the spinal tracts responsible for motor function and proprioception do not cross the spinal cord as they travel to the brain)

– Pain and temperature sensation is lost on the contralateral side (the spinal tracts responsible for conveying pain and temperature cross to the opposite side of the spinal cord as they travel to the brain)

– Functional recovery varies but is often favorable

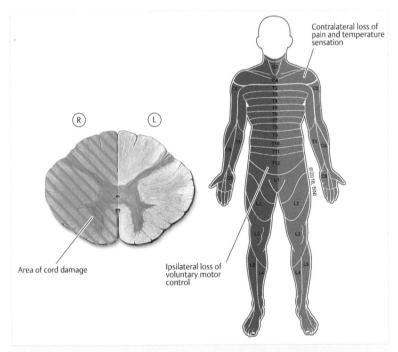

Fig. 12.6 Brown-Séquard syndrome.

○ SCI without radiographic abnormality
  – Includes SCI following a traumatic event without signs of fracture, dislocation, or ligamentous injury on plain radiography, computed tomography (CT), or myelography
  – Magnetic resonance imaging (MRI) will reveal soft tissue or spinal cord abnormalities not evident on standard radiography
  – Common in elderly patients who have stenosis of the spinal canal

---

Box 12.3 Clinical Alert: Cauda Equina Syndrome

• Symptoms of cauda equina syndrome may include any or all of the following:
  ○ Saddle anesthesia (reduced or total loss of sensation to perineum/buttocks)
  ○ Weakness in both legs
  ○ Loss of bowel or bladder control
• Report immediately if your patient develops any of these symptoms because emergency surgical decompression may be required
• Symptoms left untreated for more than 24 hours may become permanent

---

12.3 Conditions Associated with Spinal Cord Injury

12.3.1 Cervical Strain (Whiplash Injury)

• Hyperextension injury
• Common in the United States, with about 1 million cases per year from high-velocity (whiplash type) injuries
• Can occur after high- or low-velocity injuries
  ○ High-velocity injuries cause the neck muscles and ligaments to stretch due to the traumatic mechanisms that cause rapid whipping of the head
  ○ Low-velocity injuries are not as easy to attribute to one precise event and can vary from acute to chronic
• Cervical strain can be caused by unnatural cervical postures (e.g., painting overhead or sitting in the front row at the theater)
• Plain radiographs are nondiagnostic
• Treatment may include a cervical soft collar, rest, analgesics, and nonsteroidal anti-inflammatory drugs (NSAIDs)

12.3.2 Vertebral Fractures

Types of Fractures

Simple

- Usually a single break in one vertebral body, spinous process, facet, or pedicle (▶ Fig. 12.7)
- No resultant alteration in vertebral alignment
- Usually no neurologic compromise.

Compression

- Caused by axial loading (▶ Fig. 12.8)
- May be further classified as a burst (▶ Fig. 12.9), wedge, or teardrop fracture (all discussed in greater detail later).

Dislocation

- Occurs when one vertebra slides over another with disruption of one or both facets (▶ Fig. 12.10)
- May occur with or without fracture
- Subluxation
  - ○ Partial dislocation
  - ○ May cause SCI

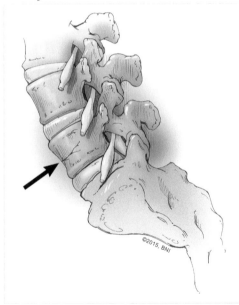

Fig. 12.7 Simple lumbar fracture.

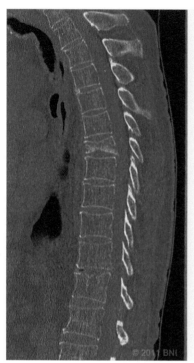

Fig. 12.8 Compression fracture.

Cervical Fractures

- A break in one or more cervical vertebrae
- Cervical fractures account for most spinal injuries and may cause injury to the spinal cord, spinal nerve, or vertebral artery

Brief Review of Anatomy

- Seven cervical vertebrae compose the cervical spine (C1 through C7)
- Occipital condyles of the skull rest upon lateral masses of C1, forming the atlanto-occipital joint; this joint allows most of the flexion and extension of the neck (about 25 degrees)
- Together, C1 (the *atlas*) and C2 (the *axis*) form the upper cervical spine
- The atlantoaxial region (i.e., the joint between C1 and C2) is uniquely shaped, extremely mobile, and stabilized by surrounding ligamentous structures
- The ring of C1 has no vertebral body; the odontoid process of C2 (also called the dens) projects up from the vertebral body to form the joint with C1 that provides most lateral head and neck rotation

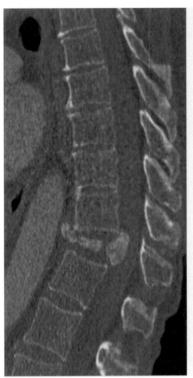

Fig. 12.9 Burst fracture.

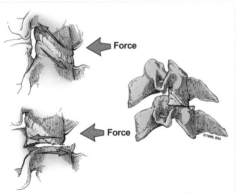

Fig. 12.10 Fracture and dislocation of the cervical spine.

Force

Force

- The vertebral artery passes through C1 and is susceptible to injury in cases of neck trauma
- C3 through C7 form the lower cervical spine
- The primary motion of the lower cervical spine is flexion-extension, but the anatomy of the cervical spine allows motion in all planes

Pathophysiology

- The cervical spine is composed of an anterior and a posterior column (▶ Fig. 12.11)
- The anterior column is responsible for load bearing and includes the posterior longitudinal ligament and all structures anterior to it
- The posterior column of the cervical spine includes the pedicles, laminae, facet joints, spinous processes, and posterior ligament complexes (ligamenta flava, interspinous ligaments, and supraspinous ligaments)
- Tension is resisted by the posterior column, which fails under extreme flexion and may be associated with injury to the anterior column

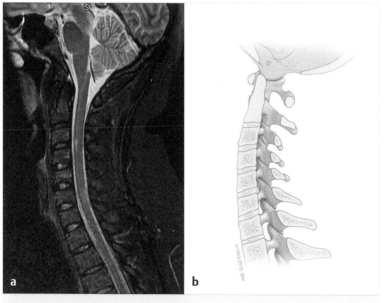

Fig. 12.11 Cervical spine.

Etiology of Cervical Fractures

- Usually caused by trauma to head and neck
- Common causes include diving into a shallow pool, high-velocity trauma from motor vehicle accidents or falls, or a sudden severe twist of neck (Box 12.4 Risk Factors for Cervical Fractures)

Clinical Manifestations of Cervical Fractures

- Limited ability to move the neck or head
- Neck pain, stiffness, or spasm
- Neck bruising and swelling
- Loss of sensation in the arms or hands
- Burning or aching pain that radiates to the shoulders or arms
- Headache or pain in the back of the head
- Weakness in extremities

Types of Cervical Fractures

- Atlanto-occipital dislocation (cervical–cranial disruption)
  - Accounts for about 1% of cervical spine injuries; occurs when a traumatic event causes severe flexion and distraction of the head and neck, resulting in instability (▶ Fig. 12.12)

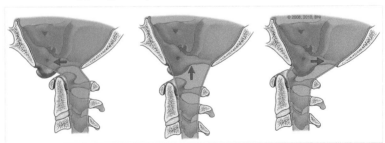

Fig. 12.12 Atlanto-occipital dislocation.

- ○ Dissociation may be complete (dislocation) or incomplete (subluxation)
- ○ Often fatal because injury to the lower brainstem frequently causes respiratory arrest
- ○ Nontraumatic atlanto-occipital subluxation may occur; this is usually related to Down's syndrome and rheumatoid arthritis; see also Chapter 11: Spinal Disorders
- ○ Treatment is a halo orthosis (e.g., halo ring and vest brace) (▶Fig. 12.19) or occipitocervical fusion
- Atlantoaxial dislocation (atlantoaxial instability)
  - ○ Caused by bony or ligamentous abnormality, results in excessive movement at the junction between C1 and C2
  - ○ Treatment may include a halo orthosis or cervical fixation
- C1 (atlas) fracture
  - ○ Jefferson's fracture of C1 (C1 burst fracture).
    - – These fractures account for 10% of cervical spine injuries and result from axial loading on the head through the occiput, leading to a burst-type fracture of C1 (▶ Fig. 12.13)
    - – Most frequently caused by diving into shallow water, being thrown against the roof of a moving vehicle, and falling directly onto one's head
    - – May include unilateral or bilateral fractures of the anterior or posterior arches of C1
    - – Elements of the posterior column can be displaced into the spinal cord
    - – Neurologic injury rarely occurs because the spinal cord is very wide at C1; however, vertebral artery injury is possible
    - – Treated with an external orthosis to immobilize the head and neck
    - – Unstable fracture that may require surgical stabilization
- C2 (axis) fractures
  - ○ Odontoid fractures
    - – Result from extreme flexion, rotation, or extension of the head and neck
    - – The odontoid process is increasingly susceptible to fracture with age (▶ Fig. 12.14)
    - – Rarely associated with SCI
    - – Occipital pain and neck muscle spasms are common symptoms (▶ Table 12.3)

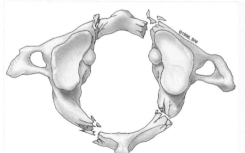

Fig. 12.13 Jefferson's fracture.

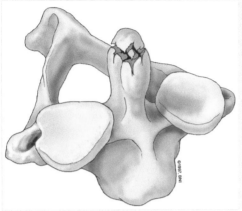

Fig. 12.14 Type I odontoid fracture.

Table 12.3 Types of odontoid fractures

Fracture type	Description	Fracture stability	Neurologic deficits	Treatment
Type I	Avulsion fracture of the tip of the dens May involve atlanto-occipital dislocation	Stable	Usually none	Immobilization with hard collar or halo orthosis
Type II	Transverse or oblique fracture through the dens Often displaced anteriorly or posteriorly	Unstable	May result in weakness or paralysis	Odontoid screw fixation or C1–C2 fusion
Type III	Fracture through the base of the dens into the body of C2	Stable	Usually none	Halo orthosis Possible traction

○ Hangman's fracture (▶ Fig. 12.15)
  – This is so named as this injury can occur as the result of hanging
  – In older adults, this type of injury can occur after falls, but it is also seen after motor vehicle accidents
  – Caused by hyperextension of the neck and axial load onto the C2 vertebra (▶ Table 12.4)
  – Involves fracture through the pedicles of C2, with or without subluxation on C3
  – The spinal cord is crushed only in cases of severe subluxation of C3 from C2

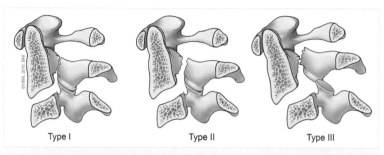

Fig. 12.15 Types of hangman's fractures.

Table 12.4 Types of hangman's fractures

Fracture type	Displacement	Fracture stability	Treatment
Type I	<3 mm subluxation	Stable	Immobilization Hard collar Halo orthosis Pedicle screw fixation
Type II	>4 mm subluxation >11 degrees of angulation	Unstable	Traction to reduce fracture Halo orthosis Posterior C2–C3 fusion if fracture cannot be reduced
Type III	Complete dislocation	Unstable	C2–C3 fusion

- Lower cervical spine fractures (subaxial fractures)
  - Involve fractures from C3 to C7
  - High-energy trauma (e.g., motor vehicle accidents, sporting activities, or violence) is the likely cause of lower cervical spine fractures in younger patients (i.e., 15–24 years)
  - Low-energy trauma (e.g., ground-level falls) is most common in patients over age 55 years
  - Age-associated cervical spondylosis narrows the spinal canal and may predispose an individual to cervical cord injury
  - Teardrop fractures
    - Named for the teardrop-shaped bone chips from the anterior edge of the vertebral body
    - Result from compression and flexion of the neck (e.g., from diving accidents or falling directly onto the head)
    - Unstable due to disruption of ligaments and disk

335

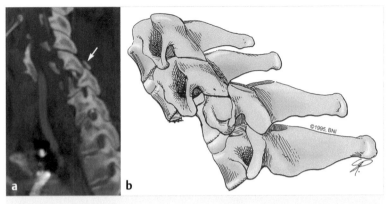

Fig. 12.16 Locked facets.

- Often results in quadriplegia from posterior displacement of bone fragments into the spinal canal
- Posterior fusion is the most common treatment
○ Locked facets (also called *perched* or *jumped facets*)
- Caused by neck flexion and distraction
- Occur when the facet joint ruptures and the facet of the superior vertebra is displaced anteriorly over the lower vertebra (▶ Fig. 12.16)
- May be unilateral or bilateral and can result in herniation of adjacent-level disk
- Often results in SCI
- Unstable fractures are usually treated with closed reduction, followed by surgical stabilization

Thoracolumbar Fractures

Brief Review of Anatomy

The thoracolumbar spine is divided into three load-bearing columns (anterior, middle, and posterior) that contribute to spinal stability. Injury to more than one column often results in instability and, ultimately, neurologic impairment.

- The anterior column includes the following:
  ○ Anterior longitudinal ligament
  ○ Anterior half of vertebral body
- The middle column includes the following:
  ○ Posterior longitudinal ligament
  ○ Posterior half of vertebral body

- The posterior column includes the following:
  - Facet joints
  - Ligamenta flava
  - Laminae
  - Spinous processes
  - Interspinous ligament

Types of Thoracolumbar Fractures

- Simple fracture
  - Single-column injuries visible on plain radiographs
  - Involves breakage of a single vertebra
  - Breaks usually occur in the spinous process, transverse process, pedicles, or facets
  - Usually causes no neurologic impairment
  - CT imaging should identify bony injury
- Wedge fracture (also called an *anterior wedge compression fracture*)
  - The most common type of thoracolumbar fracture, results from forward flexion and compression of the anterior vertebral column
  - Can cause up to 50% loss of height of anterior vertebral body
  - Usually a stable fracture
  - Rarely associated with neurologic impairment
  - Treated with thoracolumbosacral orthosis (TLSO) or lumbosacral orthosis (LSO)
- Burst fracture
  - Caused by axial loading involving loss of both anterior and posterior vertebral body height
  - Often caused by falling onto one's buttocks or feet
  - Fracture is unstable if the posterior column is involved
  - May involve nerve root, spinal cord, or vascular injury from free-floating fracture (i.e., fragments dislodged in spinal canal)
  - TLSO or LSO brace or surgical fixation with or without decompression
- Chance fracture (seat belt fracture)
  - Caused by extreme flexion and distraction
  - Also called a *seat belt fracture* because it often occurs during a head-on motor vehicle collision when the upper body is thrown forward, while the pelvis is held in place by a seat belt (▶ Fig. 12.17)
  - Often unstable, requiring surgical stabilization.

Other Spinal Fracture Etiologies

As discussed in Chapter 11: Spinal Disorders, rheumatoid arthritis can contribute to cervical spine disease. Spinal fractures may also be pathologic or osteoporotic in nature.

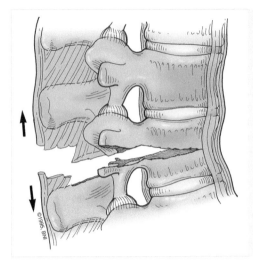

Fig. 12.17 Chance fracture.

12.3.3 Primary and Secondary Spinal Cord Injury

Primary Injury

- Physical damage to spinal cord at the time of trauma
- Extent of initial injury is related to amount of force exerted on the spine
- Initial injury may range from mild spinal cord concussion resulting in transient loss of function to severe SCI resulting in complete and permanent loss of function
- The trauma disrupts neural elements of the spinal cord (including nerve cells in the ascending and descending spinal tracts) at the level of injury
- Disruption of spinal cord vasculature may result in spinal cord hemorrhage and ischemia (▶ Fig. 12.18).

Secondary Injury

- Cascade of events that begins almost immediately after the initial trauma to the spinal cord
- Can worsen the extent of SCI by damaging the adjoining neural tissue
- Ischemia within the spinal cord at the time of primary injury can lead to additional vascular changes that disrupt spinal cord perfusion
- Cell membrane permeability increases due to dysfunction of the sodium–potassium pumps of cells, ultimately causing cellular edema and cell death
- Inflammatory response increases vascular permeability, edema, and macrophage activity, leading to additional tissue damage
- Current treatment strategies for SCI are intended to limit the severity of secondary injury

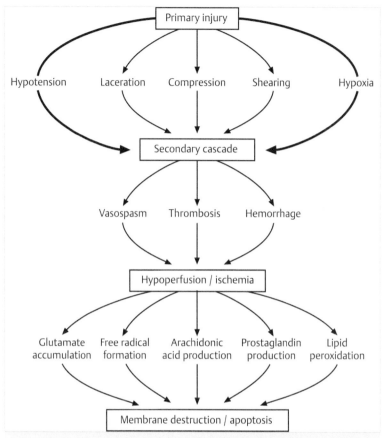

Fig. 12.18 Primary and secondary injury cascades after acute traumatic spinal cord injury.

Examples of Secondary Injury

- Spinal shock
  - Results from the concussive effect of primary injury; associated with lowered body temperature and a state of areflexia (i.e., loss of all motor, sensory, and reflex activity at the level of injury and below)
  - Duration may be several hours to several weeks after injury
  - Extent of SCI cannot be determined until spinal shock has resolved
  - Muscle spasticity and hyperreflexia become evident as spinal shock subsides
  - Return of perianal reflexes signifies resolution of spinal shock

- Neurogenic shock
  - Autonomic regulation is disrupted by the loss of sympathetic input that results from SCI
  - More common when the level of injury is at T6 or above
  - Causes loss of sensory function, muscle strength, and reflexes below the level of injury
  - The sympathetic nervous system, which originates in the thoracolumbar region of the spinal cord, is responsible for elevations in heart rate and blood pressure as well as vasoconstriction of the peripheral vascular system during stressful episodes; see also Chapter 1: Anatomy
  - Normal impulses from the brainstem are disrupted, interrupting normal sympathetic outflow and leaving vagal tone unopposed
  - Can result in bradycardia, hypotension, and decreased cardiac output
- Autonomic hyperreflexia
  - Also known as *dysreflexia*, this condition refers to the body's extreme response to pain or irritating stimuli below the level of injury, resulting in a dramatic spike in blood pressure and related symptoms (▶ Table 12.5)
  - Occurs after resolution of spinal shock in patients with SCI at or above T6
  - Urinary retention, urinary tract infection, constipation, and tight clothing are the most common causes of autonomic hyperreflexia
  - A noxious stimulus triggers a sympathetic response, resulting in vasoconstriction below the level of the SCI
  - Blood volume shifts from vasculature below the SCI to vasculature above the SCI, resulting in elevated blood pressure that causes flushing, pounding headache, and sweating
  - Impulses are blocked at the level of the SCI, allowing vasoconstriction to continue unchecked below the level of injury
  - Response continues until noxious stimulus is removed
  - Considered a medical emergency; if left untreated, could lead to retinal hemorrhage, hemorrhagic stroke, subarachnoid hemorrhage, seizures, or myocardial infarction

12.4 Spinal Cord Tumors

Spinal tumors are categorized according to their location within the spinal column. They are further classified by histology or cell type and were discussed in detail in Chapter 7: Tumors. This section describes how tumor growth within the spinal column can injure the spinal cord and spinal nerves; see also **Fig. 7.11**: Tumors of the spinal cord in Chapter 7 for a visual representation of variations in tumor growth within the spinal column.

Table 12.5 Autonomic dysreflexia

Clinical manifestations	Common causes	Nursing actions	Rationale
Severe hypertension (often >200 mm Hg) Bradycardia (patient may be unaware) Profuse sweating of face, neck, shoulders Cardiac arrhythmias Shortness of breath Visual disturbances Goosebumps Feelings of impending doom Severe headache Flushing of the skin above the level of SCI Dilated pupils Confusion Dizziness Nasal Congestion	Distended bladder Urinary tract infection Constipation Tight clothing Pressure ulcers	Check status of indwelling catheter, check for constrictions Place catheter, if one has not already been placed Avoid palpating bladder; bladder fullness can instead be checked with bedside bladder scan Send urine for culture Consider constipation or impaction Look for and remove tight or restrictive clothing or bed linens Monitor blood pressure, vital signs Place patient in upright position, with legs in dependent position Administer antihypertensives, if warranted Notify medical team immediately	All actions should be directed at identifying and removing possible causative agent Maintain safe cardiovascular parameters Nursing actions should primarily be focused on prevention

Abbreviation: SCI, spinal cord injury.

12.4.1 Intradural Intramedullary Spinal Tumors

- Located beneath the dura, growing directly into spinal cord tissue
- Common examples include ependymomas in adults and astrocytomas in children
  - Ependymomas often occur in the conus medullaris and the cauda equina
  - Astrocytomas commonly occur in the cervical and thoracic spine

12.4.2 Intradural Extramedullary Spinal Tumors

- Grow beneath the dura, between the dura and spinal cord
- Compress, but do not invade, neural tissue
- Common examples include schwannomas and meningiomas
  - Schwannomas are slightly more common in the thoracic spine
  - Meningiomas are more common in thoracic spine and in women over age 40

12.4.3 Extradural Spinal Tumors

- The most common form of spinal tumors
- Occur outside the dura
- Mostly involve vertebral bodies and are metastatic
- Weaken and destroy bone, resulting in spinal instability
- Mass effect from these tumors can compress and damage the spinal cord
- Lung cancer is the most common spinal metastatic lesion, followed by breast cancer
- Other metastatic spinal cancers include myeloma, prostate cancer, and lymphoma

12.5 Diagnosis of Spinal Cord Injury

Proper diagnosis of SCI requires a full patient history as well as a detailed account of the precipitating event (► Table 12.6). An in-depth assessment and imaging studies will facilitate or confirm suspected diagnosis.

Table 12.6 Diagnostic tests for spinal cord injury

Test	Visible structures/possible diagnoses	Nursing implications of test
Radiograph	Integrity and alignment of vertebrae Spacing of bones and joints Any abnormal movement of bony structures (instability or subluxation)	None
CT	Bony alignment, fracture locations	Assess for possible allergy to contrast agent
MRI	Soft tissues, spinal cord, nerve roots, disk spaces, CSF flow, and ligaments	Patient may need to be NPO if sedation needed (in patients with known claustrophobia) Metal screening Assess for possible allergy to contrast agent
Myelogram	Nerve compression that causes pain (radiculopathy) or weakness (myelopathy)	Usually an outpatient procedure Assess for possible allergy to contrast agent May develop postpuncture headache; if it persists, the patient may require a blood patch

Abbreviations: CSF, cerebrospinal fluid; CT, computed tomography; MRI, magnetic resonance imaging; NPO, nil per os (nothing by mouth).

12.5.1 Assessment of Spinal Cord Injury

- SCI assessment (Box 12.5 Baseline Assessment); see also Chapter 2: Assessment
- Motor function examination
  - Muscle strength grading
- Sensory evaluation
  - Dermatomes
- Reflexes
- Grading scales for SCI include the following:
  - American Spinal Injury Association (ASIA) Motor Grading Scale (▶ Table 12.7)
  - ASIA Impairment Scale (Box 12.6 ASIA Impairment Scale)

Box 12.5 Baseline Assessment

- A careful baseline neurologic examination is crucial in patients with suspected spinal injury. This initial assessment will be the basis for management of the patient and for later determination of changes in neurologic status. The baseline assessment should take place before the patient receives pain medication, sedatives, or paralytics, as medication may interfere with the accuracy of the examination

Table 12.7 American Spinal Injury Association Motor Grading Scale

Right grade	Left grade	Nerve segment	Muscle	Action to test
0–5	0–5	C5	Deltoid	Shoulder abduction
			Biceps	Elbow flexion
0–5	0–5	C6	Wrist extensors	Extend wrist
0–5	0–5	C7	Triceps	Elbow extension
0–5	0–5	C8	Flexor digitorum	Squeeze hand
0–5	0–5	T1	Hand intrinsics	Abduct fingers
0–5	0–5	L2	Iliopsoas	Flex hip
0–5	0–5	L3	Quadriceps	Straighten knee
0–5	0–5	L4	Tibialis anterior	Dorsiflex foot
0–5	0–5	L5	Extensor hallucis longus	Dorsiflex great toe
0–5	0–5	S1	Gastrocnemius	Plantarflex foot

Total possible points 50 (right grade) plus 50 (left grade) = 100.

Box 12.6 ASIA Impairment Scale

- **A = Complete:** No motor or sensory function is preserved in the sacral segments S4–S5
- **B = Incomplete:** Sensory but not motor function is preserved below the neurologic level and includes the sacral segments S4–S5
- **C = Incomplete:** Motor function is preserved below the neurologic level, and more than half of key muscles below the neurologic level have a muscle grade less than 3
- **D = Incomplete:** Motor function is preserved below the neurologic level, and at least half of key muscles below the neurologic level have a muscle grade of 3 or more
- **E = Normal:** Motor and sensory functions are normal

12.5.2 Imaging Studies

- Plain radiographs
  - Assess the integrity and alignment of vertebrae and spacing of bones and joints
  - Radiographs taken through the patient's open mouth provide views of the odontoid process of the cervical spine
  - Swimmer's view radiographs help evaluate the cervicothoracic junction
  - Flexion-extension films identify abnormal movement (instability or subluxation) of bony structures within the range of motion of the neck
- CT
  - Evaluates bony alignment, fractures, or dislocation
- MRI
  - Evaluates soft tissue such as the spinal cord, spinal nerves, and disk spaces, as well as ligament integrity and the flow of cerebrospinal fluid
  - MRI may indicate cause of neurologic injury, such as spinal cord contusion or stretching, which are not visible on plain radiographs or CT scans

12.6 Treatment of Spinal Cord Injury

12.6.1 Medical Intervention

Spinal Precautions

Spinal precautions are initiated at the trauma scene and are continued until SCI is ruled out, or until appropriate evaluation and stabilization have been established.

- The entire spine of the injured patient is immobilized to avoid additional spinal injury when the patient is moved, because about 20% of patients have SCI at multiple levels. This process includes use of a rigid cervical collar as well as a backboard with head and body straps secured and may include placement of sandbags beside the patient's head
- Log roll, keeping spine in neutral position
- Vigilant monitoring of airway and respiratory function is imperative because immobilization on a backboard decreases forced vital capacity (i.e., lung capacity) by 20%

Prevention of Secondary Injury

- Maintain adequate oxygenation
- Systolic blood pressure greater than 90 mm Hg and mean arterial pressure greater than 85 mm Hg ensure adequate spinal cord perfusion (▶ Table 12.8)
- Corticosteroid methylprednisolone is no longer recommended for routine use to control inflammation, as patient risks outweigh benefits

Spinal Stabilization

- Based on bony and soft-tissue injury type and severity, spinal stability, and neurologic examination, spinal stabilization may be the selected method of conservative treatment
- Some fractures may be treated by completely immobilizing the neck with orthoses until bone heals (usually between 8 and 12 weeks)
- Braces and collars are designed to maintain the alignment and stability of the specific spinal region (▶ Table 12.9)
- Some common spinal stabilization devices include the following:
  ○ Halo brace
    – The most rigid cervical brace includes a metal ring attached directly to the skull with pins and a hard plastic vest attached to the ring with rods and screws (▶ Fig. 12.19)
    – May be used initially to reduce a dislocation by applying traction
    – Usually worn for 8 to 12 weeks, or until healing is evident on radiographs
  ○ Philadelphia collar or Miami J Collar
    – Hard plastic cervical collar that prevents neck flexion, extension, or head rotation
  ○ Soft collar
    – Flexible cervical collar worn around the neck
    – Often used after a more rigid collar has been worn
    – Can help with cervical strain and muscle spasm, as needed (▶ Table 12.10)

Table 12.8 Pharmacology for management of spinal cord injury

Drug	Category	Indication	Nursing implications
Dopamine Dobutamine Midodrine (ProAmatine)	Vasopressor Inotropes	Hypotension due to neurogenic shock Orthostatic hypotension Increases blood pressure and cardiac output	Monitor patient's blood pressure Patient will need an arterial line, or possibly a central line
Labetalol (Trandate) Hydralazine Amlodipine (Norvasc) Nitroglycerin (nitropaste)	Vasodilator	Hypertension	Suspect autonomic hyperreflexia, identify and remove cause Monitor patient for hypotension
Enoxaparin (Lovenox) Heparin	Anticoagulant	Prevention or treatment of DVT or pulmonary embolus	Be aware of possible thrombocytopenia; monitor platelet count Use electric razors and gentle oral care to prevent bleeding
Lansoprazole (Prevacid) Omeprazole (Prilosec) Pantoprazole (Protonix) Esomeprazole (Nexium)	Proton pump inhibitor	Inhibit secretion of gastric acid	
Famotidine (Pepcid)	H2-receptor antagonist	Prevent gastric stress ulceration	Be aware of possible thrombocytopenia; monitor platelet count
Docusate sodium (Colace)	Stool softener	Prevent constipation	Initiate a bowel program as early as possible
Senna (Senokot) Bisacodyl rectal (Dulcolax suppository)	Stimulant laxative	Constipation Promote regular emptying of the colon	Monitor patient for diarrhea Ensure adequate fluid intake
Polyethylene glycol (Miralax)	Osmotic laxative	Constipation Promote regular emptying of the colon	Monitor patient for diarrhea Ensure adequate fluid intake

Table 12.8 (*continued*)

Drug	Category	Indication	Nursing implications
Diazepam (Valium) Alprazolam (Xanax) Lorazepam (Ativan)	Antianxiety	Depression of the central nervous system	Monitor sedation, oxygenation, and mood Consider alternative relaxation methods
Fluoxetine (Prozac) Sertraline (Zoloft) Paroxetine (Paxil)	Antidepressant	Depressed mood	Be vigilant for suicidal ideation Monitor patient's dietary intake and weight
Morphine sulfate Hydromorphone (Dilaudid) Oxycodone (Percocet) Hydrocodone (Vicodin, Lortab)	Opioid analgesic	Moderate to severe pain Reduces anxiety; promotes euphoria and relaxation	Assess pain score using numeric scale
Gabapentin (Neurontin) Pregabalin (Lyrica)	Neuropathic pain	Modulates excitatory neurotransmitter release; antinociceptive and antiseizure effects	
Baclofen (Lioresal) Baclofen pump (a surgically implanted reservoir that applies the drug directly to the area of spinal cord dysfunction)	Muscle relaxant	Spasticity	Monitor for signs of baclofen overdose, such as drowsiness, vomiting, weakness, dizziness, slow/shallow breaths, seizures, loss of consciousness, coma Be vigilant for signs of baclofen withdrawal (Box 12.7 Signs of Baclofen Withdrawal)

Abbreviations: DVT, deep vein thrombosis; SCI, spinal cord injury.

Table 12.9 Spinal stabilization devices

Type of device	Category	Indication	Type of spine disorder
Cervical collar (Miami J, Philadelphia)	Rigid	Prevents neck flexion, extension, or rotation	Stable fractures Cervical strain Following anterior or posterior cervical fusion procedures
Soft collar	Flexible	Neck pain/spasm	Cervical strain Following anterior fusion procedure
Halo brace	Rigid; can be used with traction	Alleviates nerve compression Realigns spine Reduces dislocation/ subluxation	Atlantoaxial dislocation Atlantoaxial rotatory dislocation Locked facets
CTO brace (Minerva, SOMI)	Rigid	Stabilizes the junction of the cervical and thoracic spine	Fractures Following spinal fixation procedure
Custom fabricated: LSO or TLSO	Rigid	Stable fracture Pain/spasm	Thoracic or lumbar compression fractures Scoliosis Following spinal fusion procedure
Lumbar corset	Flexible	Low back pain	Degenerative disk disorders Trauma Postural deformities For comfort after lumbar diskectomy or laminectomy

Abbreviations: CTO, cervical thoracic orthosis; LSO, lumbosacral orthosis; SOMI, sternal occipital mandibular immobilizer; TLSO, thoracolumbosacral orthosis.

12.6.2 Surgical Intervention

Surgery for traumatic spine injury may involve reducing or realigning spinal dislocations, decompressing compromised neural tissue, or fusing bones to stabilize fractures or dislocations. These interventions are discussed in greater detail in Chapter 15: Neurosurgical Interventions (▶ Table 12.11).

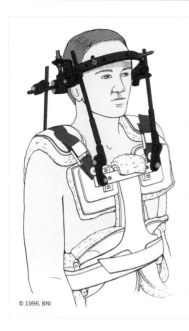

Fig. 12.19 Halo brace.

© 1996, BNI

Table 12.10 Nursing care for patients in spinal orthoses

Orthosis	Intervention	Rationale
Cervical traction	Routine pin care at every shift	Potential for infection
	Observe mobility and bed position restrictions	Potential for neurologic deterioration if the spine is unstable
	Ensure weights hang unrestricted	
	Provide prism glasses as needed	Patient's field of vision may be limited due to flat position
Halo brace	Routine pin care at every shift	Potential for infection
	Ensure that the emergency wrench is attached to the front of the halo vest	Wrench must be available for emergency removal of halo vest
	Inspect the skin for evidence of pressure ulceration	Potential for skin breakdown
	Provide comprehensive halo education to patient and family	
	Never pull on halo device to reposition patient	Potential for loosening or maladjustment of pins

Table 12.10 (continued)

Orthosis	Intervention	Rationale
Braces/collars	Ensure proper size and fit	Increases comfort and minimizes friction
	Provide good skin care, avoid lotions or powder under brace Inspect the skin for evidence of pressure ulcerations under collar	Potential for skin breakdown
	May use thick padding if the collar will be worn for several weeks Cotton t-shirt may be worn under a TLSO	Comfort
	Educate patient and family regarding brace placement and removal	Most patients require assistance with brace

Abbreviation: TLSO, thoraciclumbosacral orthosis.

12.7 Nursing Management for Patients with Traumatic Spine Injuries

Recommendations for caring for patients with traumatic spine injuries are interspersed throughout this chapter, but generalized implications appropriate for most patients with SCI are presented in ▶ Table 12.12 **and Appendix A11 Nursing Management of Patients with Spinal Cord Injury**. Nurses who are tasked with caring for this patient population must balance compassion with total familiarity of the mechanisms of SCI and sequelae. They must possess an in-depth understanding of the functional level of SCI, as well as thorough physical and neurologic examination skills.

Medical and nursing interventions should always adhere to the most current evidence-based practice guidelines. Medications should be checked against an updated drug reference source because the Food and Drug Administration frequently updates their findings on drug interactions. This chapter is intended to be a basic reference for the bedside care of neurologic patients with traumatic spine injury. To learn more about specific subjects of interest, the reader is encouraged to access the references at the end of this chapter.

12.7.1 Neurologic Assessment

- Evaluate level of consciousness
- Test motor and sensory function
- Assess cranial nerve function
- Monitor the patient for signs of autonomic dysreflexia (▶ Table 12.5)

Table 12.11 Types of surgery for cervical fractures

Procedure	Description	Indication	Implications
Traction/reduction	Halo ring or tongs are pinned to the head Weight is applied with the patient in the supine position	Odontoid type III fracture Locked facets	May not reduce fracture Should not be used for atlanto-occipital, hangman's type II, or hangman's type III fractures
Occipitocervical fusion	Posterior placement of C1 lateral mass screws and C2 pedicle screws Rods and screws connect the occiput to C1 and C2	Atlanto-occipital dislocation	30% of flexion and extension is lost 50% of head rotation is lost
C1–C2 fusion	Posterior placement of screws, rods, or wires to attach C1 to C2	Atlantoaxial instability from Jefferson's, hangman's, or odontoid fractures	50% of head rotation is lost Must wear hard collar or halo brace for about 12 wk
Odontoid screw fixation	Anterior placement of a long screw through the C2 body to the fractured dens	Odontoid type II fracture (if reduced)	No loss of head rotation
Pedicle screw fixation	Posterior placement of screws to pull the fractured isthmuses back together	Hangman's type I	No loss of head rotation

12.7.2 Respiratory Assessment

- Perform airway assessment and monitor the patient's ability to protect the airway carefully, especially in patients with high cervical injuries (C5 and above)
- Document respiratory rate and rhythm
- Measure arterial blood gases, using an O_2 saturation monitor if appropriate
- Maintain adequate oxygenation and ventilation
- Be vigilant for signs of pulmonary embolism, which can result after prolonged immobility. Pulmonary embolism may be indicated by low O_2 saturation, chest pain, shortness of breath, hypotension, fever, or elevated heart rate. Prevention of lower extremity deep vein thrombosis (DVT), discussed later, is also critical

351

Table 12.12 Spinal cord injury: what to watch for

Problem	Type of injury	Clinical manifestations	Nursing action	Rationale
Neurologic compromise	Any level	Decrease in motor or sensory function Ascending level of motor or sensory loss Loss of bowel or bladder function	Report any new finding suggestive of decreasing function	Decrease in function may result from swelling, hematoma, or infarction
	Cervical (usually C5 or above)	Decrease in respiratory effort	Ventilator support or supplemental oxygen may be indicated	Muscles needed for respiration are innervated at C4
Autonomic dysreflexia	T6 or above	Hypertension and flushing (most common symptoms)	Treat as a medical emergency Remove source of stimulus (constipation, bladder fullness, restrictive clothing)	May occur after spinal shock Often a response to noxious stimulus
Respiratory distress	Any	Increased respiratory rate Hypoxia Gasping for breath, shallow breathing Hyper- or hypotension Tachycardia	Oxygen as directed Report immediately	Immobility, intubation, or mechanical ventilation place patients at high risk for atelectasis, pneumonia, or PE
DVT/PE	Any	Pain, swelling, or redness in the calves Fever Shortness of breath/hypoxia or chest pain	Report immediately Inspect calves each shift and as needed Administer enoxaparin or heparin as directed, unless contraindicated	Immobility places patients at high risk for clots

Abbreviations: DVT, deep vein thrombosis; PE, pulmonary embolism.

- Respiratory failure
  - Atelectasis and pneumonia are common complications after SCI, regardless of the level of injury, and can contribute to deterioration in respiratory function
  - Mechanical ventilation increases the risk for morbidity (i.e., ventilator-acquired pneumonia) and mortality
  - Pulmonary hygiene (e.g., coughing, deep breathing, use of incentive spirometry) is critical
  - Mobilize and reposition the patient as often as possible
  - Elevate head of bed more than 30 degrees
  - Perform oral care with chlorhexidine and brush the patient's teeth at least twice a day

12.7.3 Cardiovascular Assessment

- Perform hemodynamic monitoring, if appropriate
- Monitor electrocardiogram for cardiac arrhythmias
- Be aware of increased risk of hypovolemic shock
  - Results from blood loss at the time of initial trauma, from dehydration, or from inadequate volume replacement
  - Signs include increased heart rate and decreased blood pressure
  - Treatment may include intravenous hydration, volume replacement, and bed rest
- Neurogenic shock
  - More common in patients with SCI at or above T6
  - Treatment may include atropine for bradycardia; vasopressors to increase heart rate, constrict blood vessels, and increase cardiac output
- Orthostatic hypotension
  - Occurs when sympathetic vascular tone and arteriole vasomotor control are lost; results in blood pooling in the abdomen and legs due to decreased peripheral vascular tone
  - Worsened by prolonged immobility and decreased intravascular volume
  - Symptoms include drop in blood pressure when patient is upright, dizziness or light-headedness, and fainting
  - Treatment may include midodrine, blood volume expanders, support hose (placed before the patient gets out of bed), an abdominal binder, elevation of feet, slow changes in position, a tilt table, or a reclining wheelchair

12.7.4 Gastrointestinal Assessment

- Spinal shock can cause gastroparesis, reduced peristalsis, and ileus
- Patients with SCI are at greater risk for gastric stress ulceration
- Administer laxatives and peptic ulcer prophylactic medications as ordered

- Establish a bowel program
  - Start bowel care during acute care and instruct the patient to continue it after discharge
  - Encourage appropriate fluids, diet, and activity
  - Establish a consistent schedule for defecation (i.e., a bowel care regimen)
  - Include use of stool softeners, fiber, chemical stimulants such as laxatives or suppositories, and mechanical stimulants such as digital stimulation of rectum

12.7.5 Genitourinary Assessment

- SCI can result in loss of normal bladder reflexes and loss of control of urination.
  - Neurogenic (atonic) bladder causes urinary retention and bladder distension
  - Urinary incontinence occurs due to overflow of urine from distended bladder (i.e., overflow incontinence)
- Increased risk of urinary tract infection, hydronephrosis, decreased renal function, or development of renal calculi (i.e., kidney stones)
- Bladder training
  - Timed voiding every 4 to 6 hours
  - Check postvoid residual by straight catheterization or bladder scan (should be < 250 mL). If postvoid residual exceeds 250 mL, then more frequent straight catheterization should be considered
  - Instruct patient about clean intermittent self-catheterization, if possible

12.7.6 Fluid and Electrolyte Assessment

- Monitor glucose levels, especially if the patient is on steroids
- Strict intake and output; see also Chapter 5: Electrolyte Disturbances

12.7.7 Integumentary Assessment

- Perform skin assessment, especially over bony prominences and under braces, at least twice daily
- Redness and blanching of skin are early signs of a pressure ulcer
- The areas most susceptible to pressure ulcer are the trochanters, ischial tuberosities, sacrum, coccyx, heels, and occiput
- The following precautions may be taken to prevent decubitus ulcers: pressure-reducing cushion; reposition every 2 hours; keep skin, clothing, and sheets clean and dry; and avoid friction during transfers

12.7.8 Immobility

- Highest risk for DVT is within the first 2 to 3 months after SCI
- Prophylactic measures against DVT should be initiated early in the patient's care

- Administer enoxaparin or heparin to prevent blood clots (unless contraindicated)
- Use sequential compression devices
- Mobilize the patient, encouraging mobilization and ambulation as early as possible
- Watch for signs and symptoms of DVT, including pain or tenderness at site (commonly a lower extremity); fever; swelling of affected limb, temperature change of affected limb; loss of peripheral pulse
- If a DVT is suspected, the medical team should be notified immediately and venography or duplex Doppler ultrasound ordered
- A full dose of anticoagulation and/or inferior vena cava filter can be used to treat DVT to prevent the development of a potentially fatal pulmonary embolism

12.7.9 Pain Management

- Administer narcotics as ordered after acute injury for acute pain, then taper off
- Administer antispasmodics (e.g., baclofen) as ordered; be vigilant for signs of baclofen withdrawal (Box 12.7 Signs of Baclofen Withdrawal
- Administer neuropathic pain medication (e.g., gabapentin) as ordered
- Consider the addition of sleep aid, anxiolytic, or antidepressant, if indicated
- Nonpharmacologic interventions (e.g., massage, repositioning, mobilization, guided imagery, relaxation, aromatherapy, cognitive behavior therapy, or counseling) may be effective alternative strategies for managing pain

---

Box 12.7 Signs of Baclofen Withdrawal

Signs of baclofen withdrawal may include the following:
- Anxiety
- Delirium and hallucinations
- Seizures
- High fever
- Hypertonia
- Muscle rigidity
- Rapid breakdown of muscle tissue (which can be quite dangerous)
- Increased, "rebound" spasticity
- Tachycardia
- Tremors
- Low blood pressure
- Organ failure
- Loss of life

12.7.10 Psychosocial Considerations, Patient and Family Teaching

- A patient with SCI will likely have an altered perception of body image and may have negative feelings about loss of independence, sexuality, control over immediate environment, economic security, and familiar lifestyle
- SCI can also put a strain on the patient's personal relationships. Encourage the patient to seek out emotional support from friends, family, and support groups
- Consult with spiritual leaders or clergy as appropriate
- Provide family education and support; encourage the family to ask questions, express their feelings, and be directly involved in the patient's care, as appropriate. Family involvement is especially critical in the rehabilitation phase; see also Chapter 17: Rehabilitation
- Encourage the patient to discuss feelings and participate in decision making about care
- Teach the patient effective coping strategies, foster promotion of healthy behaviors, and encourage the goal of return to independence (with necessary adaptations, if needed)
- Educate the patient on the use of assistive devices such as head-controlled call bells, bed controls, prism glasses, and communication boards
- Ensure that the patient and/or family completely understand discharge instructions (**Appendix B16 Sample Discharge Instructions after Baclofen Pump Placement and Appendix B17: Sample Discharge Instructions after Spinal Fracture**)

12.7.11 Collaborative Management

Patients with SCI will require a multidisciplinary treatment team, which may include members from the following specialties:

- Nursing to provide direct patient care and monitoring, to educate patients and families, and to facilitate communication between patients and other care providers
- Trauma surgeons for acute stabilization and multisystem evaluation
- Neurosurgery for surgical interventions and spinal stabilization
- Pulmonary/critical care for cardiopulmonary and ventilator management
- Respiratory therapy for ventilator care, suctioning, coughing, teaching
- Dietitian to determine nutritional requirements
- Therapies
  - Physical therapy to restore function and movement
  - Occupational therapy for life skill training and adaptive equipment to aid mobility
  - Speech therapy to evaluate swallow evaluation, and determine aspiration risk
- Rehabilitation physician (physiatrist)

- Social worker to identify resources to assist with transitioning back into the community
- Psychologist to screen for depression and to help the patient adjust to life changes

Video

Video 12.1 Traumatic spine injury.

Suggested Reading

[1] Baker L. Caring for the patient with spinal cord injuries. In: Osborn KS, Wraa CE, Watson AS, Holleran RS, eds. Medical-Surgical Nursing: Preparation for Practice. 2nd ed. Boston, MA: Pearson; 2013

[2] Christopher and Dana Reeve Foundation. 2017; http://www.christopherreeve.org. Accessed July 6, 2017

[3] Davenport M. Cervical spine fracture. 2016; http://emedicine.medscape.com/article/824380-overview#a4. Accessed June 30, 2017

[4] Dawodu ST. Cauda equina and conus medullaris syndromes. 2017; http://emedicine.medscape.com/article/1148690-overview. Accessed June 30, 2017

[5] Consortium for Spinal Cord Medicine. Early acute management in adults with spinal cord injury: a clinical practice guideline for health-care professionals. J Spinal Cord Med. 2008; 31(4):403–479

[6] Flanders A. Spine: Thoracolumbar injury. 2009; http://www.radiologyassistant.nl/en/p4906c8352d8d2/spine-thoracolumbar-injury.html. Accessed June 30, 2017

[7] Foster MR. C1 fractures. 2017; http://emedicine.medscape.com/article/1263453-overview. Accessed June 30, 2017

[8] Goodrich JA. Lower cervical spine fractures and dislocations. 2017; http://emedicine.medscape.com/article/1264065-overview. Accessed June 30, 2017

[9] Greenberg MS. Spine injuries. Handbook of Neurosurgery. New York, NY: Thieme; 2010

[10] Jandial R, Aryan HE, Nakaji P. Neurosurgical Essentials. St. Louis, MO: Taylor & Francis; 2004

[11] Johnson K, Mowrey K, Bergman MJ. Neurotrauma: spinal injury. In: Barker EM, ed. Neuroscience Nursing: A Spectrum of Care. 3rd ed. St. Louis, MO: Mosby Elsevier; 2008: 368–402

[12] Leas DP. Atlantoaxial instability. 2017; http://emedicine.medscape.com/article/1265682-overview. Accessed June 30, 2017

[13] Magnus W. Cervical strain. 2015; http://emedicine.medscape.com/article/822893-overview. Accessed July 7, 2017

[14] McIlvoy L, Meyer K, Mcquillan KA. Traumatic spine injuries. In: Bader MK, Littlejohns LR, American Association of Neuroscience Nurses, eds. AANN Core Curriculum for Neuroscience Nursing. St. Louis, MO: Saunders; 2004

[15] National Institute on Disability, Independent Living, and Rehabilitation Research (NIDILRR). http://www.acl.gov/about-acl/about-national-institute-disability-independent-living-and-rehabilitation-research. Accessed July 7, 2017

[16] National Rehabilitation Information Center (NARIC). http://www.naric.com. Accessed July 7, 2017

[17] National Spinal Association. http://www.spinalcord.org. Accessed July 7, 2017

[18] National Spinal Cord Injury Statistical Center. Spinal cord injury (SCI) facts and figures at a glance. Birmingham, AL: University of Alabama at Birmingham; 2017; https://www.nscisc.uab.edu/Public/Facts%20and%20Figures%20-%202017.pdf. Accessed July 7, 2017

[19] Newman DK, Willson MM. Review of intermittent catheterization and current best practices. Urol Nurs 2009; 29(4):239–246

[20] Paralyzed Veterans of America (PVA). http://www.pva.org. Accessed July 7, 2017

[21] Spinal Cord Society. http://www.scsus.org. Accessed July 7, 2017

[22] Strayer AL, Hickey JV. Spine and spinal cord injuries. In: Hickey JV, ed. The Clinical Practice of Neurological and Neurosurgical Nursing. 7th ed. Philadelphia, PA: Lippincott Williams & Wilkins; 2014

13 Developmental Disorders

Denita Ryan

Abstract

Developmental disorders of the central nervous system originate during fetal development. These disorders may cause neurologic symptoms that manifest when the individual is an adult and may result in cognitive impairment, sensory/motor deficits, and pain. Treatment may include observation, medical, or surgical intervention. Understanding the symptoms of developmental disorders along with their treatment and associated complications will enhance the level of care that the health care team can provide to these patients and the support they can offer to the patient's family during treatment and rehabilitation.

Keywords: arachnoid cyst, chiari malformation, encephalocele, myelomeningocele, syrinx, tethered cord

13.1 Developmental Disorders

Most developmental disorders are present at birth and are therefore diagnosed in patients when they are newborns or young children. Children with developmental disorders may still be affected by these disorders in adulthood; in other cases, disorders do not become symptomatic until a person reaches adulthood. Hydrocephalus may be a developmental disorder, or it may be acquired through other central nervous system (CNS) disorders, such as tumor, trauma, or stroke. Because of its importance in neurologic nursing, hydrocephalus is discussed in its own chapter, Chapter 4: Hydrocephalus. The present chapter addresses other developmental disorders that may be encountered in adult patients.

13.2 Arachnoid Cysts

Primary arachnoid cysts are congenital lesions that arise during embryonic development, typically in the middle cranial fossa. These sacs, which are filled with cerebrospinal fluid (CSF), are located between the brain or spinal cord and the arachnoid membrane. Although they may be large, they do not always cause symptoms (▶ Fig. 13.1).

- Form when the arachnoid membranes split during development
- Usually capable of secreting CSF
- Some contain other types of tissue, such as glial or ependymal cells
- Secondary arachnoid cysts are uncommon but may result from head injury, meningitis, tumor, or brain surgery

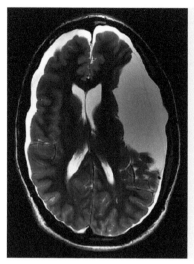

Fig. 13.1 Arachnoid cyst on magnetic resonance imaging.

13.2.1 Epidemiology of Arachnoid Cysts

- Incidence of 5 per 1,000 in autopsy studies
- Male predominance (4:1 ratio)
- Primary type typically occurs before age 20 years, especially during the first year of life

13.2.2 Clinical Manifestations of Arachnoid Cysts

- Symptoms depend on the size and location of the cyst
- Common symptoms include headache, nausea, and seizures; some patients are asymptomatic
- Decreased level of consciousness is possible
- May include symptoms of hydrocephalus (e.g., headache, nausea, sleepiness, blurred vision, irritability)

13.2.3 Diagnosis of Arachnoid Cysts

- Patient's medical history
- Imaging studies
  - Computed tomography (CT)
  - Magnetic resonance imaging (MRI)

13.2.4 Treatment of Arachnoid Cysts

Medical Treatment

- Observation for small cysts with no symptoms or minor symptoms
- Symptom relief (e.g., analgesics for pain)

Surgical Treatment

- Cyst fenestration (i.e., perforation) is the preferred treatment
- Resection via minimally invasive surgery to remove or open cyst membrane to drain CSF
- Shunt for hydrocephalus (used less frequently today than in the past)

Complications of Treatment

- Shunt failure
- Cyst reaccumulation

13.3 Chiari Malformations

Chiari malformations, sometimes called Arnold-Chiari malformations, occur when the cerebellum and medulla oblongata breach the foramen magnum and invade the spinal column. There are three types of Chiari malformation abnormalities. Types I and II are the most common, and type III is severe and is associated with a very poor prognosis. Because of its rarity, type III is not discussed in this chapter.

13.3.1 Type I Chiari Malformation

In patients with a type I Chiari malformation, the cerebellar tonsils are displaced downward below the level of the foramen magnum, without displacement of the medulla (▶ Fig. 13.2). The condition may develop when the bony space holding the cerebellum is smaller than normal, which pushes the cerebellum and brainstem downward. This displacement puts pressure on the cerebellum, which impedes CSF flow. The condition is often an incidental finding during work-up for another condition.

Epidemiology of Type I Chiari Malformation

- Average age at presentation is about 40 years
- Slight female preponderance
- May be associated with posterior fossa arachnoid cyst

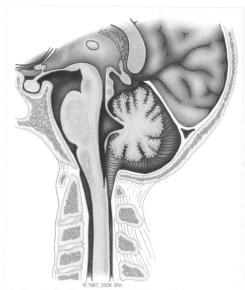

Fig. 13.2 Type I Chiari malformation.

Clinical Manifestations of Type I Chiari Malformation

- Affected persons are usually asymptomatic
- Common symptoms are wide-ranging but may include the following:
  - Headache at back of the head aggravated by coughing
  - Motor/sensory changes
  - Dizziness or ataxia

13.3.2 Type II Chiari Malformation

The type II Chiari malformation is an abnormality in which the cerebellar tonsils and brainstem are displaced downward below the level of the foramen magnum. Type II Chiari malformations are usually associated with a myelomeningocele and spina bifida (▶ Fig. 13.3).

Epidemiology of Type II Chiari Malformation

- Most common in children

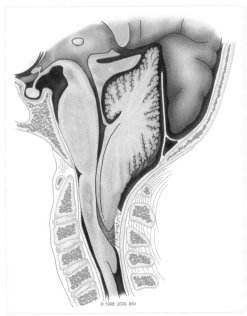

Fig. 13.3 Type II Chiari malformation.

Clinical Manifestations of Type II Chiari Malformation

- Symptoms of brainstem compression
  - Cranial nerve dysfunction, especially of the lower cranial nerves
  - Periods of apnea
- Hydrocephalus is common (from obstruction of the fourth ventricle)

Diagnosis of Type II Chiari Malformation

- Patient's medical history
- Imaging studies
  - CT
  - MRI

Treatment of Type II Chiari Malformation

Medical Treatment

- Observation in early stages
- Symptom control (e.g., analgesics for pain)

Surgical Treatment

- Placement of a shunt for hydrocephalus
- Decompression of Chiari malformation in symptomatic patients

13.4 Encephalocele

An encephalocele is a rare type of neural tube defect that may be present before or after birth. It results from failure of the neural tube to close during fetal development and involves the herniation of intracranial contents—usually meninges and brain tissue—through a defect in the skull. Most cases are diagnosed in infants immediately after birth and are associated with other deformities, but some may present later in life.

13.4.1 Clinical Manifestations of Encephalocele

The clinical manifestations of encephalocele depend on the location and size of the abnormality. An encephalocele may resemble a cyst on a prenatal ultrasound examination. Small encephaloceles (e.g., near the sinuses or nose, or on the forehead) may not be noticed immediately after birth. Encephaloceles may be associated with developmental delays and neurologic deficits.

13.4.2 Diagnosis of Encephalocele

- Patient's medical history
- Clinical assessment
- Imaging studies
  - CT
  - MRI

13.4.3 Treatment of Encephalocele

Surgical intervention is usually necessary, but a thin layer of skin covering the encephalocele can allow delay of surgery for a few months.
- Observation if surgery is not needed immediately
- Surgery if patient is symptomatic

13.5 Other Developmental Disorders

13.5.1 Syrinx

A syrinx is a long, fluid-filled cyst located within the spinal cord that occurs most commonly during fetal development, but it can also result from trauma, meningitis, hemorrhage, tumor, or arachnoiditis (▶ Fig. 13.4). It expands over

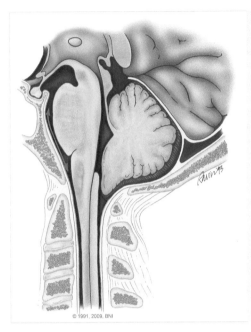

Fig. 13.4 Syrinx.

© 1991, 2009, BNI

time, damaging the spinal cord and resulting in a condition known as *syringo-myelia*.

- Associated with Chiari malformations, as well as other conditions (Box 13.1 Conditions Associated with Syrinx)
- Headaches and motor/sensory deficits are the most common symptoms
- Diagnosed by MRI
- Most common at cervical level
- Treated by surgical decompression
- If left untreated, a syrinx can progress to weakness in extremities, loss of sensation in hands, and severe chronic pain

---

Box 13.1 Conditions Associated with Syrinx

- Chiari malformation
- Spinal cord injury
- CSF obstruction
- Hemorrhage
- Infection (e.g., meningitis)
- Intramedullary tumor

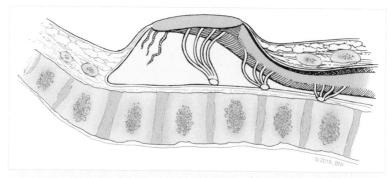

Fig. 13.5 Myelomeningocele.

13.5.2 Myelomeningocele

A myelomeningocele is a birth defect related to spina bifida that involves lack of closure of the backbone and spinal canal in the middle to lower back (▶ Fig. 13.5).

- Associated with type II Chiari malformation
- Symptoms include motor/sensory deficits, including loss of bowel and bladder control
- Occurs mainly in children
- Affects 1 in 4,000 infants

13.5.3 Tethered Spinal Cord Syndrome

In tethered spinal cord syndrome, the spinal cord becomes attached by tissue to the spinal canal, often at the conus medullaris (▶ Fig. 13.6).

- Stretches the spinal cord, causing pain and motor and sensory changes
- Usually congenital, caused by incomplete closure of the neural tube during embryonic development
- Associated with spina bifida
- Diagnosed by medical history, clinical assessment, and MRI
- May go undiagnosed until adulthood
- Treatment is usually surgical detethering
- Therapy and rehabilitation are frequently warranted

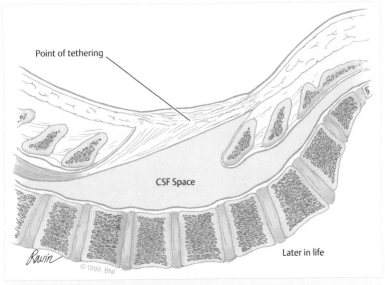

Fig. 13.6 Tethered spinal cord at the level of the conus. CSF, cerebrospinal fluid.

13.6 Nursing Management for Patients with Developmental Disorders

A thorough neurologic assessment is a necessity when caring for a patient with a developmental disorder given it could reveal neurologic changes that may dictate the course of treatment. See also Chapter 2: Assessment. Caregivers should be vigilant for symptoms of hydrocephalus in patients with developmental disorders. These patients may have other associated disorders, some of which may have been present since birth. Therefore, the whole patient must be examined and all other systems must be closely monitored (▶ Table 13.1).

13.6.1 Neurologic Assessment

- Evaluate level of consciousness; see Chapter 2: Assessment
- Watch for signs of hydrocephalus; see Chapter 4: Hydrocephalus
- Be vigilant for cranial nerve deficits, especially deficits of the lower cranial nerves in patients with Chiari malformation
- Monitor motor and sensory function

Table 13.1 Developmental disorders: what to watch for

Signs and symptoms	Indication or location	Nursing action	Rationale
Confusion Incontinence Gait disturbance Visual problems	Hydrocephalus	Complete neurologic assessment, including motor, sensory, cranial nerves, and gait assessment, if feasible	Developmental disorders may occur in patients with hydrocephalus due to obstruction in the ventricular system
Decreased performance in motor or sensory assessment	Syrinx Tethered cord	Complete neurologic assessment, including motor and sensory examination	Motor or sensory deficits may result from expansion of the syrinx
Decreased neurologic function relative to the location of the lesion	Mass effect from edema, hemorrhage, or accumulation of fluid, relative to location	Complete neurologic assessment, focusing on location of lesion Know the location of the lesion, as well as the location of any previous deficits	Lesions (e.g., arachnoid cysts, encephaloceles) may exist in areas that would cause specific deficits (e.g., an encephalocele in the region of the optic nerve would put the patient at risk for visual loss; therefore, assessing the patient's vision is of the utmost importance)

13.6.2 Respiratory Assessment

• Check for respiratory compromise due to a possible swallowing impairment
• Protect the patient's airway
• Monitor arterial blood gases

13.6.3 Gastrointestinal Assessment

• Gastrointestinal bleeding or distress is possible due to increased stress

13.6.4 Nutrition Assessment

• Start nutrition as soon as feasible

13.6.5 Management of Immobility

- Monitor for deep vein thrombosis (DVT) and pulmonary emboli; take measures to prevent DVT
- Administer enoxaparin, unless contraindicated
- Mobilize the patient as soon as possible, unless contraindicated

13.6.6 Pain Management

- Obtain a thorough pain history, including medications taken to control pain and activities or movements that relieve or exacerbate pain
- Pain management may be pharmacologic or nonpharmacologic (e.g., heat, ice, massage)

13.6.7 Patient and Family Teaching

- Provide family with support and educational material
- Provide discharge instructions for patients with Chiari malformation (**Appendix B18: Sample Discharge Instructions after Repair of Chiari Malformation**)

13.6.8 Collaborative Management

Management of patients with developmental disorders requires a team of specialists, including experts from the following specialties:

- Nursing
- Neurosurgery
- Internal medicine
- Physical therapy
- Occupational therapy
- Speech therapy
- Physiatry (i.e., specialists in rehabilitation)
- Clergy
- Palliative care
- Pain management
- Social workers or case managers

Suggested Reading

[1] Cesmebasi A, Loukas M, Hogan E, Kralovic S, Tubbs RS, Cohen-Gadol AA. The Chiari malformations: a review with emphasis on anatomical traits. Clin Anat. 2015; 28(2):184–194

[2] Greenberg MS. Handbook of Neurosurgery. 8th ed. New York, NY: Thieme Medical Publishers, 2016

[3] Mueller DM, Oró JJ. Prospective analysis of presenting symptoms among 265 patients with radiographic evidence of Chiari malformation type I with or without syringomyelia. J Am Acad Nurse Pract. 2004; 16(3):134–138

[4] National Institute of Neurological Disorders and Stroke. https://www.ninds.nih.gov. Accessed June 26, 2017

[5] Pradilla G, Jallo G. Arachnoid cysts: case series and review of the literature. Neurosurg Focus. 2007; 22(2):E7

[6] Shim KW, Lee YH, Park EK, Park YS, Choi JU, Kim DS. Treatment option for arachnoid cysts. Childs Nerv Syst. 2009; 25(11):1459–1466

[7] University of California, Los Angeles. Neurosurgery. http://neurosurgery.ucla.edu. Accessed June 26, 2017

[8] US National Library of Medicine. https://www.nlm.nih.gov. Accessed June 26, 2017

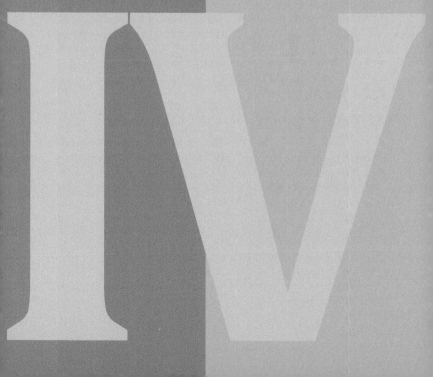

Part IV

Diagnosis and Treatment of Central Nervous System Disorders

14 Neuroradiology and Neuroendovascular Interventions

Manuel F. Mejia, Jr.

Abstract

Neuroradiology is an area of radiology that focuses exclusively on radiology used to diagnose and characterize neurologic diseases, disorders, and injuries. Neuroradiologic examinations may include noninvasive measures such as plain radiographs, computed tomography, and magnetic resonance imaging; they may also encompass more invasive procedures such as cerebral angiograms and myelograms. Neuroendovascular interventions are procedures carried out by neuroradiologists and neurosurgeons who specialize in this type of treatment, including angioplasty, embolization, and stenting. Nurses caring for these patients must possess specific knowledge of these procedures and their indications in order to provide patients with the specialized care they require.

Keywords: cerebral angiography, computed tomography, embolization, magnetic resonance imaging, myelography, radiography, stenting

14.1 Neuroradiology

Neuroradiology is a discipline of radiology that focuses on diagnosis of, and intervention for, abnormalities of the central and peripheral nervous systems. This field comprises many imaging and diagnostic modalities, some of which are discussed in this chapter. Neuroendovascular procedures to treat abnormalities of the nervous system are also described herein.

14.2 Imaging

14.2.1 Radiography

Radiographs, commonly referred to as *plain films* or *X-rays*, are gross two-dimensional structural images obtained without the use of a contrast medium.
- Most fundamental radiologic modality
- Decreasing role in neuroradiology due to advances in computed tomography (CT) and magnetic resonance imaging (MRI)

Indications for Radiography

- Lesions or fractures of bony structures, including the following:
  - Skull or spine fractures
  - Facial trauma

- Abnormal structure or positioning of bones, as in flexion-extension injuries
- Sinusitis

Contraindications

- None (pregnancy is considered a relative risk; potential risk must be weighed against possible benefit)

Method

- Screening per hospital policy
- Noninvasive

Complications

- None

14.2.2 Myelography

Myelography is an imaging technique that uses a contrast agent to reveal abnormalities within the spinal cord.

- The subarachnoid space is accessed via insertion of a spinal needle between L3 and L4 or L4 and L5
- Contrast medium is injected directly into the subarachnoid space, and radiographs are taken of relevant spinal levels (cervical, thoracic, or lumbar)

Indications for Myelography

- Disk herniation
- Spinal stenosis
- Bone displacement
- Spinal cord compression secondary to tumor or vascular malformation

Contraindications

- Actual or suspected intracranial mass (with or without increased intracranial pressure), as this introduces the potential for brain stem herniation. See also Chapter 3: Principles of Intracranial Pressure
- Noncommunicating hydrocephalus
- Coagulopathies
- Impaired renal function
- Known allergic reaction to contrast agents

Method

- Informed consent required
- Review of previous laboratory studies, including coagulation profile
- Review of medications (anticoagulants such as warfarin should be suspended several days before myelogram)
- Patient should be nil per os (NPO), or nothing by mouth, for 2 hours before procedure
- Patient should be sedated
- Take precautions for patients with contrast agent allergy per institutional policies and procedures, if warranted (Box 14.1 Hospital Policy and Procedure)

Box 14.1 Hospital Policy and Procedure

- Follow institutional guidelines, policies, and protocols regarding contrast allergy prep and anticoagulation reversal. A regular CT can be completed with or without contrast, but computed tomography angiography (CTA) is always performed with contrast. Patients with contrast allergies may undergo any neuroradiologic modality, as long as they are properly prepared

---

Complications

- Headaches (i.e., positional or "low-pressure" headache)
  - Worse when patient is in an upright position
  - Usually improves with time, rest, and hydration
  - Epidural blood patch may be helpful
  - Infection
- Reaction to sedation or contrast medium
- Extravasation of contrast (Box 14.2 Clinical Alert: Metformin and Contrast Agents)

Box 14.2 Clinical Alert: Metformin and Contrast Agents

- Metformin should not be given to patients receiving radiologic contrast agents
- May cause renal failure

14.2.3 Computed Tomography

CT is the most commonly used neuroimaging modality in the neurosciences. In CT imaging, X-ray beams are projected into the body in a single slice. A

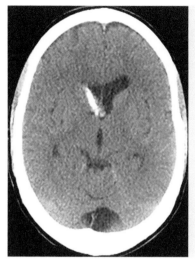

Fig. 14.1 Axial computed tomogram of the head.

stationary detector then measures and reconstructs signals from multiple points of view, and images are generated from those signals and the attenuation of the radiation (▶ Fig. 14.1).

Computed Tomography Angiography

CTA is a computed tomogram of the vascular system that combines the CT procedure described above with injected contrast material. The resulting CT angiogram provides detailed images of the patient's blood vessels.

Attenuation

As it applies to imaging techniques, the term *attenuation* refers to the intensity of a radiation beam as it passes through matter.
- Greater density equals greater attenuation, so objects with greater density will have greater attenuation and therefore will appear whiter/lighter
- Conversely, less density equals less attenuation, resulting in a darker/blacker appearance on CT (▶ Table 14.1)

Indications for Computed Tomography and Computed Tomography Angiography

- Acute intracranial hemorrhage
- Space-occupying lesions
- Bony structural abnormalities

Table 14.1 Attenuation

Substance	Appearance on CT
Bone	White (+ + +)
Blood (acute)	White (+ +)
Gray matter (brain parenchyma)	Light gray (+ +)
White matter (brain parenchyma)	Gray (+ + +)
Water or CSF	Dark gray/light black (+ +)
Air	Black (+ + +)

Abbreviations: CSF, cerebrospinal fluid; CT, computed tomography.
+++ represents full appreciation of stated color; ++ represents moderate appreciation of stated color.

- Bony alignment, fractures, or dislocation of the spine
- Hydrocephalus
- Ischemic or hemorrhagic stroke (CTA is the gold standard for management of stroke)

Contraindications

- Pregnancy is a relative risk
- Contrast allergy, requires a contrast allergy work-up per institutional policy and protocol (Box 14.1 Hospital Policy and Procedure)
- Impaired renal function (a contraindication only if contrast is ordered)

Method

- Noninvasive, no preparation is required for basic nonenhanced CT
- Follow institutional guidelines and policies regarding administration of contrast agent and testing for allergy to contrast agent
- Patient is placed on a flat surface and rolled into scanner up to the level to be examined
- Test usually takes less than 5 minutes
- Cross-sectional images can be viewed in sagittal, axial, and coronal views

Complications

- Delayed allergic reaction to contrast agent
- Acute renal failure secondary to contrast-induced nephrotoxicity
  - Occurs in about 2% of general population, in 4.1% of patients with renal insufficiency (whose serum creatinine is >1.5 mg/dL), and in 12% of patients with both renal insufficiency and diabetes mellitus
- Extravasation of contrast material, which can damage tissue or cause compartment syndrome

14.2.4 Magnetic Resonance Imaging

Magnetic resonance imaging is a sophisticated noninvasive imaging technique that combines radiofrequency waves with magnetic fields to visualize various anatomical structures, providing valuable details about their composition and location.

MRI involves creation of a magnetic field that aligns the hydrogen ions in the body, which are otherwise randomly organized in the absence of a magnetic stimulant. Radio waves are introduced into the field, and signal energy from excitation of the ions to resting is measured and reconstructed into a visual matrix that features different shades of gray. Water and cerebrospinal fluid (CSF) are dark on T1-weighted MRI (▶ Fig. 14.2) and are white on T2-weighted MRI (▶ Fig. 14.3). Enhancement is the result of shortened T1, which is induced by the addition of a contrast agent (Box 14.3 T1-Weighted MRI and T2-Weighted MRI).

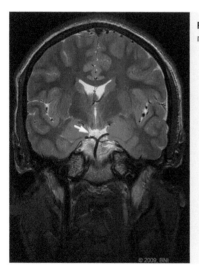

Fig. 14.2 T1-weighted coronal magnetic resonance image of the head.

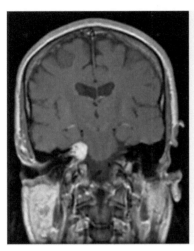

Fig. 14.3 T2-weighted coronal magnetic resonance image of the head.

Box 14.3 T1- and T2-Weighted MRI

- T1 and T2 are defined as constant measurement of time that represents the relaxation time needed for magnetized substance to return to equilibrium
  - T1 = longitudinal relaxation time
  - T2 = transverse relaxation time

Types of Magnetic Resonance Imaging

Different types of MRI may be indicated depending on the type of information sought. These types include the following:
- Magnetic resonance angiography (MRA)
  - Noninvasive imaging study that uses a combination of radiofrequency waves and magnetic fields to define cerebral vasculature (▶ Fig. 14.6)
  - May require the use of gadolinium (a contrast agent)
  - Images are obtained by changing the protocol of signal acquisition to enhance the vasculature of the brain
- Magnetic resonance venography
  - MRI of the venous system (▶ Fig. 14.5)
- Magnetic resonance spectroscopy
  - MRI used to define the compounds within the brain tissue that contain protons

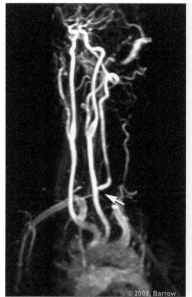

Fig. 14.4 Magnetic resonance angiography shows postoperative patency of anastamosis (arrow).

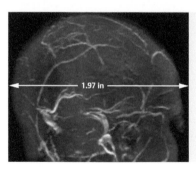

Fig. 14.5 Magnetic resonance venography.

- ○ Differentiates between abscess and neoplasm, tumor and multiple sclerosis plaques, tumor and radiation treatment necrosis, postoperative enhancement and tumor recurrence
- Diffusion-weighted imaging
  - ○ Differentiates between vasogenic edema, cytotoxic edema, and acute ischemic brain tissue or cells
- Perfusion-weighted imaging
  - ○ Evaluates microvascular circulation

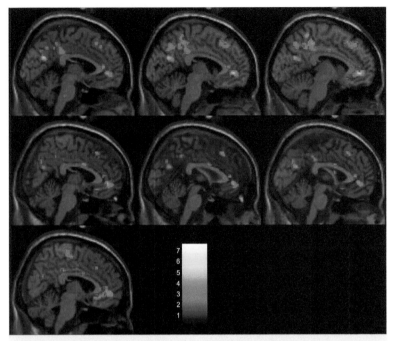

Fig. 14.6 Sagittal functional magnetic resonance image of the head.

- Functional MRI
  - Tool for preoperative brain mapping to identify eloquent areas of the brain, such as speech and motor cortices (▶ Fig. 14.6)
- MRI with navigation systems
  - Allows the surgeon to visualize the anatomical target in relation to surrounding normal structures
  - Improves accuracy of lesion localization

Indications for Magnetic Resonance Imaging

- Tumor
- Infection
- Stroke
- Vascular abnormalities
- Demyelinating processes
- Hydrocephalus
- Inflammatory processes
- Visualization of soft tissue (e.g., spinal cord, spinal nerves, disk spaces, CSF flow, ligament integrity) (▶ Fig. 14.7)

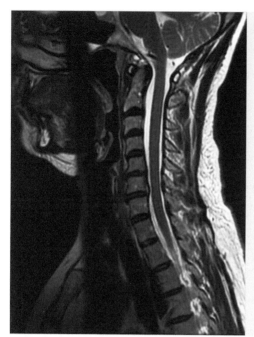

Fig. 14.7 Sagittal magnetic resonance image of cervical spine.

Contraindications

- Pregnancy is relatively contraindicated (potential risk must be weighed against possible benefit)
- Implanted metallic devices, such as pacemakers, defibrillators, spinal cord stimulators, or medication pumps; foreign bodies such as removable or permanent body piercing (dermal anchor piercing) (▶ Table 14.2)
- Clinical instability (potential risk must be weighed against possible benefit; Box 14.4 Clinical Alert: Clinical Instability and MRI)

Table 14.2 Devices compatible with magnetic resonance imaging

Compatibles[a]	Incompatible
Programmable shunt valves	Pacemakers
	Spinal cord stimulators
Deep brain stimulators	Metal workers (anyone with history of working with metal should have orbital films done prior to MRI)
Most intrathecal pumps	
Most surgical clips, plates	Jewelry, body piercings (including dermal implants)
	Bullets, shrapnel

Abbreviation: MRI, magnetic resonance imaging.
Note: This is a partial list only. For a complete list of compatible devices, see http://www.mrisafety.com, the official site of the Institute for Magnetic Resonance Safety, Education, and Research.
[a]Settings may become altered during MRI and should be checked afterward.

- Clinically unstable patients may not be candidates for MRI for the following several reasons:
  - Need for mechanical ventilation
  - Use of infusion pumps (antiarrhythmic or vasopressor drugs)
  - Very difficult to assess condition while patient is in cylinder
    - Rapidly deteriorating neurologic status
    - Difficulty maintaining airway

Method

- Screening form per hospital policy (Box 14.5 MRI Safety)
- Sedation for patients with known claustrophobia
- NPO for patients undergoing sedation for 6 hours prior to MRI, or for as long as indicated by institutional policy and protocol
- Comprehensive metabolic profile with glomerular filtration rate per institutional policy; renal function screening if gadolinium will be administered
- Follow institutional guidelines for patient safety and patient selection

Box 14.5 MRI Safety

- Nursing obligation is first-level screening only
- MRI safety falls on the MRI technician and the radiologist
- For more information on materials allowed in MRI scanners, see the following:
  - http://www.MRIsafety.com
  - http://www.IMRSER.org

Complications

- Allergic reaction to contrast agent

14.2.5 Diagnostic Cerebral Angiography

Cerebral angiography has long been considered the best tool for diagnosis and evaluation of cerebrovascular anomalies (▶ Fig. 14.8).

Digital Subtraction Angiography

- Digital subtraction angiography (DSA) is a modification of the standard cerebral angiography process

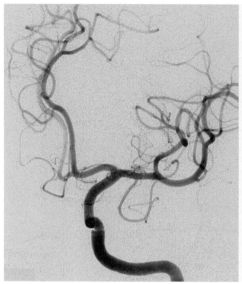

Fig. 14.8 Normal cerebral angiogram.

- DSA allows for visualization of a specific artery by eliminating surrounding structures from view, facilitating treatment such as embolization, stenting, angioplasty, clot removal, and thrombolytic therapy (discussed in greater detail below)

Indications for Digital Subtraction Angiography

- Evaluation of vascular malformations
  - Fistulas (▶ Fig. 14.9)
  - Aneurysms
  - Arteriovenous malformations (AVMs)
- Vascular flow studies (pre- or postoperatively)
  - Vascular flow studies may reveal stenosis, occlusion, or vasospasm
- DSA is the gold standard for evaluation of the vasculature of the brain and neck
- Used for the intervention or treatment of vasospasm, arterial or venous trauma, stroke, aneurysms, fistulas, vascular tumors, AVMs, and stenosis.

Contraindications

There are no absolute contraindications for DSA. Rather, the risk versus benefit must be considered for each patient. Relative contraindications may include the following:
- Known allergic reaction to the contrast medium used
- Coagulopathies

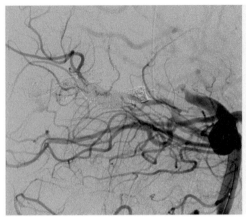

Fig. 14.9 Fistula draining into a venous pouch on digital subtraction angiography.

- Pregnancy
- Acute or chronic renal failure
- Ehlers-Danlos syndrome
- Marfan's syndrome
- Clinical instability

Method

- Patient must remain NPO for 4 to 6 hours, or as long as stipulated by institutional policy
- Informed consent required
- Review of previous laboratory studies, including coagulation profile
- Arterial or venous system can be accessed via the femoral artery or by a vein (preferred method). Any artery or vein, including the brachial and radial arteries or veins, may be used if its diameter can accommodate the catheter sheath
- Fluoroscopic guidance is used to navigate the catheter through the vascular system
- In a traditional diagnostic four-vessel cerebral angiogram, the anterior circulation is accessed by placing the catheters in the right and left common carotid arteries or in the right and left internal carotid arteries
- The posterior circulation is accessed by inserting the catheter in the right or left vertebral artery
- A six-vessel cerebral angiogram includes the right and left external carotid arteries
- The catheter sheath is removed and manual pressure is maintained for 15 to 30 minutes to allow maturation of a clot to establish hemostasis. Alternatively, a vascular closure device may be deployed

Complications

- Allergic reaction to contrast agent
- Extravasation of contrast agent
- Renal failure
- Hematoma or bleeding at the catheter insertion site
- Partial blockage of blood flow to the leg, resulting in discoloration or signs of decreased perfusion
- Formation of a pseudoaneurysm or arteriovenous fistula
- Infection
- Retroperitoneal hemorrhage (Box 14.6 Focus on: Retroperitoneal Hemorrhage)
- The DSA catheter can damage the arterial wall, blocking blood flow and resulting in a stroke (this is a rare complication)

Box 14.6 Focus On: Retroperitoneal Hemorrhage

- Retroperitoneal hemorrhage is a rare but potentially life-threatening complication of femoral angiography
- It is usually caused by poor puncture technique, location, or unusual vascular anatomy
- Symptoms usually occur within 48 hours and include the following:
  - Significant drop in hemoglobin
  - Abdominal, flank, or back pain
  - Hypotension
- CT can help identify presence and location of hematoma
- May require blood transfusion, volume replacement, or urgent vascular surgery to repair the damaged artery

---

14.3 Other Diagnostic Modalities

14.3.1 Lumbar Puncture

Although not considered a radiologic procedure, a lumbar puncture (LP) is an important diagnostic tool for patients with neurologic disorders. It serves both therapeutic and diagnostic purposes.

Indications for Lumbar Puncture

- Evaluation of CSF
  - Diagnosis of infection
  - Diagnosis of neurologic disease (i.e., demyelinating, infectious, or neoplastic)

- Measurement of CSF pressure
- Drainage of CSF
- Administration of medications (i.e., antibiotics or chemotherapeutic agents) or diagnostic agents (e.g., spinal anesthetic)

Contraindications

- Actual or suspected intracranial mass (with or without increased intracranial pressure), given this introduces the potential for brain stem herniation. See also Chapter 3: Principles of Intracranial Pressure
- Noncommunicating hydrocephalus
- Coagulopathies

Method

- Informed consent required
- Results of previous laboratory studies reviewed, including coagulation profile
- Large-bore peripheral IV is used for sedation or contrast medium
- May use fluoroscopic guidance if necessary
- LP is always a sterile procedure
- Local anesthesia administered (1% or 2% lidocaine)
- Spinal needle is inserted into the subarachnoid space between L3 and L4 or L4 and L5 (► Fig. 14.10)
- Opening pressures are measured and one to four tubes of CSF are collected
- CSF is sent to the laboratory for testing, including the following:
  - Glucose
  - Total protein
  - Cell count (number of cells per mm^3) on first and last tubes collected
  - Culture and sensitivity: if an infectious etiology is in the differential diagnosis, at least 10 mL must be collected in a single tube for culture and sensitivity
  - Other testing may be requested by treating physician. Normal values for CSF testing are summarized in Chapter 10, **Table 10.1**

Complications

- Headaches (i.e., positional or "low-pressure" headaches)
  - Worse when patient is in an upright position
  - Usually improve with time, rest, and hydration
  - Epidural blood patch may be helpful
- Infection

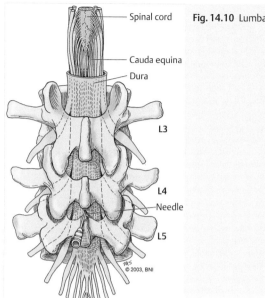

Fig. 14.10 Lumbar puncture.

Spinal cord

Cauda equina

Dura

L3

L4

Needle

L5

© 2003, BNI

14.4 Neuroendovascular Interventions

Neuroendovascular procedures may be performed by neurosurgeons, neuro-radiologists, or neurologists specially trained in the field. Neuroendovascular interventions and cerebral angiography may have similar beginnings and endings, but the intraoperative portion of the procedure differs significantly.

14.4.1 Embolization

Embolization is a therapeutic intervention for certain neurovascular malformations and tumors. The goal of embolization is to permanently obstruct or occlude blood flow to the lesion (▶ Fig. 14.11).

Indications for Embolization

- Intracranial and extracranial aneurysms
- AVMs
- Arteriovenous fistulas
- Some vascular tumors

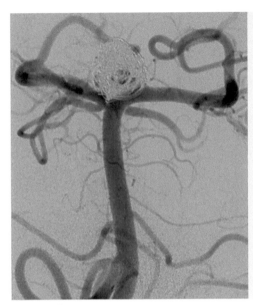

Fig. 14.11 Coiled aneurysm on cerebral angiogram.

Method

Depending on the type and location of the lesion, different types of embolic agents may be used. These may include the following:

- Detachable metal coils
- Balloons
- Tissue adhesives (glues)
- Particles (e.g., polyvinyl alcohol)
- Ethylene-vinyl alcohol copolymer dissolved in dimethyl sulfoxide liquid agent (e.g., Onyx [ev3 Neurovascular, Irvine, CA])
- Stents (e.g., Neuroform [Stryker Corp., Kalamazoo, MI], Wingspan [Stryker Corp.], Enterprise [Johnson & Johnson, Raynham, MA])
- Flow diverters; endoluminal devices; self-expanding, flow-directed microstents (e.g., PipeLine [ev3 Neurovascular, Irvine, CA] or Silk [Balt Extrusion, Montmorency, France])

Technique

- The vascular system is accessed by selective catheterization of the appropriate vessels. This involves the same technique used for cerebral angiography
- Catheters are positioned near the aneurysm, and detachable metal coils or other embolic agents are inserted into the aneurysm to embolize it

Patient and Family Education

Preprocedure

- Patient may be required to take a chlorhexidine shower the night before and the day of the procedure
- Patient must be NPO for at least 6 hours before the procedure
- Informed consent required

Intraprocedure

- Procedure may be performed in an operating room or in an interventional suite
- Patient will be placed under general anesthesia and intubated

Postprocedure

- After the procedure, the patient will be moved to a recovery room or postprocedure unit until fully recovered from anesthesia
- Embolization requires a one-night stay in the intensive care unit
- See **Appendix B19: Sample Discharge Instructions after Cerebral Angiogram for Cerebral Aneurysm Embolization or Coiling**

Complications

- Intracerebral hemorrhage (occurs in roughly 6.8% of cases)
- Infarction (embolic stroke)
- Vasospasm
- Wound infection

14.4.2 Angioplasty or Percutaneous Transluminal Angioplasty or Stent Placement

Percutaneous transluminal angioplasty is the revascularization (opening) of stenotic blood vessels. Stenosis may have many causes, natural or acquired (Box 14.7 Causes of Vascular Stenosis).

- A stent is a device placed in the lumen of a vessel or passageway to maintain patency and structural integrity (▶ Fig. 14.12)
- Before the use of stents, stenotic lesions were primarily managed medically or with "open" surgery (Box 14.8 Use of Intracerebral Stents)

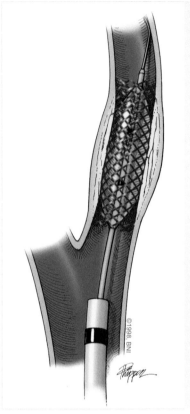

Fig. 14.12 Stent.

Box 14.7 Causes of Vascular Stenosis

- Atherosclerosis
- Radiotherapy
- Graft strictures
- Inflammation
- Traumatic or spontaneous intimal dissection
- Pseudoaneurysms
- Aneurysms
- Vasospasm

Box 14.8 Use of Intracerebral Stents

- The use of stents in cerebrovascular circulation has only been reported in the medical literature since 1999
- Their use is considered innovative medicine and many medical centers that offer cerebrovascular stent placement as a treatment modality are participating in clinical trials
- The use of percutaneous transluminal angioplasty and metallic stent placement is widely accepted in the cardiac and general interventional radiology arenas, but their use in the cerebrovascular circulation is still not widely accepted due to the lack of large multicenter studies specifically designed for intracranial lesions

Categories of Stenting Procedures

- Stent deployment is separated into two categories: primary and secondary stenting
- Characterized by presence or absence of angioplasty to facilitate stent deployment
- Primary stenting deploys stent without initial angioplasty
- Secondary stenting begins with balloon dilation of the vessel lumen before the stent is placed due to decreased available space for instrumentation (Box 14.9 Intra-arterial Drugs)

Box 14.9 Intra-Arterial Drugs

- The intra-arterial use of nicardipine (Cardene) or papaverine hydrochloride (Papaverine) for treatment of cerebral vasospasm is considered off-label use
- Use of intra-arterial agents varies by medical institution

Indications

- Severe atherosclerosis
- Radiation therapy
- Graft strictures
- Inflammation
- Traumatic or spontaneous intimal dissection
- Pseudoaneurysms
- Some aneurysms
- Vasospasm

Technique

- The vascular circulation is accessed with selective catheterization of appropriate vessels, using the same technique as for cerebral angiography (▸ Fig. 14.13, ▸ Fig. 14.14)
- Catheter with an attached balloon is navigated into affected vessel
- Balloon is inflated with mixture of saline and contrast medium for about 5 seconds. This provides visualization under fluoroscopy
- At the same time, pressure inside the vessel is monitored with a manometric device
- Balloon may be inflated up to three times within the vessel during one treatment session

Complications

- Restenosis of vessel
- Occlusion of stent (Box 14.10 Complications of Stent Placement and Angioplasty)

Box 14.10 Complications of Stent Placement and Angioplasty

- The placement of a stent may commit the patient to 3 to 6 months or a lifetime of oral anticoagulant or antiplatelet therapy for prevention of restenosis or stent occlusion

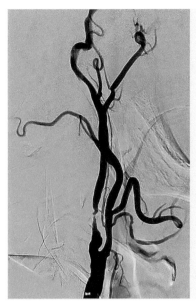

Fig. 14.13 Preoperative cerebral angiogram of stenosed right common carotid artery.

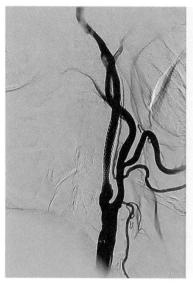

Fig. 14.14 Postoperative cerebral angiogram of a right common carotid artery stent.

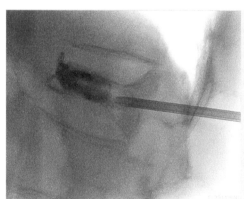

Fig. 14.15 Vertebroplasty.

14.4.3 Vertebroplasty

Vertebroplasty is an image-guided, minimally invasive procedure intended to stabilize certain vertebral body fractures and improve back or radicular pain caused by spinal nerve compression (Box 14.11 Vertebroplasty and Kyphoplasty and ▶ Fig. 14.15).

> ## Box 14.11 Vertebroplasty and Kyphoplasty
>
> • The use of vertebroplasty and kyphoplasty appears to be losing favor, because given conservative treatment alone (i.e., bracing and analgesic use) has demonstrated adequate pain relief at both 6- and 12-month patient follow-up.

Indications

Stabilization and relief of pain due to the following causes:
• Fractures at lumbar or thoracic levels
  ○ Osteoporotic fractures (most common use)
  ○ Compression fractures
  ○ Pathologic fractures (e.g., due to multiple myeloma, hemangiomas, metastases)
• Vertebral body instability
• Pain resulting in significant activity impairment, refractory to conservative measures

Technique

• Local anesthesia
• Image-guided procedure
• Posterior approach
• Percutaneous access to vertebral body obtained via large-gauge needle; each level treated requires a separate puncture
• Vertebral body is filled with 2 to 20 mL of liquid bone cement (polymethylmethacrylate), which gradually becomes solid within the vertebral body
• Patient should remain supine for the first hour, then may be elevated to 30 degrees for the second hour

Complications

• Decreased motor or sensory function of lower extremities
• Increase in intensity or type of pain from baseline
• Pulmonary embolism due to migration of liquid bone cement

14.4.4 Kyphoplasty

Kyphoplasty is considered an augmented version of the vertebroplasty procedure. It differs from vertebroplasty in its ability to restore or gain vertebral body height.

Indications

- Vertebral body fractures (i.e., osteoporotic, compression, and some pathologic fractures)
- Conditions for which the goal of treatment is to restore or gain vertebral body height
- Application is limited to larger vertebral bodies of the midthoracic and lumbar spine (due to the use of larger instrumentation and the two required access puncture sites)

Technique

- Same as for vertebroplasty
- Height is gained in the vertebral body by the inflated balloon compressing the fracture and creating a cavity. This cavity is then filled with cement

Complications

- Same as for vertebroplasty

14.5 Nursing Management for Patients Undergoing Neuroendovascular Intervention

Neuroendovascular intervention continues to evolve from its infancy into a primary, reliable, and evidence-based practice that offers a minimally invasive alternative to open surgery. Neuroendovascular intervention can give hope to patients who have been denied traditional open surgical intervention because of advanced age, an inoperable location, or multiple comorbidities. Neuroendovascular intervention is not only an adjunctive intervention to supplement open surgery, but can also provide a definitive cure (▶ Table 14.3).

It is extremely likely that most, if not all, neurosurgical patients will undergo at least one neuroradiologic procedure during hospitalization and possibly many during their disease course. The nurse must be familiar with neuroendovascular intervention, including preparation, monitoring, technical aspects, and symptoms of possible complications. A nurse may be called to assist with some procedural aspects and must always be available to provide support and education for patients and their families.

Patients undergoing neuroradiologic or neuroendovascular procedures frequently have serious neurologic problems. Neuroendovascular procedures also carry risks; therefore, patients must be educated about the risks, benefits, and options of this type of treatment. Nurses who are familiar with these procedures can help minimize the patient's fear and apprehension, as well as offer information about the risks associated with these treatment modalities (▶ Table 14.4).

Table 14.3 Neuroendovascular interventions

Procedure	Nursing action	Rationale
Preprocedure Embolization Angioplasty	Check recent laboratory values, specifically coagulation profile and CMP	Patients previously on warfarin (Coumadin) or clopidogrel (Plavix) must have an INR and/or a clopidogrel inhibition assay at acceptable levels prior to the procedure
	Check medications, ascertain that patient has stopped taking warfarin and/or clopidogrel if appropriate	Coagulation reversal may be undertaken, rather than postponing the procedure
	Check for allergies, noting any allergy to contrast agent (or to iodine or shellfish), reporting confirmed allergy and instituting allergy prep as ordered	Note contrast allergy and have appropriate prep instituted if warranted
	Ascertain if patient has been taking metformin, and if so, report	Use of metformin (Glucophage) in the presence of contrast material may cause renal failure
Postprocedure	Monitor neurologic assessment at least hourly for the first 4 h, then as directed. Follow postprocedure protocol	Potential for neurologic deterioration due to intracerebral hemorrhage, infarction, or vasospasm
	Patients must be kept flat and immobile for 4 h after procedure, or longer if sheath is left in. Follow postprocedure protocol	Patient could experience a "low pressure" or spinal headache with head elevated
	Monitor puncture site for bleeding or hematoma, monitor patient for abdominal or flank pain	Possibility of bleeding from puncture site, including retroperitoneal hemorrhage
	Monitor circulation of lower extremity on side of puncture Check pedal pulses Monitor color and temperature of lower extremity Document findings	Possibility of clot at puncture site, causing circulatory occlusion
	Monitor cardiovascular hemodynamic trends (blood pressure, heart rate)	Blood pressure should be maintained in appropriate range; hypertension and hypotension should be avoided
	Triple-H therapy (induced hypertension, hypervolemia, and hemodilution) may be required if patient has had an SAH; see Chapter 8: Vascular disorders	Patient with SAH at risk for vasospasm
Specific to angioplasty for vasospasm	Maintain ordered MAP (MAP usually > 60 mm Hg)	Helps to maintain with cerebral perfusion

Abbreviations: CMP, comprehensive metabolic panel; INR, international normalized ratio; MAP, mean arterial pressure; SAH, subarachnoid hemorrhage.

Table 14.4 Nursing management of patients undergoing neuroradiologic procedures

Diagnostic procedure	Nursing action	Rationale
LP	Informed consent	
	Review laboratory studies, especially coagulation studies	Coagulopathies GFR (if contrast agent is used)
	Review medications, ensure that patient has stopped warfarin (Coumadin) or clopidogrel (Plavix) for approximately 4 d prior to examination	Coagulopathy due to warfarin or clopidogrel
	Educate patient regarding procedure and what to expect	Alleviate fear or apprehension about examination
	Assist practitioner in positioning patient properly	
	Encourage patient to maintain bed rest for approximately 4 h, or as ordered	Possible headache due to low intracranial pressure, exacerbated by elevating head position
	Encourage fluid intake Medicate for headache or discomfort as ordered	
	CSF to laboratory for diagnostic tests	Monitor for infection, other abnormality
Myelogram	Same as for LP	
	Maintain NPO status for 6 h prior to examination	
	Establish IV access with large-bore IV	Administration of contrast
	Review allergy list, ascertain that patient is not allergic to contrast, notify ordering physician if patient has contrast allergy and initiate protocol	Allergy to contrast requires prep prior to procedure
	Note if patient is taking metformin	Metformin may cause or exacerbate renal failure
CT	Educate patient on what to expect during procedure	Alleviate patient's fear and apprehension about test
	Start IV line if contrast study	Administration of contrast agent
MRI	Educate patient about what to expect during procedure, including length of time patient must be immobile and the closed nature of the imaging tube	Claustrophobia is common; patient may require sedation Alleviate patient's fear and apprehension about examination

Table 14.4 (*continued*)

Diagnostic procedure	Nursing action	Rationale
	Start intravenous line for sedation or contrast agent	Administration of contrast agent and/or sedation
	Keep patient NPO if sedation is required	Prevent nausea
	MRI screening form	Patient safety regarding exposure to metal
Cerebral angiography	Obtain informed consent	Cerebral angiography should be approached with the same diligence as an open surgical procedure
	Review laboratory studies, especially coagulation studies	
	Review patient's medications, including warfarin; ascertain that patient has stopped taking it for at least 5 d prior to examination, or as ordered	
	Review patient's allergies, including to contrast agents, notify physician if patient is allergic to contrast	
	Educate patient regarding procedure and what to expect, including use of sedation during examination	
	Keep patient NPO for appropriate amount of time	
	After procedure, keep patient on bed rest for approximately 4 h, or as ordered	
	Perform neurologic assessments as ordered, or per hospital protocol	
	Encourage fluid intake	
	Monitor injection site for hematoma, bleeding, bruising, or redness	
	Monitor pedal pulse on side of injection, color of extremity and capillary refill; and record observations and report if abnormal	Hemorrhage or hematoma at site of puncture Possible retroperitoneal hemorrhage
	Medicate for headache or discomfort, as ordered	

Table 14.4 (*continued*)

Diagnostic procedure	Nursing action	Rationale
Any diagnostic study in which patient receives contrast medium	Prior to test, ascertain that patient is not allergic to contrast agent (or to iodine). Notify physician or radiologist immediately if patient states possible allergy to any of these things If patient has a known or suspected allergy to contrast material, follow hospital guidelines regarding preparation, as ordered Monitor patient for signs of allergic reaction (i.e., nausea, vomiting, flushing, rash, diaphoresis, anaphylactic reaction)	
	Check BUN and creatinine	Monitor renal function
	Do not give metformin after contrast agent for prescribed number of days	May exacerbate or cause renal failure

Abbreviations: BUN, blood urea nitrogen; CSF, cerebrospinal fluid; CT, computed tomography; GFR, glomerular filtration rate; IV, intravenous; LP, lumbar puncture; MRI, magnetic resonance imaging; NPO, nil per os (nothing by mouth).

This chapter is intended as a basic reference for bedside care of the patient undergoing a neuroradiologic procedure or a neuroendovascular intervention. For further information, references are included at the end of this chapter, and the reader is encouraged to use these resources to learn more about subjects of interest.

14.5.1 Neurologic Assessment

- Level of consciousness
- Watch for signs of increased intracranial pressure
- New onset of stroke symptoms following angiography; see Chapter 8: Vascular Disorders
- Motor and sensory assessment
- Cranial nerve assessment
- Report new findings immediately

14.5.2 Respiratory Assessment

- Airway assessment
- Monitor respiratory rate and rhythm
- O_2 saturation, monitor if appropriate
- Results of the respiratory assessment will be related to the findings of the neurologic assessment and accompanying trauma or comorbidities

14.5.3 Cardiovascular Assessment

- Determine cardiovascular status of patients scheduled for MRI, given the magnet may interfere with patient monitors
- Infusion pumps regulating antiarrhythmic or vasopressor drugs may not be MRI-compatible
- Watch angiogram groin wound puncture site for hematoma, bruising, or bleeding
- Monitor circulation of lower extremity distal to angiogram puncture site, including assessment of pedal pulses, temperature, capillary refill, and color
- Results of the cardiovascular assessment will be related to the findings of the neurologic assessment

14.5.4 Pain Management

- Assess pain using pain scale and nonverbal cues
- Administer medication as appropriate
- Encourage patient to remain flat after LP, myelogram, or angiogram
- Encourage hydration
- Report headache that increases with change of position (standing up, or raising head of bed)

14.5.5 Patient and Family Teaching

- Educate patient and family about the following procedures:
  - Approximate length of test
  - If and when patient must remain NPO
  - Activity restrictions after test
- Determine patient allergies, especially to iodine or shellfish (contrast allergy)
- Review patient medications, especially metformin, if patient is to receive contrast or any antiplatelet or anticoagulation agent (Box 14.12 Antiplatelet Medications That May Be Used Before, During, and After Surgery)
- Let family know the location of imaging department and how long patient is expected to be there

- Metal screening for patients having an MRI
- Discharge instructions
  - Cerebral angiogram for aneurysm embolization or coiling (**Appendix B19: Sample Discharge Instructions after Cerebral Angiogram for Cerebral Aneurysm Embolization or Coiling**)
  - Kyphoplasty (**Appendix B20: Sample Discharge Instructions after Kyphoplasty**)
  - Vertebroplasty (**Appendix B21: Sample Discharge Instructions after Vertebroplasty**)

Box 14.12 Antiplatelet Medications That May Be Used Before, During, and After Surgery

- Aspirin
- Clopidogrel (Plavix)
- Prasugrel (Effient)
- Ticlopidine (Ticlid)
- Abciximab (ReoPro)
- Tirofiban (Aggrastat)
- Aspirin/dipyridamole (Aggrenox)
- Dipyridamole (Persantine)

14.5.6 Collaborative Management

Various specialties may be called upon to help support patients undergoing neuroendovascular procedures. These may include the following:

- Nursing
- Neuroradiology, neuroendovascular surgery, neurointerventional radiology
- Neurosurgery for primary disorder (e.g., tumors, aneurysms, AVM, spine disorders)
- Specialists associated with specific disorder (e.g., stroke, neurologic oncology, medical oncology)
- Therapies
  - Physical therapy
  - Occupational therapy
  - Speech therapy
- Physiatrists (rehabilitation)
- Pain management
- Case management and social work

Suggested Reading

[1] Bader MK, Littlejohns LR. AANN Core Curriculum for Neuroscience Nursing. St. Louis, MO: Saunders; 2010

[2] Benjamin I, Griggs RC, Wing EJ, Fitz G. Andreoli and Carpenter's Cecil Essentials of Medicine. 9th ed. St. Louis, MO: Saunders; 2015.

[3] Brenner DJ, Hall EJ. Computed tomography—an increasing source of radiation exposure. N Engl J Med. 2007; 357(22):2277–2284

[4] Castillo M. Myelography. Neuroradiology Companion: Methods, Guidelines, and Imaging Fundamentals. Philadelphia, PA: Lippincott Williams & Wilkins; 2012

[5] Destrebecq A, Terzoni S, Sala E. Post-lumbar puncture headache: a review of issues for nursing practice. J Neurosci Nurs. 2014; 46(3):180–186

[6] Fenton DS, Czervionke LF. Image-guided Spine Intervention. 2nd ed. New York: Springer; 2010.

[7] Greenberg MS. Handbook of Neurosurgery. New York, NY: Thieme; 2010

[8] Harris C. Neuromonitoring indications and utility in the intensive care unit. Crit Care Nurse. 2014; 34(3):30–39, quiz 40

[9] Hickey JV. Diagnostics for patients with neurological disorders. In Hickey JV, ed. The Clinical Practice of Neurological and Neurosurgical Nursing, 7th ed. Philadelphia, PA: Lippincott Williams & Wilkins; 2014

[10] Illescas FF, Baker ME, McCann R, Cohan RH, Silverman PM, Dunnick NR. CT evaluation of retroperitoneal hemorrhage associated with femoral arteriography. AJR Am J Roentgenol. 1986; 146(6):1289–1292

[11] Jones RW, Littlejohns LR. Hydrocephalus. In: Bader MK, Littlejohns LR, eds. AANN Core Curriculum for Neuroscience Nursing. 4th ed. St. Louis, MO: Saunders; 2004

[12] Lundén M, Lundgren SM, Persson LO, Lepp M. Patients' experiences and feelings before undergoing peripheral percutaneous transluminal angioplasty. J Vasc Nurs. 2013; 31(4):158–164

[13] Marks MP, Do HM. Endovascular and Percutaneous Therapy of the Brain and Spine. Philadelphia, PA: Lippincott Williams and Wilkins; 2002

[14] Nadgir R, Yousem DM. Neuroradiology: The Requisites. 4th ed. Amsterdam, Netherlands: Elsevier; 2016

[15] Sartor K. Diagnostic and Interventional Neuroradiology. New York, NY: Thieme; 2002

[16] Weissleder R, Wittenberg J, Harisinghani M, Chen JW. Primer of Diagnostic Imaging. St. Louis, MO: Mosby; 2011

15 Neurosurgical Interventions

Nancy White, Tammy Tyree, and Joseph M. Zabramski

Abstract
Neurosurgery is a rapidly growing field that includes surgery of the brain and spinal cord. Nursing for patients who have undergone neurosurgical interventions encompasses preoperative care, such as preparing a patient for surgery; intraoperative care, such as positioning and monitoring; and postoperative care, such as preventing complications and controlling pain. Awareness of the patient's positioning during the surgical procedure, as well as the surgical approach used, will help nurses prepare for postoperative outcomes and anticipate possible complications.

Keywords: craniotomy, intensive care unit, patient positioning, postanesthesia care unit, spine surgery, surgical approaches

15.1 Neurosurgical Interventions

Despite recent advances in the field, the prospect of neurosurgery is still a major source of anxiety for patients and families. This chapter describes common neurosurgical procedures undergone by many patients with neurologic disorders. These procedures may be the selected treatments for disorders discussed in previous chapters.

Caring for neurosurgical patients may involve preoperative care, intraoperative responsibilities, postoperative implications, and potential complications. For nurses who work in the surgical suite, or for those interested in what transpires behind the doors of the operating room, this chapter features a section on intraoperative care (i.e., patient positioning, prevention of skin breakdown, and implications of various surgical approaches). Neurosurgery is usually classified into two main groups: brain surgery and spine surgery.

15.2 Brain Surgery

Various brain surgery procedures are described below. Standard descriptive terms are used to communicate the purpose of a given procedure. Such terms may include *clipping/obliteration*, *debridement*, *debulking*, *decompression*, *evacuation*, *excision*, *replacement*, and *resection*.

The term *craniotomy* refers to the surgical opening of the skull to allow access to intracranial contents. It is usually performed to facilitate removal of a space-occupying lesion (e.g., blood, infection, or tumor) or to treat a vascular abnormality

403

(Box 15.1 Indications for Craniotomy). Although craniotomy is a basic component of many brain surgeries, not all brain surgery requires craniotomy.

Box 15.1 Indications for Craniotomy

- Tumor
- Hematoma
- Infection/abscess
- Vascular malformation procedure
  - Aneurysm clipping
  - Arteriovenous malformation resection
  - Revascularization surgery (i.e., bypass)
- Decompression
- Hydrocephalus
- Seizures

15.2.1 Craniotomy

Classification of Craniotomies

Craniotomies are defined as either above or below the tentorium; see also Chapter 1: Anatomy (▶ Fig. 15.1).
- The term *supratentorial* refers to the region above the tentorium
- The term *infratentorial* refers to the region below the tentorium

Common Terms Related to Craniotomy

Biopsy

- Surgical excision of a tissue sample to establish diagnosis
- Useful for diagnosis of brain tumor, infection, or degenerative disease

Burr Holes

- Small openings created in the cranium with a twist drill to access the subdural space (▶ Fig. 15.2)
- Least invasive way to gain access to the brain
- Often performed to drain a chronic subdural hematoma; see also Chapter 9: Traumatic Brain Injury
- Used emergently to drain acute fluid collections in patients with life-threatening herniation syndromes
- May serve as a temporary decompressive measure until craniotomy can be performed

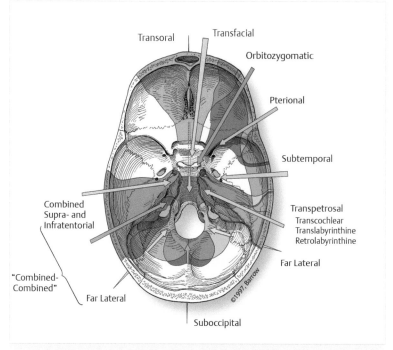

Transoral

Transfacial

Orbitozygomatic

Pterional

Subtemporal

Combined
Supra- and
Infratentorial

Transpetrosal
Transcochlear
Translabyrinthine
Retrolabyrinthine

Far Lateral

"Combined-
Combined"

Far Lateral

Suboccipital

©1997 Barrow

Fig. 15.1 Approaches for craniotomy. (Used with permission from Barrow Neurological Institute, Phoenix, AZ.)

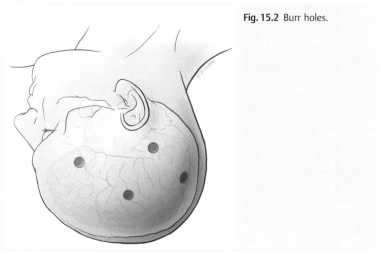

Fig. 15.2 Burr holes.

405

Craniectomy

- Removal of a portion of the skull (the removed portion is referred to as a *bone flap*)
- Relieves severe brain swelling
- May be carried out to remove infected bone
- In a craniectomy, the bone flap is not replaced right away

Cranioplasty

- Repair of a skull defect (from trauma, malformation, or craniectomy)
- Restores the contour and integrity of the skull
- May be carried out to replace a bone flap; usually performed in the weeks or months after craniectomy
- Timing of replacement or repair depends on the reason for the initial bone flap removal

Hemicraniectomy

- Removal of part or half of the skull
- Serves as an aggressive treatment option for patients whose persistent intracranial hypertension is refractory to conservative measures
- May reduce mortality in some patients with nondominant hemisphere strokes

Microsurgery

- Any surgery performed with the aid of an intraoperative microscope or a loupe magnifying glass (▶ Fig. 15.3)
- Magnifies the operative field, enhancing visualization of small or hard-to-see structures

Navigational Systems

- Used for image-guided or stereotactic surgery
- Allow the neurosurgeon to identify the exact location of a lesion by providing its three-dimensional coordinates
- Patients scheduled for this type of procedure will undergo preoperative stereotactic magnetic resonance imaging (MRI) or computed tomography (CT); see also Chapter 14: Neuroradiology and Neuroendovascular Interventions
- These preoperative images are loaded into a navigational system computer that generates a three-dimensional map of the brain intraoperatively

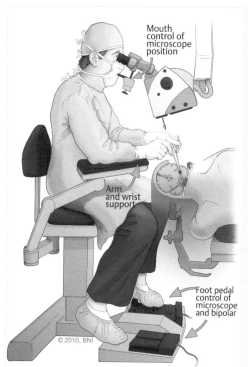

Fig. 15.3 Microsurgery.

Mouth
control of
microscope
position

Arm
and wrist
support

Foot pedal
control of
microscope
and bipolar

© 2010, BNI

15.2.2 Other Types of Brain Surgery

Amygdalohippocampectomy

- Surgical interruption of seizure pathways
- Common treatment for patients with temporal lobe epilepsy refractory to medical treatment
- Usually reserved for patients who do not respond to pharmacologic intervention for seizures; see also Chapter 6: Seizures

Deep Brain Stimulation

- Insertion of stimulators into targeted areas of the brain (▶ Fig. 15.4)
- Used to treat epilepsy, Parkinson's disease, and some chronic pain syndromes

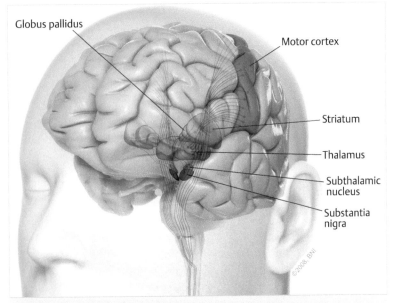

Fig. 15.4 Common anatomical structures targeted in deep brain stimulation.

Microvascular Decompression

- Treatment designed to relieve pressure on a cranial nerve (CN); the most commonly affected CNs include CN V, CN VII, CN IX, CN X, and CN XI
- The pressure is caused by a vessel pulsating against the CN, resulting in a range of conditions including trigeminal neuralgia, hemifacial spasm, and glossopharyngeal neuralgia
- A microscope or endoscope is used to identify and reposition the vessel or to place padding (e.g., Teflon or cotton) between the vessel and the compressed nerve (▶ Fig. 15.5)

Revascularization Procedures

- Include direct and indirect procedures (▶ Fig. 15.6)
  - Artery-to-artery bypass is an example of direct bypass
  - Temporalis muscle overlay is an example of indirect bypass
- Used as treatment for some cerebrovascular diseases (e.g., moyamoya disease) or skull base tumors

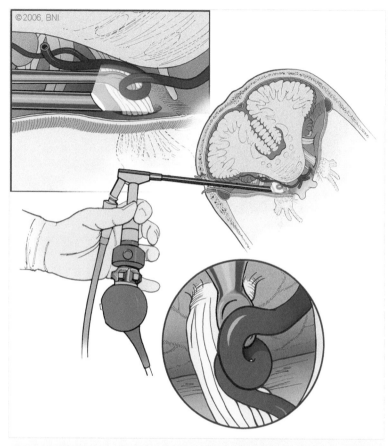

Fig. 15.5 Microvascular decompression.

Ventriculoperitoneal, Lumboperitoneal, or Ventriculoatrial Shunt

- Shunts placed to divert excess cerebrospinal fluid (CSF) away from the ventricular system
- Used to treat hydrocephalus or benign intracranial hypertension (i.e., pseudotumor cerebri); see also Chapter 4: Hydrocephalus

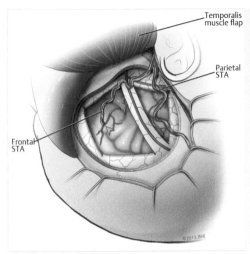

Fig. 15.6 Combined direct (arrowhead) and indirect bypass procedures. STA, superficial temporal artery.

Temporalis muscle flap

Parietal STA

Frontal STA

©2013 BNI

15.3 Spine Surgery

Indications for spinal surgery may include normal degenerative processes or traumatic events (Box 15.2 Indications for Spine Surgery). Many of these conditions were discussed in Chapter 11: Spinal Disorders and Chapter 12: Traumatic Spine Injury.

Box 15.2 Indications for Spine Surgery

- Abscess
- Degenerative disk disease
- Herniated disk
- Kyphosis
- Myelopathy
- Radiculopathy
- Spinal instability
- Spondylolisthesis
- Spondylolysis
- Spondylosis
- Stenosis
- Tumor
- Vascular lesion

15.3.1 Common Types of Spine Surgery

Anterior Lumbar Interbody Fusion

- Removal of disk material followed by placement of a cage device between the two vertebral bodies
- Cage device is packed with autograft and/or allograft bone (Box 15.3 Types of Grafts)
- Procedure may be combined with posterior lumbar spinal fusion to stabilize the spine

---

Box 15.3 Types of Grafts

- Autograft: Refers to harvest of bone from patient's own body (e.g., iliac crest bone from the pelvis)
- Allograft: Refers to use of cadaver bone or synthetic material

---

Diskectomy

- Excision and removal of disk material or the entire herniated disk (▶ Fig. 15.7)
- In a microdiskectomy procedure, the surgeon uses a microscope or magnifying eyeglasses to view the operative field and remove disk material

Fusion

- Addition of bone (allograft and/or autograft) to a specific area of the spine, either with or without a cage (▶ Fig. 15.8)
- Fosters ossification and solidification in the space between bones
- Limits range of motion at that level, thereby decreasing pain

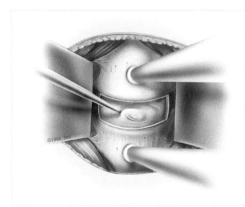

Fig. 15.7 Anterior cervical diskectomy.

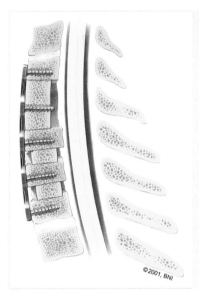

Fig. 15.8 Cervical fusion.

Interspinous Process Device

- Device placed between lumbar spinous processes, placing the spine in a slightly flexed position, which widens the spinal canal and the nerve root foramen
- Alternative to laminectomy for treatment of lumbar spinal stenosis

Laminectomy

- Also referred to as *open decompression*
- Removal of spinous process and bilateral laminae (▶ Fig. 15.9)
- Used to treat spinal stenosis and foraminal narrowing, usually at multiple levels

Laminotomy

- Lamina is opened to relieve pressure on the nerve root or the spinal canal
- Used to treat spinal stenosis at a single level, usually on one side

Pedicle Screws and Rods

- Screws are placed through the pedicles and into the vertebral bodies at the consecutive spine segments being fused (two or more segments may be fused at a time)
- The screws are attached to a rod, preventing motion at the fused segments (▶ Fig. 15.10)

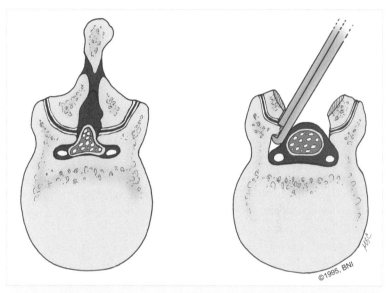

Fig. 15.9 Laminectomy.

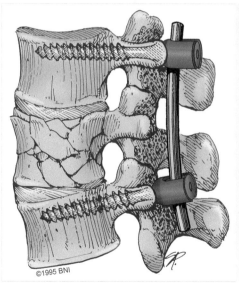

Fig. 15.10 Pedicle screws and rods.

Plating

- Most common in anterior cervical procedures after anterior cervical microdiskectomy and fusion device placement between vertebral bodies (▶ Fig. 15.11)
- Decreases motion, secures fusion device, and provides additional stabilization until fusion is complete
- Prevents anterior or posterior migration of the fusion device

Posterior Lumbar Interbody Fusion

- After diskectomy, a cage device containing autograft and/or allograft bone is inserted into the disk space (▶ Fig. 15.12)
- The desired outcome is a biological response: solid bony fusion between the two vertebrae, stopping motion at that segment

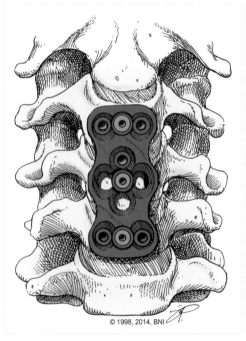

Fig. 15.11 Anterior cervical plating.

© 1998, 2014, BNI

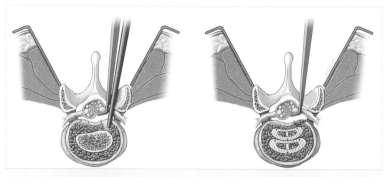

Fig. 15.12 Posterior lumbar interbody fusion.

15.4 Preoperative Nursing Care

In elective surgeries, the care team may have days or weeks to complete the preoperative steps that ensure optimal outcomes. However, surgeries may be emergent or scheduled during the current hospitalization, with little time to prepare. Regardless of the timeline or other circumstances surrounding the procedure, certain preoperative measures must be taken. These may include the following:

- Medical clearance (i.e., Is the patient's condition stable enough to withstand surgery?)
- Review of current medications
- Discontinuation of certain medications prior to surgery, especially anticoagulants such as clopidogrel, warfarin, and aspirin (Box 15.4 Clinical Alert: Anticoagulation/Antiplatelet Drugs)
- Laboratory tests (▶ Table 15.1)
  - ○ Coagulation profile
  - ○ Complete blood cell count (CBC)
  - ○ Electrolytes
  - ○ Pregnancy test, if appropriate
  - ○ If the patient is taking clopidogrel, a platelet aggregation panel and clopidogrel inhibition assay must be drawn to assess platelet function (Box 15.5 Preoperative Management of Coagulopathies)
  - ○ Blood type and screen or crossmatch (autologous blood donation may be used for large-scale spine procedures, if this is the patient's preference and if time permits)
- Informed consent
- Advanced directives

Table 15.1 Preoperative checklist: normal laboratory values

Test	Normal values
CBC	
Hemoglobin	12.9–16.1 g/dL
Hematocrit	37.7–51.3%
White blood cells	3.6–11.1/μL
Platelets	150–450 × 10^3/μL
BMP	
Sodium	135–145 mmol/L
Potassium	3.6–5.3 mmol/L
BUN	8–25 mg/dL
Creatinine	0.65–1.25 mg/dL
Glucose	65–99 mg/dL
Coagulation profile	
Prothrombin time	9.3–12.9 s
PTT	21–31 s
INR	0.8–1.2
TEG	55–73 mm
Platelet inhibition assay	Depends on physician preference and type of surgery to be performed

Abbreviations: BMP, basic metabolic profile; BUN, blood urea nitrogen; CBC, complete blood cell count; INR, international normalized ratio; PTT, partial thromboplastin time; TEG, thromboelastography.
Note: Normal laboratory values are slightly different at every laboratory/institution.

- Patient/family teaching of expected preoperative, intraoperative, and postoperative course
- Some cases of tumor resection may require wand-guided MRI or CT for intraoperative navigation

Box 15.4 Clinical Alert: Anticoagulation/Antiplatelet Drugs

Patients who take antiplatelet medications or warfarin should discontinue these medications several days before surgery, as determined by the surgeon. Preoperative laboratories should include CBC and a coagulation profile, including a platelet aggregation panel/assay for patients receiving antiplatelet medications. The surgeon should be notified immediately of any abnormal laboratory values.

Box 15.5 Preoperative Management of Coagulopathies

Coagulopathies must be corrected before surgery

- Platelet dysfunction
  - A medication the patient is taking (e.g., aspirin or clopidogrel) may be causing platelet dysfunction. The platelet count may be normal, but platelet function is altered
  - Patient may need a platelet transfusion, which will give the patient functioning platelets capable of clotting
  - Platelet transfusion may be carried out pre-, intra-, and/or postoperatively, as needed
- Thrombocytopenia
  - Patients with a low platelet count will require a preoperative platelet transfusion, and may require additional intra-, and/or postoperative transfusion
- Elevated INR
  - Patients receiving warfarin with elevated INR are treated with vitamin K (Aquamephyton), fresh frozen plasma, or both
  - Oral vitamin K may be preferred over subcutaneous or intravenous vitamin K
    - Oral vitamin K may correct excessive anticoagulation more effectively than subcutaneous vitamin K
    - Intravenous vitamin K has been associated with anaphylactic reactions
- Bleeding prophylaxis
  - Tranexamic acid
    - Tranexamic acid inhibits multiple plasminogen-binding sites, decreasing fibrinolysis and plasmin formation
- Elevated PTT
  - Patients receiving heparin with a prolonged PTT need to be treated with protamine sulfate

15.4.1 Patient and Family Teaching

For all surgeries emergent and planned, it is critical to educate and support the patient and family. Important information to relay includes the following:

- Type of surgery (as listed on surgical consent), including the approach and the area of planned incision
- Location of operating room and waiting room for family members
- Anticipated duration of surgery
- Location of recovery room and anticipated length of stay in the hospital
- Expected location of patient's room after recovery unit

- Intensive care unit (ICU) information
  - Visiting hours
  - Restrictions (e.g., whether children are allowed, acceptable number of visitors)
  - Increased stimulation in ICU (noise, alarms, increased frequency of assessments)
  - Expected length of stay in ICU, if appropriate

15.4.2 Informed Consent

The nurse is occasionally called upon to assist with obtaining informed consent for surgery. Informed consent should be obtained after the physician discusses the following with the patient and/or family:

- Reason for proposed surgery
- Alternative treatments, if any
- Potential consequences/risks of surgery
- Potential consequences/risks of foregoing surgery

The adult patient should sign the consent. If the patient's medical condition renders the patient unable to sign, a surrogate decision maker, usually the next of kin or the medical power of attorney, may be called upon to sign the informed consent.

It is important that all questions are answered and the patient and/or family have the information needed to consent to surgery. Informed consent forms must include the following details:

- Patient's full name
- Attending surgeon's full name
- Complete descriptive name of intended surgical procedure, including site (left or right), with all words spelled out completely. Abbreviations are not acceptable on informed consent forms

15.4.3 Advanced Directives

Advanced directives are personalized legal documents that define and clarify the patient's wishes for health care and end-of-life issues. These documents direct specific care. If the patient is rendered unable to participate in decisions regarding his or her own medical care, the advanced directives should be consulted to determine the next step. Ideally, these forms are completed prior to hospital admission, but they can be completed during the admitting process, during hospitalization, or just before surgery. Ensuring the inclusion of the patient's advanced directives in the medical chart is an important element of preoperative nursing care.

Durable Power of Attorney for Health Care

- The durable power of attorney for health care is the person designated to make health care decisions in the event when the patient is unable to make decisions regarding his or her own care

Living Will

- A living will is a document that specifies what treatments the patient does or does not want to receive at the end of life
- It applies only if medical treatment in question is necessary to prolong life and the patient is unable to speak for himself
- Hospital chaplains are excellent resources who are usually available to assist with writing living wills and naming the medical power of attorney

15.4.4 Preoperative Nursing Checklist

Prior to surgery, the nurse should review the following checklist to ensure that the patient is properly prepared. Policies and procedures may vary among institutions. This preoperative nursing checklist can also be found in **Appendix C: Preoperative Nursing Checklist**.

- Informed consents
  - Surgical consent
  - Blood consent or refusal of blood/blood products
  - Anesthesia consent
- Preoperative teaching
  - Patient and family education about the procedure, the expected timeline, and expected outcomes
- History and physical examination
- Allergies, including reactions
- Laboratory tests as ordered. These may include the following:
  - CBC
  - Coagulation profile
  - Urinalysis
  - Blood tests
    - Type and screen
    - Crossmatch
    - Number of units ordered and availability
    - Pregnancy test, if appropriate
  - Comprehensive metabolic profile or basic metabolic profile
- Electrocardiogram
- Chest radiograph
- Old chart, if available

- Special preparatory measures, if ordered
- Identification bracelet
- Compliance with orders for nil per os (NPO), or nothing by mouth, and ordered duration
- Removal of undergarments
- Removal of bobby pins, combs, wig, hairpiece, and false eyelashes
- Removal of jewelry, watches, and/or religious medals. Document placement (e.g., with a specific family member or with hospital security staff)
- Rings taped
- Removal of dentures (bridge, plates, partials), container labeled
- Removal of prostheses, with documentation of placement. Prostheses may include the following:
  - Artificial eye (if removal is necessary for surgical access)
  - Contact lenses
  - Glasses
  - Hearing aids
  - Prosthetic limbs
  - Other
- Identification labels with chart
- Face sheet, or a one-page sheet that summarizes important patient information, attached to chart
- Measures to prevent deep vein thrombosis (DVT)
  - Sequential compression devices or antiembolism stockings, unless contraindicated
- Documentation of the time of last void or catheter placement
- Compliance with necessary isolation precautions
- Medication reconciliation on chart
  - List of medications administered preoperatively, with documented drug/dose/time
- Time of last dose of β-blockers, if applicable
  - For patients receiving β-blocker therapy at home, the β-blocker must be administered 24 hours before surgery or within the perioperative period (within 6 hours of the end of surgery for patients going directly to ICU postoperatively)
    - Document whether a β-blocker was given within 24 hours of surgery
    - Document whether a β-blocker was not administered before surgery
- Safety
  - Side rails up
  - Call light within reach
- Vital signs, including the following:
  - Blood pressure
  - Temperature
  - Pulse

- ○ Respiration rate
- ○ Oxygen saturation
- Special comments and considerations for operating room and recovery room nurses
- Communication of patient limitations
  - ○ Sight
  - ○ Motion
  - ○ Hearing
  - ○ Speech
  - ○ Other
- Measure patient's height and weight
- Test bedside blood glucose level (for patients with diabetes mellitus or on steroids).
  - ○ Document last dose of insulin or oral hypoglycemic agent.
    - – Include type and amount
- The night before or day of surgery
  - ○ Preoperative shower/shampoo (preferably with chlorhexidine)

15.5 Intraoperative Nursing Care

15.5.1 Patient Positioning

Effective patient positioning should offer ideal operative exposure for the neurosurgeon; maintain adequate cerebral circulation; promote optimum cardiovascular, hemodynamic, and respiratory function; and prevent position-related injury.

Although it may sound trivial, precise patient positioning must not be overlooked because it can prevent significant pre-, intra-, and postoperative complications and contribute to positive outcomes for neurosurgical patients. Preparing the operating room with the correct positioning equipment before the patient is brought in for surgery is an efficient way to prevent position-related injuries. This section describes three positions commonly used to access the brain and spine (supine, prone, and lateral) and covers some variations of these positions.

15.5.2 Surgical Approaches: Indications, Concerns, and Implications

Craniotomy: Supine Position

- Head position is determined by surgeon preference, but the most common positions are the following:
  - ○ Mayfield 3-point head holder
  - ○ Horseshoe head rest
  - ○ Gel or foam donut head rest

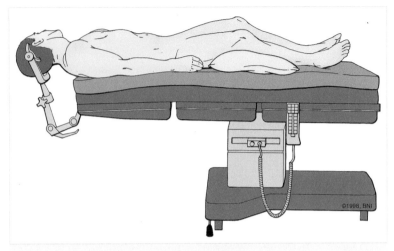

Fig. 15.13 Supine position for craniotomy.

- Right arm wrapped circumferentially in egg crate and tucked at the patient's side with safety strap or 3-inch-wide adhesive tape wrapped around the entire torso, arms, and operating table three times (▶ Fig. 15.13). The wrist and fingers, as well as the median, ulnar, and radial nerves, should be protected
- Left arm rests on egg crate or padded arm board for anesthesia access
- Pillow under the knees
- Foam padding between the ankles and the knees
- Small towel under the lordotic curve of the lower back
- Padded safety strap across the anterior thighs

Frontal/Bifrontal Approach

This approach, through the forehead, allows access to the frontal lobe of the brain (▶ Fig. 15.14). Patients undergoing a procedure via this approach are usually positioned with the head in a neutral position.

Indications

- Abscess
- Aneurysm
- CSF fistula
- Frontal lobe tumor
- Intracerebral hematoma

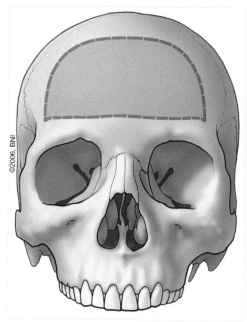

Fig. 15.14 Bifrontal craniotomy.

- Lesion of the frontal sinus
- Malignant intracranial hypertension
- Olfactory groove lesion
- Parasagittal meningioma
- Sellar tumor, including craniopharyngioma and planum sphenoidale meningioma
- Tumor/lesion of the third ventricle or hypothalamus

Common Surgical Procedures

- Bifrontal decompressive craniectomy
- Burr hole for endoscopic third ventriculostomy
- Burr holes for placement of deep brain stimulators
- Endoscopic wand-guided cyst fenestration
- Eyebrow incision for endoscopic tumor resection
- Frontal craniotomy for biopsy, debulking, and/or tumor removal

Postoperative Nursing Concerns

- Sagittal sinus injury
- Venous infarction

- Hematoma due to inadequate hemostasis
- CSF leak (frontal sinus)
- Anterior cerebral artery injury
- Superior facial nerve branches may be injured if skin incision is extended too far
- Seizure
- Incisional edema
- Behavioral changes (e.g., loss of inhibition, disorientation)

Frontotemporal Approach

This approach facilitates access to the frontal and temporal lobes of the brain.

Indications

- Most aneurysms of the anterior circulation
- Tumor of the anterior fossa, middle fossa, frontal lobe, or temporal lobe
- Suprasellar lesion
- Lesion involving the anterior midbrain

Common Surgical Procedures

- Pterional craniotomy (▶ Fig. 15.15)
- Orbitozygomatic craniotomy (▶ Fig. 15.16)
  - Full
  - Modified
  - Miniature

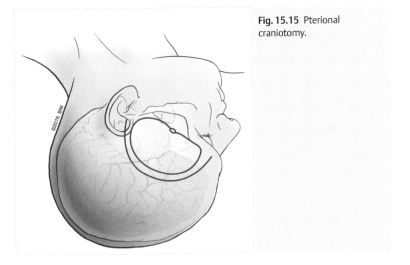

Fig. 15.15 Pterional craniotomy.

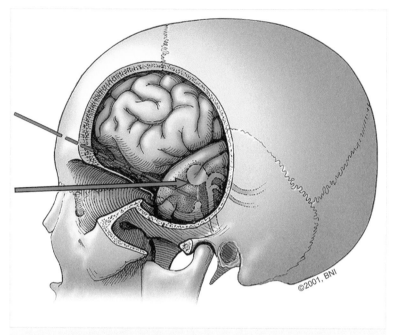

Fig. 15.16 Orbitozygomatic craniotomy.

Postoperative Nursing Concerns

- Orbital or periorbital edema and ecchymosis
- Orbital muscle entrapment (partial ophthalmoplegia)
- Optic nerve entrapment (blindness)
- Injury to the frontalis nerve (ipsilateral forehead paralysis)
- Hematoma
- CSF leak

Parietal Approach

The parietal approach allows access to the parietal lobe of the brain (▶ Fig. 15.17).

Indications

- Tumor, vascular lesion, infection, or hemorrhage of the parietal lobe
- Tumor or lesion surrounding the superior sagittal sinus

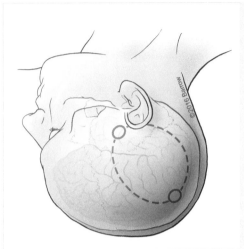

Fig. 15.17 Parietal approach.

Common Surgical Procedures

- Biparietal craniotomy (for a tumor or lesion surrounding the superior sagittal sinus)
- Superior parietal lobe approach

Postoperative Nursing Concerns

- Intraoperative injury to superior sagittal sinus
- Hematoma related to inadequate hemostasis
- Cerebral infarction (venous or arterial)

Postoperative Nursing Implications

- Motor and sensory examination
- Visual fields should be assessed and compared with preoperative assessment
- Assess presence of seizures, monitor antiepileptic drug (AED) levels
- Assess speech function (both receptive and expressive speech)

Temporal Approach

This approach allows access to the temporal lobe of the brain (▶ Fig. 15.18).

Indications

- Seizure monitoring or resection of seizure focus
- Tumor or arteriovenous malformation (AVM) of the medial or lateral temporal lobe
- Vascular lesion of the temporal lobe

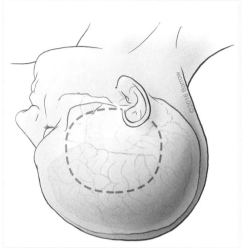

Fig. 15.18 Temporal approach.

Common Surgical Procedures

- Anterior temporal lobectomy
- Craniotomy for placement of grid/depth electrodes for seizure monitoring
- Decompressive hemicraniectomy
- Selective amygdalohippocampectomy

Postoperative Nursing Concerns

- Language or speech impairment, especially after surgery on the left hemisphere of the brain
- Neck pain related to intraoperative positioning of head
- CSF leak
- Deficits of CN III or CN VII
- Visual field defect
- Hemiparesis
- Seizure
- Trapped temporal horn of the lateral ventricle resulting in uncal herniation syndrome

Subtemporal Approach (Intradural or Extradural)

The subtemporal approach allows access to the posterior edge of the temporal lobe (▶ Fig. 15.19).

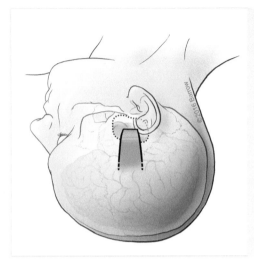

Fig. 15.19 Subtemporal approach.

Indications

- Acoustic neuroma
- Aneurysm of the posterior cerebral artery
- Aneurysm of the superior cerebellar/basilar artery
- Cavernous sinus lesion
- Complex large or giant basilar apex aneurysm

Common Surgical Procedures

- Tumor resection
- Evacuation of hematoma
- Aneurysm clipping (Video 15.1)
- Middle fossa approach for tumors along CN XII or CN XIII

Postoperative Nursing Concerns

- Seizure
- CSF leak
- Temporal lobe edema
- Stroke (may result from injury to the branches of the basilar artery)
- Diplopia (may result from injury of CN III and/or CN IV)
- Infarction (may result from injury to the venous sinuses)
- Facial nerve injury
- Unilateral eye dryness (may result from injury to the greater superior petrosal nerve)

Craniofacial Approaches to the Skull Base

The craniofacial approaches refer to gaining access to the brain via various parts of the face.

Indications

- Nasopharyngeal tumor
- Olfactory groove tumor
- Skull base tumor
- Sphenoid sinus mass
- Suprasellar tumor

Common Surgical Procedures

- Sublabial approach
- Supraorbital craniotomy (also called an *eyebrow craniotomy*)
- Transfacial approach (levels 1–6) (▶ Fig. 15.20)

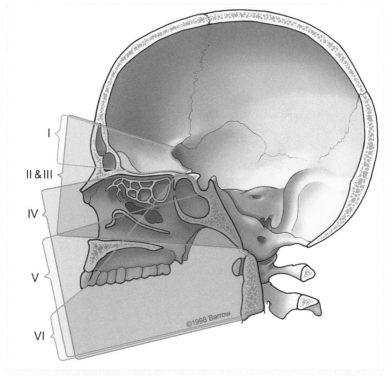

Fig. 15.20 Transfacial approach levels.

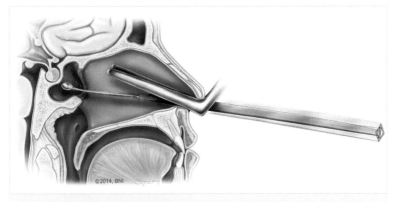

Fig. 15.21 Transsphenoidal approach.

- Transoral approach
- Transsphenoidal approach (▶ Fig. 15.21)

Postoperative Nursing Concerns

- CSF leak
- Infection (a common complication of manipulation of the paranasal sinuses)
- Wound healing, wound infection
- CN deficits
- Injury to internal carotid artery
- Tongue edema (with transoral/transpharyngeal approach)
- Diabetes insipidus; see Chapter 7, Table 7.5 Pituitary Apoplexy
- Nasal packing (Box 15.6 Transsphenoidal Surgery)

Box 15.6 Transsphenoidal Surgery

- During transsphenoidal surgery, the dura is excised and the sphenoid sinus is accessed. A fat pad is placed over the dura in closure to help prevent postoperative CSF leak
- After undergoing transsphenoidal surgery, patients should not use an incentive spirometer, nasal/facial bilevel positive airway pressure (BiPAP), or drinking straws because these increase the risk of fat pad displacement and can result in pneumocephalus and/or a CSF leak

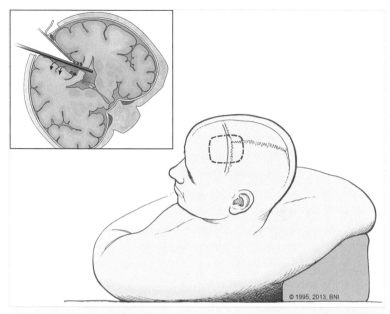

Fig. 15.22 Interhemispheric approach.

Interhemispheric Approach

The interhemispheric approach refers to gaining access to the intracranial contents via the top of the skull (▶ Fig. 15.22).

Indications

- Hypothalamic tumor
- Lateral ventricle lesion
- Third ventricle tumor

Common Surgical Procedures

- Corpus callosotomy
- Transcallosal approach
- Interforniceal approach

Postoperative Nursing Concerns

- Intraoperative sagittal sinus injury
- Injury to anterior cerebral arteries
- Hydrocephalus

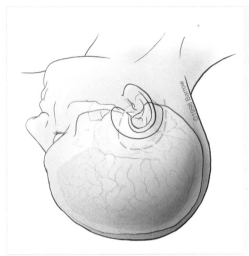

Fig. 15.23 Petrosal approach.

Postoperative Nursing Implications

- Ventricular drain care
- Memory deficits

Transpetrosal Approach

This approach involves accessing the skull just above and behind the ear (▶ Fig. 15.23).

Indications

- Acoustic neuroma
- Cerebellopontine angle tumor (tumor resected to preserve hearing)
- Lower basilar trunk aneurysm
- Petrous meningioma of superior, anterior, or medial posterior fossa
- Trigeminal neuralgia (this approach allows access to CN V)
- Vertebral artery aneurysm
- Vertigo and dizziness (this approach allows access to CN VIII)

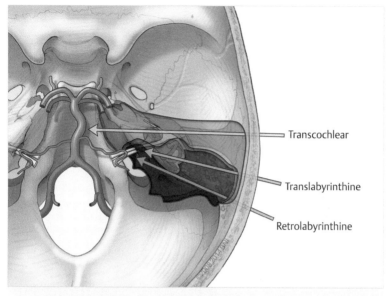

Fig. 15.24 Translabyrinthine approach.

Common Surgical Procedures

- Presigmoid approach
- Transcochlear approach
- Retrolabyrinthine approach
- Translabyrinthine approach (▶ Fig. 15.24)

Postoperative Nursing Concerns

- CSF leak
  - CSF leak is of particular concern for procedures using the translabyrinthine approach, and so a surgeon may choose to place a drain for 24 to 48 hours postoperatively (Box 15.7 Lumbar Drains)
  - Meningitis related to CSF leak
- Neck pain related to intraoperative positioning of the head
- Deficits of CN VII or CN VIII
- Brainstem stroke (may result from arterial, venous, or sinus occlusion)
- Ataxia related to cerebellar edema

Box 15.7 Lumbar Drains

- A lumbar drain alleviates or treats CSF leak by creating an alternate drainage route for CSF
  - The following elements are components of a lumbar drain:
    - Informed consent is required
    - Lumbar puncture performed under sterile conditions
    - Tubing is attached and secured to the skin, to the transducer, and to the drainage bag (as for external ventricular drain [EVD])
    - Drain is placed at desired lumbar level (per physician's orders)
    - Drainage is monitored closely and recorded hourly
  - Management of a lumbar drain is the same as that of an EVD; see also Chapter 3: Principles of Intracranial Pressure
  - A patient with a lumbar drain should be in the ICU

Craniotomy: Prone Position

- Mayfield head clamp and table attachment are used (▶ Fig. 15.25)
- Gel rolls under the patient, parallel to the length of the operating room table. One draw sheet is placed under the gel rolls and one is placed on top; the top draw sheet secures the gel rolls

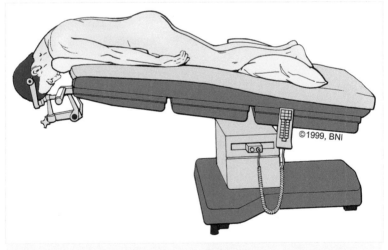

©1999, BNI

Fig. 15.25 Prone position for craniotomy.

- Draw sheets are brought together and secured around the patient's back; safety strap or 3-inch-wide adhesive tape encircles the patient and table three times
- Arms are wrapped circumferentially in egg crates and tucked at sides, thumbs down, under the top draw sheet
- Abdomen free from pressure to prevent decrease in epidural venous pressure and lessen intraoperative bleeding
- Foam padding under the knees
- Pillows under the shins, toes free from pressure
- Genitalia free from pressure
- Mild reverse Trendelenburg position assists with venous drainage
- Safety strap across the posterior thighs

Suboccipital/Posterior Fossa Approach

This approach allows access to the posterior fossa and the base of the occiput (► Fig. 15.26).

Indications

- Cerebellar or high spinal cord lesion/tumor/hematoma
- Chiari malformation
  - Fourth ventricle tumor
  - Tentorial meningioma

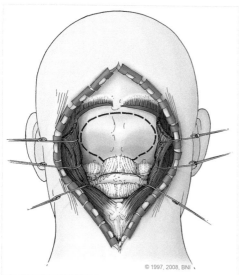

Fig. 15.26 Suboccipital/ posterior fossa approach.

© 1997, 2008, BNI

Common Surgical Procedures

- Chiari decompression
- Brain tumor resection

Postoperative Nursing Concerns

- Injury to occipital nerve (may result in new visual field deficits)
- Delayed venous infarct

Far-Lateral Approach to the Skull Base

The far-lateral approach is the favored approach for access to the skull base (▶ Fig. 15.27).

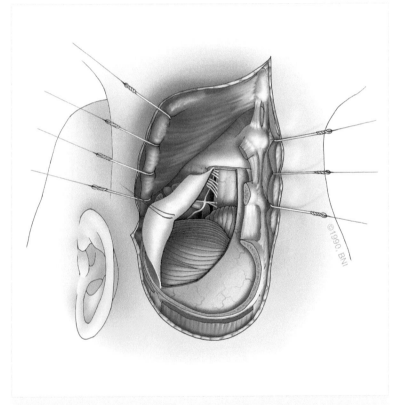

Fig. 15.27 Far-lateral approach.

Indications

- Anterolateral upper cervical spine lesion
- Cervicomedullary junction lesion
- Foramen magnum lesion
- Lower clivus lesion

Common Surgical Procedures

- Far-lateral craniotomy
- Suboccipital craniotomy

Postoperative Nursing Concerns

- Hydrocephalus; may require EVD
- CSF leak
- Deficits associated with damage to lower CNs, including the following:
  - Dysphagia
  - Poor airway protection
- Vertebral artery injury

Postoperative Nursing Implications

- Swallow evaluation, if patient is experiencing dysphagia
- Consultation from ears, nose, and throat specialist in patients with pre- or postoperative vocal cord paralysis

Supracerebellar–Infratentorial Approach

This approach offers access to structures in the posterior temporomedial area of the brain (▶ Fig. 15.28).

Indications

- Dorsal midbrain lesion
- Pineal region tumor
- Some lesions of the cerebellar peduncle
- Thalamic lesion

Common Surgical Procedures

- Lateral approach
- Midline approach
- Transtentorial approach

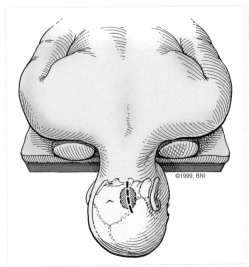

Fig. 15.28 Supracerebellar–infratentorial approach.

Postoperative Nursing Concerns

- Superior sagittal sinus and transverse sinus are at increased risk for intraoperative injury
- Hematoma related to inadequate hemostasis
- Venous infarction
- Cortical blindness
- Cerebral edema due to poor venous drainage (symptoms are similar to those of patients with pseudotumor cerebri)
- Posterior fossa syndrome (Box 15.8 Posterior Fossa Syndrome)

Box 15.8 Posterior Fossa Syndrome

- Mimics symptoms of meningitis, including nuchal rigidity
- Negative CSF cultures
- Seen in patients who have undergone surgery in the posterior fossa and have blood in the CSF

Craniotomy: Lateral Position

- Mayfield 3-point head holder is used
- The patient is usually positioned laterally (▶ Fig. 15.29), although the surgeon may instead prefer that the patient be in supine position, with a gel roll under the shoulder to tilt the patient away from the side of the pathologic lesion

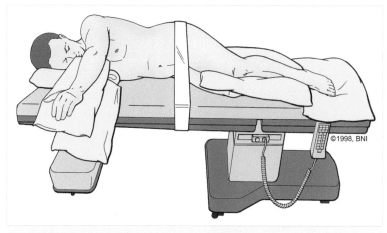

Fig. 15.29 Lateral position for craniotomy.

- If the patient is positioned in the true lateral position, he or she may be positioned atop a "bean bag." This pad covers the entire table, and once the patient is positioned, excess air is sucked from the bag, allowing it to contour to the patient's body and stabilize him or her in the lateral position
- Axillary roll under dependent arm
- May use airplane arm support, depending on the preference of the anesthesiologist and surgeon
- Arms are flexed at 90/90 position on padded arm boards, with the axillae padded
- Pillows between knees, ankles, and arms for support
- Foam padding under flexed knees and ankles
- Genitalia free from pressure
- Padded safety strap around lateral superior thigh, or safety strap or 3-inch-wide adhesive tape with padding against the skin at the hips and thighs

Lateral Suboccipital/Retrosigmoid Approach

This approach allows the surgeon to access the intracranial contents from just behind the ear (▶ Fig. 15.30).

Indications

- Access to CN V, CN VII, CN VIII, CN IX, CN X, and CN XI
- Cerebellopontine angle tumor (procedure performed to preserve hearing)
- Microvascular decompression for
  ○ Trigeminal neuralgia
  ○ Hemifacial spasm
  ○ Glossopharyngeal neuralgia

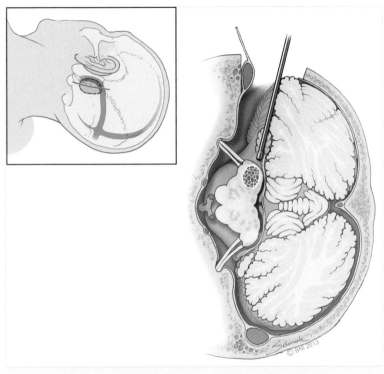

Fig. 15.30 Lateral suboccipital/retrosigmoid approach.

Common Surgical Procedures

- Lateral supracerebellar–infratentorial craniotomy
- Retrosigmoid craniotomy

Postoperative Nursing Concerns

- CSF leak
  - Meningitis or pseudomeningocele may lead to intracranial abscess or osteomyelitis of the bone flap
- Hydrocephalus
- Deficits of CN V, CN VII, CN VIII, CN IX, CN X, and CN XI
- Cerebellar edema; ataxia
- Brainstem stroke from venous, arterial, or sinus occlusion

Spine Surgery: Supine Position

- Mayfield 3-point head holder is used
- Pillow under the knees
- Foam padding between the ankles and the knees
- Small towel under the lordotic curve of the lower back
- Padded safety strap across the anterior thighs

Transoral Approach

The transoral approach involves using the mouth as a way to access the cranio-vertebral junction and the cervical spine (▶ Fig. 15.31).

Indications

- Anterior craniovertebral junction tumor/lesion
- Atlantodental synovial cyst
- Basilar invagination
- Midline anterior lesion between the clivus and the lower body of C2
- Odontoid fracture
- Rheumatoid arthritis

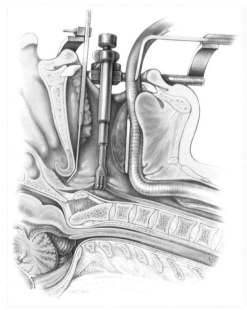

Fig. 15.31 Transoral approach.

Common Surgical Procedures

- Anterior odontoid screw fixation
- Removal of tumor or cyst

Postoperative Nursing Implications

- A feeding tube is usually placed intraoperatively (avoiding the posterior pharyngeal incision) to provide nutritional support, as the oral mucosa require at least 4 days to heal
- Observe oral mucosa for healing and for complications such as dehiscence, CSF leak, or retropharyngeal abscess
- Prescribed medications may include the following:
  - Intravenous antibiotics to prevent infection
  - H2 blocker or proton pump inhibitor to decrease reflux
  - Steroids to control inflammation
- Patient may experience dysphagia resulting from incisional edema and/or from the tongue obstructing the airway
- Patient may remain intubated for 1 to 3 days, due to edema
- Patient may be fitted for a hard cervical collar, or possible halo fixation. See Chapter 12, **Table 12.9**: Spinal Stabilization Devices, and **Table 12.10**: Nursing Care for Patients in Spinal Orthoses

Anterior Cervical Approach

This approach is used to gain access to the cervical spine through patient's anterior side (▶ Fig. 15.32).

Indications

- Anterior cervical tumor
- Anterior osteophyte formation
- Cervical cord compression from ossification of the posterior longitudinal ligament
- Cervical fracture (compression/burst) with instability
- Cervical spinal stenosis
- Cervical spondylosis with radiculopathy and/or myelopathy
- Herniated cervical disk with radiculopathy and/or myelopathy
- Posterior osteophyte formation

Common Surgical Procedures

- Anterior cervical corpectomy with fusion and plating
- Anterior cervical diskectomy or microdiskectomy with or without fusion and plating

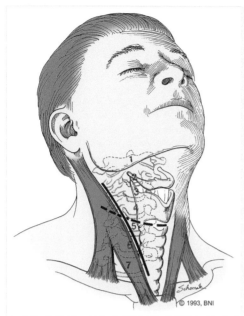

Fig. 15.32 Anterior cervical approach.

Fusion Options

- Autograft hip graft
- Allograft fibular strut
- Trabecular metal (Zimmer Biomet, Warsaw, Indiana)
- Synthetic cage

Postoperative Nursing Concerns

- Hoarseness due to laryngeal nerve injury
- Tracheal deviation due to hematoma (may cause airway emergency)
- Pneumothorax
- Dysphagia due to local tissue edema (from prolonged tissue retraction)
- Patient may need a hard cervical collar for uninstrumented or multilevel instrumented cases
- Patient may need a soft cervical collar for single-level instrumented cases (for comfort only)
- CSF leak
- Altered mental status may indicate carotid artery or vertebral artery injury

Spine Surgery: Prone Position

- Arms wrapped circumferentially in egg crate and tucked at sides, thumbs down
- Foam padding placed under the knees
- Pillows under the shins, toes free from pressure
- Genitalia free from pressure
- Padded safety strap across the posterior thighs

Suboccipital Approach

The suboccipital approach offers access to the cervical spine as well as the foramen magnum and posterior fossa (▶ Fig. 15.33).

Indications

- Chiari malformation/decompression with removal of arch of C1
- Occipital-to-cervical fusion

Common Surgical Procedures

- Occipitalcervical instrumentation and fusion
- Posterior cervical laminectomy
- Suboccipital decompression for Chiari malformation
- Transarticular screws/fusion

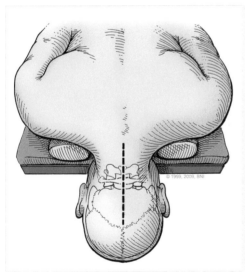

Fig. 15.33 Suboccipital approach.

Postoperative Nursing Concerns

- CSF leak or pseudomeningocele may contribute to poor wound healing, dehiscence, or infection
- Headache from CSF leak or posterior fossa syndrome
- Cranial nerve deficits
- Vertebral artery injury or stroke
- Pulmonary complications due to prone position
- Hemovac drain (Zimmer Biomet) or Jackson-Pratt drain for occipitalcervical fusion

Posterior Cervical Approach

This approach is used to gain access to the cervical spine through patient's posterior side (▶ Fig. 15.34).

Indications

- Central cord syndrome
- Cervical radiculopathy or myelopathy
- Cervical spine stabilization

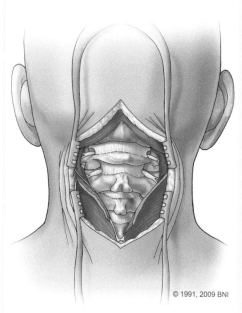

Fig. 15.34 Posterior cervical approach.

© 1991, 2009 BNI

- Cervical stenosis
- Chiari malformation
- Ossification of posterior longitudinal ligament
- Spinal tumor
- Spinal vascular malformation
- Syrinx
- Tethered cord

Common Surgical Procedures

- Posterior cervical diskectomy
- Posterior cervical laminectomy/hemilaminectomy or laminotomy with decompression
- Posterior fossa decompression with suboccipital craniectomy and C1 laminectomy, instrumentation, and fusion
- Selective dorsal rhizotomy

Fusion Options

- Allograft
- Autograft posterior iliac crest

Postoperative Nursing Concerns

- CSF leak or pseudomeningocele may lead to the following:
  - Poor wound healing or dehiscence
  - Infection
- Intramedullary hematoma
- Occlusion of intramedullary arteries, leading to spinal cord infarction
- Possible cranial nerve deficits
- Possible spinal cord or nerve root injury
- Possible vertebral artery injury or stroke
- Pulmonary function may be decreased due to prone position

Postoperative Nursing Implications

- Soft cervical collar for comfort; should be removed to accommodate air circulation needs
- Posterior neck heat and moisture may provide environment conducive to bacterial growth. Facilitate air flow to posterior neck by positioning the patient on his or her side with the head and neck supported
- Hemovac drain (Zimmer Biomet) or Jackson-Pratt drain for occipitalcervical fusion

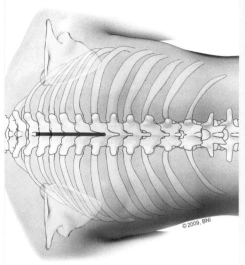

Fig. 15.35 Posterior thoracic approach.

Posterior Thoracic Approach

This is the standard approach for access to the thoracic vertebrae (▶ Fig. 15.35).

Indications

- Arthrodesis
- AVM
- Compression fracture
- Cordotomy
- Deformity
- Foraminal stenosis
- Instrumentation
- Syrinx
- Tethered cord
- Thoracic myelopathy
- Thoracic radiculopathy
- Thoracic stenosis
- Trauma
- Tumor (intradural-extramedullary, intradural-intramedullary, extradural, or of the vertebral body)

Common Surgical Procedures

- Dorsal root entry zone
- Intradural/epidural removal of tumor
- Kyphoplasty/vertebroplasty
- Lateral mass rods and screws or lateral mass plates for stabilization
- Posterior thoracic fusion
- Posterior thoracic hooks and rods
- Selective posterior rhizotomy
- Syringopleural shunt
- Thoracic decompressive laminectomy
- Transpedicular laminectomy

Postoperative Nursing Concerns

- Pulmonary function may be decreased due to prone position
- Hemovac drain (Zimmer Biomet)
- Nerve root injury
- Spinal cord injury
- CSF leak or dural tear
- Prolonged prone position may cause orbital/facial edema
- Iliac crest hematoma, if autograft was harvested

Postoperative Nursing Implications

- Pre- or postoperative steroids may be prescribed for patients undergoing decompression surgery
- Patient may be on intravenous (IV) antibiotics for 24 hours, or until Hemovac is discontinued
- Assess patient for eye injury/blindness from prone position

Posterior Lumbar Approach

The posterior lumbar approach allows access to the lumbar spine when the patient is in the prone position (▶ Fig. 15.36). Patients undergoing certain types of lumbar surgery (e.g., laminectomy, microdiskectomy) may be placed on a Wilson frame to keep them in a position of slight flexion (▶ Fig. 15.37).

Indications

- Cauda equina syndrome
- Deformity
- Instrumentation
- Lumbar spinal stenosis
- Lumbosacral cyst
- Spinal instability
- Tumor
- Vascular malformation

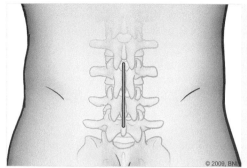

Fig. 15.36 Posterior lumbar approach.

© 2009, BNI

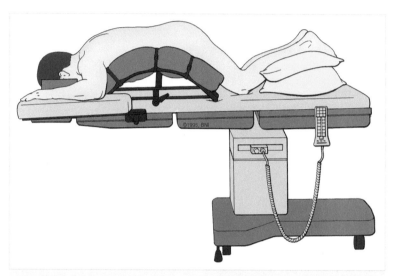

Fig. 15.37 Lumbar surgery on Wilson frame.

Common Surgical Procedures

- Decompressive lumbar laminectomy
- Lumbar microdiskectomy with or without foraminotomy
- Lumbar pedicle screw/rod fixation
- Posterior lumbar interbody fusion
- Transforaminal lumbar interbody fusion

Postoperative Nursing Concerns

- Patient will be unable to void
- Pulmonary function may be decreased due to prone position
- Hemovac drain (Zimmer Biomet)
- Nerve root injury
- Vascular injury (iliac artery/vein)
- Bowel/ureteral injury
- Possible instability related to facet joint removal without instrumentation
- CSF leak or dural tear
- Prolonged prone position may cause orbital/facial edema
- Iliac crest hematoma, if autograft was harvested
- Steroids may be considered for 24 to 48 hours if neurologic deficit or significant nerve root manipulation was required intraoperatively

Postoperative Nursing Implications

- Pre- or postoperative steroids may be prescribed for patients undergoing decompression surgery
- Patient may be on IV antibiotics for 24 hours, or until Hemovac is discontinued
- Assess patient for eye injury/blindness from prone position
- Pain control
  - Consider patient-controlled analgesia for patients who have undergone instrumentation procedures
- Encourage early ambulation

Spine Surgery: Lateral Position

- Foam head cradle or pillow
- Axillary roll under dependent arm
- Pillows between the arms, the knees, and the ankles
- Genitalia free from pressure
- Padded safety strap across lateral superior thigh

Transthoracic Thoracotomy

This procedure usually requires collaboration with a thoracic surgeon for incision and exposure.

Indications

- Herniated thoracic disk
- Infection/osteomyelitis
- Palliative decompression for metastatic disease

- Thoracic fracture (compression/burst) with instability
- Tumor; biopsy or removal of vertebral or paraspinal lesion

Common Surgical Procedures

- Debulking or removal of a thoracic lesion, with instrumentation and stabilization
- Thoracic corpectomy and fusion
- Thoracic diskectomy

Postoperative Nursing Concerns

- Respiratory distress
- Pleural/lung injury
- Pneumothorax
- Hematoma

Postoperative Nursing Implications

- Neurologic assessment and assessment of nerve root/spinal cord function for appropriate level should be compared with results of preoperative assessment
- Spine radiographs may be needed to view instrumentation and/or graft position
- Body mechanics instruction for patient
- Chest tubes (usually placed two levels below rib resection) to water seal drainage unit. These tubes will require close observation and meticulous care from the nurse
  - Cephalad placement for air
  - Caudal placement for fluid
  - Antibiotics are required until chest tube removal
  - Chest tube removal is based on output and chest radiograph
- Smoking cessation will improve pulmonary recovery and degree of bone fusion
- Lumbar drain with concurrent drain care should be considered if a dural tear is not adequately repaired or sealed intraoperatively
- Initial pain management may include patient-controlled analgesia, IV, or oral medication
- Bowel care regimen should be established. Patient may be prescribed a stool softener due to constipation concerns related to prescribed opiates

Retropleural Thoracotomy

This approach allows anterolateral access to the mid and lower thoracic spine, and one- to three-segment access to thoracolumbar junction.

Indications

- Compression/burst fracture
- Deformity
- Herniated thoracic disk
- Infection/osteomyelitis
- Vertebral body tumor

Common Surgical Procedures

- Debulking or removal of a lesion with instrumentation and fusion
- Thoracic corpectomy with instrumentation and fusion
- Thoracic diskectomy

Postoperative Nursing Concerns

- Rib is removed for surgical access
- Intercostal neuralgia
- Pneumothorax is a concern; chest radiograph should be carried out in postanesthesia care unit (PACU) and on postoperative day (POD) 1
- Hematoma may result from vascular injury

Postoperative Nursing Implications

- Thoracolumbosacral orthosis (TLSO) may be required for patients who have undergone corpectomy or instrumentation
- Chest tube may be placed if a pleural tear occurs intraoperatively
- Antibiotics should be continued until drains are removed
- Spine radiographs may be needed to visualize instrumentation and/or graft placement

Costotransversectomy

This approach allows posterolateral access to the thoracic spine.

Indications

- Biopsy of paraspinal or vertebral body lesion
- Corpectomy, decompression, or instrumentation
- Debulking of metastatic lesion
- Herniated thoracic disk
- Infection or osteomyelitis

Common Surgical Procedures

- Debulking or removal of a lesion with instrumentation and fusion
- Herniated thoracic disk

Postoperative Nursing Concerns

- Rib is removed for surgical access
- Hematoma
- Pain or intercostal neuralgia
- Hemovac drain (Zimmer Biomet)
- Respiratory distress and pneumothorax are concerns associated with this approach; chest radiograph should be carried out in PACU and on POD 1

Postoperative Nursing Implications

- Chest tube may be placed if a pleural tear occurs intraoperatively
- Continue antibiotics until drains discontinued
- TLSO may be required for patients who have undergone corpectomy or instrumentation
- Spine radiographs may be needed to visualize instrumentation and/or graft placement

Retroperitoneal Approach

This approach allows anterolateral access to the lumbar spine from L2 to L5 (▶ Fig. 15.38).

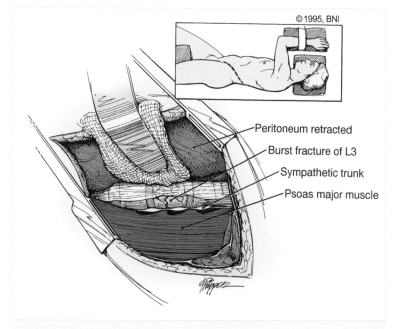

©1995, BNI

Peritoneum retracted
Burst fracture of L3
Sympathetic trunk
Psoas major muscle

Fig. 15.38 Retroperitoneal approach.

Indications

- Anterior lumbar fusion
- Burst fracture
- Deformity
- Lumbosacral fusion
- Osteomyelitis
- Tumor of the vertebral body

Common Surgical Procedures

- Corpectomy and fusion
- Laparotomy for anterior lumbar interbody fusion

Fusion Options

- Allograft
- Autograft

Postoperative Nursing Concerns

- Nerve root injury
- Intraoperative vascular, bowel, or ureteral injury

Postoperative Nursing Implications

- Antibiotics treatment until drain removal
- TLSO or lumbosacral orthosis if the patient undergoes corpectomy or instrumentation

Thoracoscopic Approach

This minimally invasive approach allows access to the thoracic cavity via operative ports (▶ Fig. 15.39).

Indications

- Thoracic disc herniation (T2–T12, possibly L1)

Common Surgical Procedures

- Bilateral sympathectomy
- Biopsy of thoracic lesion
- Right thoracoscopic resection of extradural schwannoma
- Thoracoscopic diskectomy
- Vertebrectomy with reconstruction

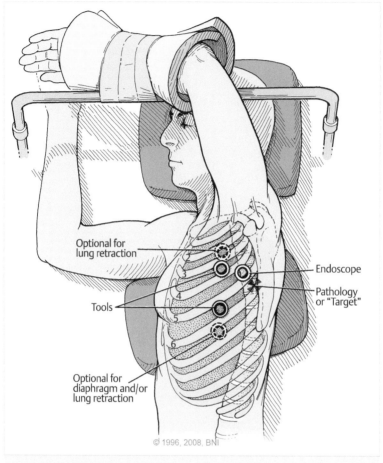

Fig. 15.39 Thoracoscopic approach.

Postoperative Nursing Concerns

- CSF fistula (resulting from CSF leak)
- Hematoma (hemothorax) or vascular injury
- Pneumothorax, pleural injury, or lung injury
- Procedure necessitates placement of chest tube connected to a water seal drainage unit

455

- ○ Chest radiograph should be obtained in PACU and on POD 1
- ○ Wean chest tube based on output. Surgeon will remove when less than 150 cc in a 24-hour period
- ○ Antibiotic therapy is required for 24 hours, or until chest tube removal

Postoperative Nursing Implications

- Wound care is required for the three trocar incisions (for the camera, retractor, and instruments)

15.5.3 Nerves Susceptible to Position-Related Injury

Brachial Plexus Nerve

- May occur in prone, supine, or lateral position
- Arm mobility should be limited to 90 degrees at shoulder and elbow to prevent stretch injury
- If the arms are placed laterally along the patient's sides, anatomical position should be observed (thumbs anterior, palms against side)
- In supine position, the arm board should be level with the table to prevent dorsal arm extension
- Lateral position may place excessive weight on abducted, internally rotated arm. If the upper arm is positioned above head, stretch injury may result
- Brachial nerve stretch is decreased when the head is in neutral position

Ulnar Nerve

- Elbows should be padded and positioned at the level of the table
- Excessive elbow extension should be avoided, given that it may compress the ulnar nerve
- Ulnar nerve injury may result from intermittent compression from blood pressure cuff if it is placed too close to the elbow

Radial Nerve

- The arm and wrist, including the fingers, should be padded in anatomical position and secured with the palm against the side at the level of the table
- The palm should face upward on a padded arm board at the level of the table

Median Nerve

- Elbow hyperextension or extension beyond the patient's normal range should be avoided. The arm should not hang unsupported off the bedside
- Avoid leaning against the patient's arm during surgery

Peroneal Nerve

- Avoid excessive pressure to the lateral distal knee when placing safety straps across the thighs. An egg crate should be placed under the safety strap
- Padding should be placed under the lateral aspect of the dependent knee in the lateral position, protecting the fibular head
- Avoid hip flexion with knee extension (stretch injury)
- Pillows should be used to provide support behind the knees instead of firm knee supports

Sciatic (Notch) Nerve

- Avoid hip flexion with knee extension (stretch injury)

Supraorbital Nerve

- The anesthesiologist frequently repositions the head while the patient is in prone position to avoid damage to the supraorbital nerve

Recurrent Laryngeal Nerve

- Patient should have an appropriately sized laryngeal mask
- The nerve should be retracted and dissected with the utmost precision and care

Facial Nerve

- Caution should be used during mask ventilation because excessive pressure on the face may damage the facial nerve

15.5.4 Common Position-Related Skin Breakdown Points

Bony Prominence and Soft-Tissue Injury Prevention/ Assessment

Supine Position

- Occiput
- Face, ears, nose, and eyes
- Scapulae, shoulder, elbow, wrist, hand, and fingers
- Sacrum and coccyx
- Hip
- Ischial tuberosity
- Knee, patella, distal femur, proximal tibia, and fibula protuberances
- Heels, ankles, and toes

Prone Position

- Forehead, eyes, mouth, nose, ears, and chin
- Clavicle
- Shoulder, elbow, wrist, hand, and fingers
- Iliac crest
- Knee, patella, distal femur, proximal tibia, and fibula protuberances
- Heels, ankles, and toes

Lateral Position

- Dependent ear, eye, and cheek
- Scapulae, shoulder, elbow, wrist, hand, and fingers
- Dependent hip
- Dependent lateral knee
- Dependent lateral heel, ankle, and toes

Documentation of Postoperative Skin Condition

Pressure ulcer development falls into one of four stages:
- Stage I: Blanchable hyperemia
- Stage II: Extension through epidermis
- Stage III: Full-thickness skin loss
- Stage IV: Full-thickness wounds with extension into muscle, bone, or supporting structures
  - If burn eschar or slough overlies the wound, the wound cannot be classified according to this categorization system
  - Deep tissue injury should be suspected if the area is discolored or if the skin is blistered

15.6 Postoperative Nursing Care

15.6.1 PACU

- The PACU, or the recovery room, is the first stop after surgery, unless the patient is admitted directly to the ICU
- Patient will remain in the PACU until discharge criteria are met (patient may be discharged to the ICU or to a standard care floor bed). Those criteria may vary based on institution, but they usually include the following:
  - Acceptable neurologic status (as deemed by surgeon)
  - Stable respiratory and cardiovascular status
  - Pain and nausea are controlled and/or appropriate medications are prescribed
  - Patient is normothermic
- Some patients bypass the PACU and are transferred directly from the operating room to the ICU

15.6.2 ICU

- Patients are kept in the ICU until they are stable
- Admission to ICU depends on several factors, including the following:
  - Duration of surgery
  - Type of surgery (i.e., cranial or extensive spine procedure)
  - Intraoperative blood loss
  - Patient's medical condition, including comorbidities
- Patients in the ICU are closely supervised and assessed often
- The ICU offers advanced monitoring techniques, including intracranial pressure (ICP) monitoring, blood pressure via arterial line, central venous pressure monitoring, and other hemodynamic monitoring, as needed

15.7 Surgical Complications

15.7.1 Neurologic Complications

Craniotomy

Cerebral Edema

- Risk increases in prolonged procedures (> 6 hours), prolonged brain retraction, and repeat intracranial surgery
- Edema is most commonly seen in tumor resection procedures (especially resection of malignant tumors), but it can occur with other types of procedures that require craniotomy
- Signs and symptoms of cerebral edema may include change in neurologic status or exacerbation of preexisting focal neurologic deficits; see also Chapter 2: Assessment

Increased ICP

- May be caused by edema, hemorrhage, hydrocephalus, or pneumocephalus; see also Chapter 3: Principles of Intracranial Pressure

Cerebral Infarction

- May occur during periods of decreased cerebral blood flow
- Possible causes include surgical retraction injury, hypotension, or cerebral edema
- Signs and symptoms depend on the area of the brain affected by decreased or absent blood flow
- The goal of treatment is to prevent secondary injury and to salvage the penumbra by minimizing cerebral edema and providing adequate cerebral perfusion pressure

Cranial Nerve Injury

- Potential for cranial neuropathies depends on the type and location of surgery; see also Chapter 2: Assessment

Pneumocephalus

- Refers to the presence of air in the cranial vault. It may be observed on CT after craniotomy or it may be the result of traumatic penetrating injury
- Large amounts of air in the fixed space of the cranial vault may function in the same way that a space-occupying lesion would, resulting in increased ICP and/or pain (e.g., headache)
- Some studies have shown more rapid absorption of postoperative pneumocephalus when patients are given 100% oxygen by nonrebreather mask as opposed to breathing room air, but this practice remains controversial

Hydrocephalus

- Can occur in patients who have undergone craniotomy
- Common in patients with subarachnoid hemorrhage
- May be managed by drainage of CSF via lumbar drain or EVD
- May require ventriculoperitoneal shunt for long-term management; see also Chapter 4: Hydrocephalus

Seizures

- Can occur in any patient postoperatively, but seizures are a more common complication of surgical procedures focused near the motor area of the brain. See also Chapter 6: Seizures

Spine Surgery

Decreased Motor/Sensory Function

- May result from the following causes:
  - Hematoma
  - Infarction
  - Intraoperative manipulation
  - Postoperative edema

Bowel/Bladder Dysfunction

- May result from the following causes:
  - Hematoma
  - Infarction

- ○ Postoperative edema
- ○ Intraoperative nerve/cord/canal manipulation
- ○ Cauda equina syndrome; see also Chapter 12: Traumatic Spine Injury
- ○ Narcotics
- ○ Anesthesia

Gastrointestinal

- Ileus, an obstruction of the intestines, may be caused by the following factors:
  - ○ Surgical approach
  - ○ Narcotics
  - ○ Immobility

Nausea/Vomiting

- Multiple possible causes
  - ○ Increased ICP
  - ○ Pressure on the floor of the fourth ventricle in the medulla, which controls vomiting
  - ○ General anesthetic agents
  - ○ Narcotics for pain control
- Nausea and vomiting are common after posterior fossa craniotomy
- Patients with compromised swallowing or impaired gag reflex are at risk for aspiration
- Nausea and vomiting may be prevented with antiemetics
  - ○ Antiemetics should be administered with caution, given that some (e.g., promethazine) can cause depression of the central nervous system and altered level of consciousness (LOC)

CSF Leak

- May occur with any disruption of the dura during spinal or cranial surgery
- May heal without treatment, or may require a lumbar drain to divert CSF to the path of least resistance (Box 15.7 Lumbar Drains)
- Surgical repair of CSF leak may be warranted if it does not resolve on its own
- A dural defect with a long-standing CSF leak increases the risk of infection or meningitis

Hemorrhage

- Preventive measures are taken during cranial and spinal surgery to prevent intra- and postoperative hemorrhage; however, hemorrhage may still occur
- Abnormal bleeding inside the cranial vault may increase ICP and can result in neurologic deterioration

- Any change in neurologic status (as determined by neurologic assessment) should be reported immediately
- Hemorrhage can be confirmed by noncontrast CT or MRI (CT is the best imaging technique for demonstrating bleeding)
- Emergent surgery may be required, depending on the findings of CT and the patient's clinical status

15.7.2 Respiratory Complications

Airway Compromise

- Dysfunction of lower cranial nerves (i.e., CN IX, CN X, and CN XII) may result in impaired swallowing and gag reflexes, making it difficult for patients to protect the airway
- Decrease in LOC may compromise the airway
- Close observation of airway and respiratory status is required, and some patients need assistance in clearing secretions (via suctioning). Appropriate patient positioning can help prevent respiratory distress

Pneumonia/Atelectasis

- These complications are associated with immobility, intubation, and mechanical ventilation

15.7.3 Infection

Meningitis

- May occur when microorganisms invade CSF or the meninges; see also Chapter 10: Infectious Diseases
- May be caused by contamination during surgery, ventriculostomy, lumbar drains, or dural tear and resultant CSF leak
- Prophylactic intraoperative antibiotics may help prevent postoperative nosocomial meningitis

Abscess or Empyema

- May result from penetrating traumatic injury, IV drug usage, or surgery
- Symptoms depend on the location and severity of abscess or empyema
- A CT scan with contrast is usually sufficient to diagnose brain abscess; abscess appears as a ring-enhancing lesion on imaging
- Close observation and antibiotics are indicated for patients with cranial or spinal abscess
- Open craniotomy or craniotomy with stereotactic guidance may be necessary to drain a cranial abscess or empyema and obtain specimens for culture

Wound Infection

- Wound infection is a possible complication of any surgical procedure
- Antibiotics should be administered within 1 hour of the initial surgical incision and repeated intraoperatively during prolonged surgical procedures as indicated

15.7.4 Fluid and Electrolyte Abnormalities

- More common after craniotomy, especially when pituitary function is altered
- Common in patients with
  - Subarachnoid hemorrhage
  - Skull fractures
  - Craniofacial trauma or surgery
  - Hypothalamic or pituitary surgery
  - Brain tumors
- Hyponatremia is the most common electrolyte abnormality in postoperative neurosurgery patients; see also Chapter 5: Electrolyte Disorders
- Diabetes insipidus is also common in patients who have undergone pituitary surgery; see also Chapter 5: Electrolyte Disorders

15.7.5 Deep Vein Thrombosis and Pulmonary Embolus

- Common in patients with malignancies (e.g., brain tumors)
- Patients with history of deep vein thrombosis or pulmonary embolus are at greater risk
- Caution should be used when initiating anticoagulation therapy after surgery

15.8 Nursing Management for Patients Undergoing Neurosurgery

This chapter is intended as a basic reference for bedside care of neurologic patients undergoing neurosurgical intervention (▶ Table 15.2, ▶ Table 15.3, **Appendix A12: Nursing Management of Patients Undergoing Craniotomy**, and **Appendix A13: Nursing Management of Patients Undergoing Neurosurgery**). Neurosurgery is a vast, complex, and ever-changing topic, and individuals caring for these patients are tasked with staying abreast of new developments and treatment strategies. The reader is encouraged to consult the references at the end of this chapter to learn more about subjects of interest.

Table 15.2 Postoperative craniotomy: what to watch for

Problem	Indication	Nursing action	Rationale
Decline in neurologic function	Cerebral edema Hemorrhage Pneumocephalus	Perform complete neurologic assessment Compare to previous documented assessment Report any new decrease in examination	Declining neurologic function may be an indication of cerebral edema, hemorrhage, or infarct
Respiratory distress	Respiratory failure	Perform respiratory assessment, including respiration rate and pattern, oxygen saturation, ABGs, and pulmonary auscultation Prepare for intubation and mechanical ventilation Provide supplementary oxygen as indicated	Decreased LOC or a medical event, such as pulmonary embolus, pneumothorax, or myocardial infarction may increase the likelihood of respiratory failure
Seizure	Irritation of meninges, possibly from hematoma	Report if seizure is a new event for the patient Administer AEDs as ordered Check blood level of AED, if appropriate	Depending on the diagnosis, preoperative seizures may not be uncommon. They may also occur postoperatively

Abbreviations: ABGs, arterial blood gases; AED, antiepileptic drug; LOC, level of consciousness.

15.8.1 Neurologic Assessment

- Assess LOC; see also Chapter 2: Assessment
- Monitor for signs of increased ICP; see also Chapter 3: Principles of Intracranial Pressure
- Perform motor, sensory, CN, and cerebellar assessments
- Compare assessment findings with those of previous examinations, report any change

15.8.2 Respiratory Assessment

- Monitor respiratory rhythm and rate
- Monitor oxygen saturation levels
- Assess and protect airway
- Perform pulmonary auscultation

Table 15.3 Postoperative spinal surgery: what to watch for

Problem	Nursing action	Rationale
Decrease in motor or sensory function/gait	Neurologic assessment, including motor and sensory assessment	Neurologic function may worsen as a result of edema, hemorrhage, or infarction
Urinary retention	Strict intake and output Check PVR Timed voiding (every 4–6 h) Notify medical team for new symptoms of retention or incontinence	Common complication of lumbar surgery, also a result of opioid use Urinary retention or incontinence could be a symptom of cauda equina syndrome, a medical emergency that requires immediate treatment
Pain	Administer analgesic and muscle relaxants as ordered and as determined by the patient's pain level Assess the patient's response to the medications Use alternative pain relief methods when possible (e.g., ice or heat, massage, and repositioning)	Increased pain may cause the patient to refrain from activity Severe pain could indicate an unintended consequence of surgery (i.e., increased swelling, bleeding, disk fragment)
Patient/family teaching	Assessment of risk factors, such as smoking, excess weight, lack of exercise Education of proper body mechanics Appropriate exercise program Smoking cessation education	Many spinal disorders, such as DDD and disk herniation, are aggravated by poor body mechanics Smoking is not only detrimental to general health, but it also negatively affects bone health and slows healing

Abbreviations: DDD, degenerative disk disease; PVR, postvoid residual.

- Perform frequent oral care to prevent ventilator-acquired pneumonia
- Monitor chest tube output, as directed
- Encourage patient to use incentive spirometer, if he or she is not mechanically ventilated
- Assist with intubation as necessary

15.8.3 Cardiovascular Assessment

- Perform hemodynamic monitoring as indicated, including central and arterial lines
- Monitor blood pressure
- Monitor electrocardiogram for heart rate and arrhythmias

- Monitor laboratory values (especially CBC to monitor blood loss and leukocytosis)
- Perform examination of extremities, observing color, sensation, and pulses

15.8.4 Gastrointestinal Assessment

- Assess for bowel sounds, advance diet as tolerated by the patient
- Administer antiemetics as ordered
- Administer stool softeners to prevent constipation, and monitor frequency of bowel movements
- Administer H2 blockers or proton pump inhibitors as ordered to prevent gastrointestinal bleeding

15.8.5 Fluid, Electrolyte, and Nutrition Assessment

- Intake and output as indicated
- Monitor serum electrolytes
- Be aware of foods and medications that may affect sodium levels
- Use Chemsticks to monitor glucose levels
- Administer insulin as ordered
- Start diet as soon as bowel sounds are appreciated
- Advance diet (as tolerated by the patient and as ordered by the physician)

15.8.6 Integumentary Assessment

- Monitor incision for signs and symptoms of infection, excessive edema, hematoma, and adequate circulation
- Monitor incision for CSF leak
- Assess skin for signs of breakdown related to intraoperative positioning

15.8.7 Immobility

- Advance activity as indicated
- Encourage the patient to ambulate as early as possible; use sequential compression devices until that time
- Administer enoxaparin as indicated
- Assess patient for signs of DVT at every shift change

15.8.8 Pain Assessment

- Assess for presence and severity of pain using pain scale
- Administer medications as directed, taking care to avoid oversedation
- Use nonpharmacologic methods (e.g., ice/heat, massage, repositioning, reduction of environmental stimulus) to relieve pain (Box 15.9 Focus on: Postoperative Pain Control for the Elderly)

Box 15.9 Focus On: Postoperative Pain Control for the Elderly

Although older patients report the same levels of pain as younger patients, older patients tend to be undertreated. This may result in the following:
- Anxiety
- Delirium
- Depression
- Complications related to decreased activity
  - Pulmonary complications
  - Decreased functional status
  - Longer hospital stays

Older patients experience a higher peak and longer duration of effects from opioids. Therefore, when controlling postoperative pain in an elderly patient, the caregiver must do the following:
- Monitor the cumulative effects of all prescribed analgesics
- Be mindful that the patient may be satisfied with incomplete treatment of pain
- Consistently use a pain scale to have the patient indicate pain intensity
- Remember that cognitively impaired patients may require nonverbal behavior scales to measure pain intensity

15.8.9 Patient and Family Teaching

- Offer preoperative teaching as indicated
- Ensure completion of advanced directives
- Provide and review discharge instructions; see the sample discharge instructions for the patient's specific procedure in **Appendix B: Sample Discharge Instructions**

15.8.10 Collaborative Management

- Nursing
- Neurosurgery
- Neurology for management of neurologic manifestations (e.g., seizures)
- Neuroanesthesia (for anesthesia tailored to patients undergoing neurosurgical procedures)
- Neuropathology for tumor diagnosis
- Trauma surgery for management of coexisting conditions resulting from trauma
- Critical care intensivists/pulmonary specialists for management of critical care issues, including intubation and mechanical ventilation

- Internal medicine for management of generalized medical issues
- Infectious disease
- Therapies
  - Physical therapy
  - Occupational therapy
  - Speech therapy for swallow or cognitive evaluation
- Rehabilitation specialists or physiatrists
- Clergy
- Palliative care or hospice workers
- Social workers or case management personnel
- Other specialists as appropriate, depending on the underlying neurologic condition (e.g., brain tumor, epilepsy, stroke, or endocrine issues associated with pituitary lesions)

Video

Video 15.1 Aneurysm treated with clipping.

Suggested Reading

[1] American Association of Neuroscience Nurses. Cervical Spine Surgery: A Guide to Preoperative and Postoperative Patient Care. Chicago, IL: American Association of Neuroscience Nurses; 2007

[2] American Association of Neuroscience Nurses. Lumbar Spine Surgery: A Guide to Preoperative and Postoperative Care. Glenview, IL: American Association of Neuroscience Nurses; 2006

[3] Association of Perioperative Registered Nurses. Guidelines for Perioperative Practice. 2017 ed. Denver, CO; Association of Perioperative Registered Nurses; 2017

[4] Bader MK, Littlejohns LR, Olson DM, eds. AANN Core Curriculum for Neuroscience Nursing. 6th ed. Chicago, IL: American Association of Neuroscience Nurses; 2016

[5] Barker EM. Neuroscience Nursing: A Spectrum of Care. St. Louis, MO: Mosby Elsevier; 2008

[6] Barker FG, II. Efficacy of prophylactic antibiotics against meningitis after craniotomy: a meta-analysis. Neurosurgery. 2007; 60(5):887–894, discussion 887–894

[7] Beals SP, Joganic EF, Hamilton MG, Spetzler RF. Posterior skull base transfacial approaches. Clin Plast Surg. 1995; 22(3):491–511

[8] Connolly ES Jr, McKhann GM II, Huang J, Choudhri TF, Komotar RJ, Mocco J. Fundamentals of Operative Techniques in Neurosurgery. 2nd ed. New York, NY: Thieme Medical Publishers, Inc.; 2010

[9] Dezee KJ, Shimeall WT, Douglas KM, Shumway NM, O'Malley PG. Treatment of excessive anticoagulation with phytonadione (vitamin K): a meta-analysis. Arch Intern Med. 2006; 166(4):391–397

[10] Freeman WD, Brott TG, Barrett KM, et al. Recombinant factor VIIa for rapid reversal of warfarin anticoagulation in acute intracranial hemorrhage. Mayo Clin Proc. 2004; 79(12):1495–1500

[11] Gilroy J. Basic Neurology. 3rd ed. New York, NY: McGraw-Hill; 2000

[12] Gore PA, Maan H, Chang S, Pitt AM, Spetzler RF, Nakaji P. Normobaric oxygen therapy strategies in the treatment of postcraniotomy pneumocephalus. J Neurosurg. 2008; 108(5):926–929

[13] Greenberg MS. Handbook of Neurosurgery. 8th ed. New York, NY: Thieme Medical Publishers; 2016

[14] Gullo A, ed. Anaesthesia, Pain, Intensive Care and Emergency Medicine—A.P.I.C.E.: Proceedings of the 22st Postgraduate Course in Critical Medicine Venice-Mestre, Italy—November 9–11, 2007. Springer-Verlag Milan; 2008

[15] Hickey JV. Clinical Practice of Neurological and Neurosurgical Nursing. 7th ed. Philadelphia, PA: Lippincott Williams & Wilkins; 2013

[16] Kamada H, Yu F, Nito C, Chan PH. Influence of hyperglycemia on oxidative stress and matrix metalloproteinase-9 activation after focal cerebral ischemia/reperfusion in rats: relation to blood-brain barrier dysfunction. Stroke. 2007; 38(3):1044–1049

[17] Kaye AH, Black PM. Operative Neurosurgery. London, UK: Churchill Livingstone; 1999

[18] Kim D, Vaccaro A, Dickman C, Cho D, Lee S, Kim I, eds. Surgical Anatomy and Techniques to the Spine. 2nd ed. Philadelphia, PA: Elsevier Saunders; 2013

[19] Kosier MB, Minkler P. Nursing management of patients with an implanted Ommaya reservoir. Clin J Oncol Nurs. 1999; 3(2):63–67

[20] Lalwani A. Current Diagnosis and Treatment: Otolaryngology—Head and Neck Surgery. 3rd ed. New York, NY: McGraw-Hill Education; 2012

[21] Lexicomp Drug Information Handbook for Advanced Practice Nursing: A Comprehensive Resource for Nurse Practitioners, Nurse Midwives, and Clinical Specialists, Including Selected Disease Management Guidelines. 16th ed. Hudson, OH: Wolters Kluwer Clinical Drug Information, Inc; 2015

[22] McQuay N, Jr, Cipolla J, Franges EZ, Thompson GE. The use of recombinant activated factor VIIa in coagulopathic traumatic brain injuries requiring emergent craniotomy: is it beneficial? J Neurosurg. 2009; 111(4):666–671

[23] Nettina SM, ed. Lippincott Manual of Nursing Practice. 10th ed. Philadelphia, PA: Lippincott Williams & Wilkins; 2014

[24] Papadakis MA, McPhee SJ, Rabow MW, eds. Current Medical Diagnosis and Treatment 2017. 56th ed. New York, NY: McGraw-Hill Education; 2017

[25] Park TS, Bourgeois BF, Silbergeld DL, Dodson WE. Subtemporal transparahippocampal amygdalohippocampectomy for surgical treatment of mesial temporal lobe epilepsy. Technical note. J Neurosurg. 1996; 85(6):1172–1176

[26] Patel RS, Yousem DM, Maldjian JA, Zager EL. Incidence and clinical significance of frontal sinus or orbital entry during pterional (frontotemporal) craniotomy. AJNR Am J Neuroradiol. 2000; 21(7):1327–1330

[27] Pritchard C, Radcliffe J. General principles of postoperative neurosurgical care. Anaesth Intensive Care Med. 2008; 9(6):231–236

[28] Rhoton AL, Jr. Rhoton's Cranial Anatomy and Surgical Approaches. Philadelphia, PA: Lippincott Williams & Wilkins; 2007

[29] Rothrock JC. Alexander's Care of the Patient in Surgery. 15th ed. St. Louis, MO: Elsevier Mosby; 2015

[30] Rozet I, Vavilala MS. Risks and benefits of patient positioning during neurosurgical care. Anesthesiol Clin. 2007; 25(3):631–653

[31] Seçkin H, Avci E, Uluç K, Niemann D, Başkaya MK. The work horse of skull base surgery: orbitozygomatic approach. Technique, modifications, and applications. Neurosurg Focus. 2008; 25(6):E4

[32] St-Arnaud D, Paquin MJ. Safe positioning for neurosurgical patients. AORN J. 2008; 87(6):1156–1168, quiz 1169–1172

[33] Tighe SM. Instrumentation for the Operating Room: A Photographic Manual. 9th ed. St. Louis, MO: Elsevier Mosby; 2016

[34] Tummala RP, Coscarella E, Morcos JJ. Transpetrosal approaches to the posterior fossa. Neurosurg Focus. 2005; 19(2):E6

16 Radiotherapy

Maeve Dargush and Bryan Lee

Abstract

Radiotherapy refers to the use of high-energy X-rays or charged particles to treat lesions that are radiosensitive. It is typically used as an adjuvant therapy once pathology is determined for lesions of the brain or spine. Different types of radiotherapy are associated with different courses of treatment. The type of treatment used is determined by radiation oncologists. Regardless of the type of treatment, nurses and other health care providers assist patients in their treatment journey, and they must be aware of the possible effects and complications the patients might encounter along the way.

Keywords: brachytherapy, CyberKnife, external beam radiotherapy, Gamma Knife, radiation oncology, radiobiology, stereotactic radiosurgery

16.1 Radiation Therapy

Surgery is the first step of treatment for many patients with benign tumors or vascular lesions and for all patients with malignant tumors. In most cases, however, surgery alone is not enough—adjuvant therapy is also indicated. The term *radiation therapy* refers to the use of high-energy X-rays or charged particles to treat benign and malignant tumors and certain functional conditions. It is often performed after surgery or in patients whose tumors are unresectable or can only be partially resected. Radiation therapy can also serve as the primary treatment for radiosensitive lesions or for lesions located in an eloquent area of the brain.

Ionizing radiation disrupts atomic structures by ejecting orbiting electrons. These electrons break chemical bonds and ultimately effect biological change.

- If radiation has sufficient energy, it ejects one or more electrons from the atom or molecule in a process known as *ionization*. When radiation therapy is used as sole or adjuvant treatment, it is ionizing radiation
- The idea to apply ionizing radiation in cancer treatment was realized soon after the discovery of X-rays
- Radiation is thought to kill tumor cells by inducing lethal DNA damage
- Ionizing radiation is composed of electromagnetic radiation (e.g., X-rays and γ-rays) and particulate radiation (e.g., electrons, protons, neutrons, and α-particles)

Radiation can be produced by megavoltage machines and by radionuclides. Megavoltage machines, used for external beam radiotherapy (EBRT), include linear accelerators, cobalt-60 machines, and cyclotrons, which produce protons or neutrons. Radionuclides are natural radioactive sources that emit radiation in the form of particles or γ-rays, and they emit energy characteristic of that particular radionuclide. Types of therapy that use radionuclides include brachytherapy and radiopharmaceutical therapy (Box 16.1 Measurement of Radioactivity).

Radiation oncology is the medical specialty that uses ionizing radiation to eradicate malignancies as well as to treat some benign diseases.

- A treatment regimen is centered around a dose of radiation high enough to cure or control the tumor/disease but not so high as to seriously damage normal surrounding tissue
- The *tissue tolerance dose* is the amount of radiation that normal tissue can withstand while continuing to function

---

Box 16.1 Measurement of Radioactivity

- The unit of measurement for radioactivity is the *gray* (Gy)
- *RAD* is an older term that may still be used. It stands for *radiation absorbed dose* and is synonymous with centigray (cGy)
- 1 Gy =100 cGy = 100 RAD
- Activity of radioactive sources is measured in curies (Ci) or becquerel (Bq)

16.1.1 Principles of Radiobiology

Radiobiology is the study of events that occur after ionizing radiation is absorbed by a living organism.

- Radiation works at cellular level by breaking chemical bonds, eventually leading to tissue change
- Probability of cell death is higher if critical sites, such as DNA, are damaged by radiation
- Both normal and cancerous cells are susceptible to the effects of radiation
- Rapidly dividing cells are the most radiosensitive cells

The "Five Rs" of radiobiology—Repair, Redistribution, Reoxygenation, Repopulation, and Radiosensitivity—play a major role in a patient's response to radiation therapy and in tumor growth fraction and cell loss factor (Box 16.2 The "Five Rs" of Radiobiology). Different types of radiation therapy may be indicated depending on the disease and the patient. In this chapter, we discuss various types of radiotherapy, addressing the indications, standard dosing, and typical patient response for each.

> ## Box 16.2 The "Five Rs" of Radiobiology
>
> - **Repair** (of sublethal damage): Time period required for healthy cells to repair
> - **Redistribution**: Process of waiting for surviving tumor cells to enter more sensitive phases of the cell cycle, so that future radiation doses can kill them
> - **Reoxygenation** (of tumor cells): Occurs in tumor cells, but not in normal tissue. Tumor cells are generally hypoxic, but tumor cells with high intracellular oxygen concentration are more susceptible to radiation. During fractionated radiation treatment, oxygenated tumor cells are killed by early doses. The oxygen freed by this process can then diffuse to the radiation-resistant cells, oxygenating them and making them easier to kill at the next round of treatment
> - **Repopulation** (of normal tissue): Repopulation of stem cells and mature cells by surviving stem cells is a key factor in regaining tissue function after treatment
> - **Radiosensitivity**: Sensitivity or susceptibility of different cell types to X-rays or other sources of ionizing radiation

16.2 Types of Radiotherapy

16.2.1 External Beam Radiation Therapy

External beam radiotherapy delivers radiation from a distance to a defined target.

- Can be administered postoperatively or as an alternative to surgery
- May be given concurrently with chemotherapy
- Indicated in most types of malignancies
- Involves daily treatment over the course of several weeks to deliver radiation to the affected area
- Specific indications for radiotherapy in the central nervous system (CNS) are discussed later in this chapter

External Beam Radiotherapy Techniques Used in the Central Nervous System

- Craniospinal irradiation (CSI)
  - Irradiates the entire subarachnoid space
  - Technically challenging
  - Frequently used in management of pediatric patients with tumors of the CNS

- Whole brain irradiation (WBI)
  - Irradiates the entire brain
- Partial brain irradiation
  - Radiation directed at the primary tumor site and edema, plus an additional margin determined by protocol or by the treating physician
  - Most commonly used in adult patients with tumors of the CNS

Different techniques are used to plan the treatment course for tumors of the CNS. Modern computer technology has made three-dimensional (3D) treatment planning possible.

- Conformal radiotherapy (CRT)
  - Also known as 3D-CRT
  - Refers to the use of a patient's 3D geometry to select beam directions, determine doses, design beam apertures, evaluate plans, and verify effectiveness of treatment
- Intensity-modulated radiation therapy (IMRT)
  - Uses the same technology as in CRT, but creates beams of varying intensities, compared with the uniform doses contained in each 3D-CRT beam
- Both 3D-CRT and IMRT are intended to apply a lethal dose of radiation to the tumor while sparing normal surrounding tissue. These methods are used to treat most tumors of the CNS

16.2.2 Fractionation

Fractionation of treatment takes the total required dose of radiation and separates it into a number of equal daily treatments. Fractionation can reduce both acute side effects and late reactions to radiation.

- Spares normal tissue, as cells can repair and repopulate between doses of radiation
- May increase cancer cell damage due to reoxygenation of tumor cells between cycles. Reoxygenated tumor cells are more responsive to radiation treatment than hypoxic tumor cells
- Time between doses allows for reassortment of tumor cells into more radiosensitive cell cycles
- High-dose fractionation administered in a short period of time is likely to produce severe acute side effects, which may jeopardize completion of the radiation treatment
- Conventional fractionation usually involves one treatment per day, 5 days per week, at a dose of 1.8 to 2.2 Gy/fraction
- Hyperfractionation is a type of treatment designed to reduce late side effects. Patients undergoing hyperfractionation usually receive two treatments per day, roughly 6 hours apart

- Accelerated fractionation, also called *hypofractionation*, decreases overall treatment time but can increase acute effects both to tumor tissue and normal tissue

16.2.3 Stereotactic Radiosurgery

The word *stereotactic* refers to precise localization of a specific target point based on 3D coordinates derived either from imaging or from external devices. Stereotactic radiosurgery (SRS) is a treatment strategy in which narrow beams of radiation are focused on a precise target and deliver a high dose of localized radiation to that target (Box 16.3 Stereotactic Radiosurgery).

- If the dose gradient (i.e., the degree to which beams are focused on the target and spare surrounding tissues) is very steep at the edges of target, a single dose can cause tumor necrosis
- Fractionated SRS refers to stereotactically guided high-dose radiation administered to a precisely defined target over the course of two to five separate treatment sessions

There are many different modalities for SRS, including Gamma Knife (Elekta Instruments, Inc., Crawley, UK), LINAC-based SRS, CyberKnife (Accuray, Sunnyvale, CA), and proton beam SRS.

Box 16.3 Stereotactic Radiosurgery

- Types of lesions/disorders
  - Arteriovenous malformation
  - Benign or malignant tumor
  - Brain metastasis
  - Trigeminal neuralgia
  - Vestibular schwannoma
- Indications
  - Adjuvant to surgery or EBRT
  - Alternative to surgery
  - Primary management in selected patients
  - Recurrent lesions
  - Subtotal resection of lesions
- Key requirements for optimal stereotactic irradiation
  - Accurate radiation delivery
  - Exclusion of sensitive structures
  - High conformity of lesion
  - Sharply defined target
  - Small target/volume

Gamma Knife

- The Gamma Knife system is a machine that contains 192 sources of cobalt-60 radiation (Video 16.1)
- Radiation sources are oriented in such a way that all beams converge at a single point, referred to as the *isocenter*
- Target accuracy is between 0.1 and 1 mm
- A rigid head frame is used to limit motion during treatment. This frame, which is essential for treatment, means that Gamma Knife treatment is limited to targets in the head or upper cervical spine
- Frame-based methodologies such as Gamma Knife are the gold standard for SRS

LINAC-Based Stereotactic Radiosurgery

- Similar to Gamma Knife, but multiple noncoplanar arcs of radiation are used instead of cobalt sources
- Multiple arcs of radiation intersect at the isocenter, resulting in high doses at the beam convergence with the surrounding normal tissue receiving only a minimal dose

CyberKnife

- Device that uses an image-guided robotic system with a mobile linear accelerator
- Uses the skeletal structure of the body as a reference frame for targeting, instead of a rigid head frame

Proton Beam Therapy

- This type of therapy involves the use of protons instead of X-rays to target tumors. These charged particles (i.e., protons) cause the most ionization at energy-dependent depth
- Almost no exit dose; therefore, a smaller volume of normal tissue is exposed
- This is a very expensive technology and is currently only available at a limited number of centers

16.2.4 Internal Radiation

Internal radiation, or brachytherapy, involves surgical implantation of a radioactive source in or beside a tumor.

- Implanted during surgery or through a device (i.e., a catheter)
- Delivers a large dose of radiation to the tumor volume, with rapid fall-off in surrounding tissues

- Source works by releasing low-dose radiation for duration of the life of the isotope
- The isotope most commonly used in internal radiation procedures is iodine-125
- Interest in brachytherapy has waned with the advent of IMRT, 3D-CRT, and SRS, as these treatment options offer greater radiobiological and dosimetric advantages compared with brachytherapy
- Studies have failed to demonstrate the efficacy of brachytherapy in the treatment of malignant gliomas

16.3 Indications for Radiation Therapy in the Central Nervous System

Radiation therapy may be used to treat both benign and malignant conditions of the CNS; see also Chapter 7: Tumors.

- Tumors of the brain, supporting structures, and spine vary widely from benign to malignant
- Primary and metastatic tumors arising from or affecting these structures are of great interest to radiation oncologists, due to their sensitivity to radiation therapy (▶ Table 16.1)
- Even tumors that are pathologically benign may be life threatening due to their location or effect on surrounding structures. See Box 7.3: Benign Tumors in Chapter 7: Tumors
- Normal tissue in the CNS is often incapable of regeneration, which may make complete surgical resection or high doses of radiation unsafe
- Tumors of the spinal cord may be treated differently than tumors of the brain due to the increased dose tolerance of the spinal cord and its location

Table 16.1 Types of central nervous system lesions treated with radiation/radiosurgery

Malignant tumors	Benign tumors	Functional disorders
Astrocytoma: grades I–IV	Meningioma	Trigeminal neuralgia
Oligodendroglioma	Pituitary adenoma	
Oligoastrocytoma	Arteriovenous malformation	
Ependymoma	Cranial nerve and spinal cord schwannoma	
Medulloblastoma	Neurofibromatosis	
Primitive neuroectodermal tumor	Craniopharyngioma	
Chordoma/chondrosarcoma	Glomus jugulare	
Primary CNS lymphoma	Paraganglioma	
Hemangiopericytoma (solitary fibrous tumor)	Hypothalamic hamartoma	
Pineal region tumor		
Metastatic tumor		

Abbreviation: CNS, central nervous system.

16.3.1 Dosing

Most primary adult tumors are treated with partial brain irradiation using conventional fractionated EBRT (e.g., IMRT, 3D-CRT).

- General guidelines call for doses of 50 to 54 Gy for benign/low-grade lesions of the CNS and 60 Gy for malignant primary lesions of the CNS
- Dosage to the optic nerves, optic chiasm, brainstem, and spinal cord is a limiting factor as injury can occur after high doses. More sophisticated technologies and novel fractionation may be indicated
- Prior CNS surgery or radiation therapy, comorbidities, advanced age, smoking history, and tumor location may be contraindications for radiation therapy, given they may increase the risk for radiation-induced injury
- The decision to treat a specific tumor is based on many factors, including the following:
  - Patient's age
  - Patient's medical history
  - Tumor pathology and location
  - Extent of tumor resection
  - Physician judgment (▶ Table 16.2)
- Radiation dose constraints are based on many factors, including the following:
  - Patient's history
  - Tumor pathology and location
  - Physician's judgment (▶ Table 16.3)
- Patients may receive a combination of both EBRT and SRS

16.4 Preparation for Treatment

Whether the patient is undergoing intracranial or extracranial radiation treatment, the patient must undergo treatment simulation. The treatment planning session usually takes place a few days before the start of therapy, unless radiation must occur in an emergent manner. With some SRS techniques (e.g., Gamma Knife), planning and treatment occur on the same day.

16.4.1 Simulation

Patients undergoing EBRT require treatment simulation. This establishes a reproducible treatment position upon which daily radiation treatments will be modeled. This is a necessary part of any radiation treatment to ensure the accurate dose is delivered to the intended target.

- The ability to reproduce the position at each treatment session is critical to ensure the tumor receives the maximum radiation dose and normal surrounding tissue suffers only minimal damage

Table 16.2 Treatment recommendations for specific types of lesions/tumors

Type of lesion/tumor	Radiation treatment recommendations
Glioblastoma multiforme	EBRT up to 60 Gy, concurrent with chemotherapy using temozolomide (Temodar)
Anaplastic astrocytoma	EBRT to 60 Gy, concurrent with chemotherapy
Anaplastic oligodendroglioma	EBRT to 60 Gy, either sequential to (standard) or concurrent with chemotherapy
Low-grade astrocytoma	EBRT to 54 Gy vs. observation if GTR of tumor
Oligodendroglioma	EBRT vs. chemotherapy vs. observation
Pituitary adenoma	Nonfunctioning: observation vs. SRS or EBRT up to 45–50 Gy Functioning (secretory): observation vs. medical management vs. SRS or EBRT
Meningioma	Grade I: Observation vs. SRS to residual Grade II or anaplastic: EBRT or SRS to residual Inoperable: EBRT or SRS alone Recurrence: EBRT or SRS as salvage
Ependymoma (including anaplastic)	If GTR: radiotherapy up to 54–60 Gy Subtotal resection with positive CSF culture: CSI up to 36 Gy, with additional dose to gross disease up to 54–60 Gy, if needed Recurrence: EBRT if no prior radiotherapy; SRS for salvage
Metastases	WBI up to 30–37.5 Gy vs. SRS alone for fewer than four metastatic lesions Spine: EBRT up to 30–45 Gy Recurrence: SRS as salvage vs. repeat WBI
Arteriovenous malformation	SRS as adjuvant therapy (or when surgical resection/embolization are not possible)
Vestibular schwannoma	SRS for small lesions, adjuvantly for residual tumor or recurrence
Primary CNS lymphoma	Chemotherapy vs. WBI up to 45 Gy (radiotherapy is rarely undertaken due to potential neurotoxicity, but may be used in cases of recurrence)
Medulloblastoma	Standard risk: reduced-dose CSI concurrent with chemotherapy up to 23.4 Gy with additional dose to posterior fossa to 54 Gy, if needed High risk: CSI up to 36–39 Gy with posterior fossa and metastases boosted to 54 Gy, plus chemotherapy

Abbreviations: CNS, central nervous system; CSF, cerebrospinal fluid; CSI, craniospinal irradiation; EBRT, external beam radiotherapy; GTR, gross total resection; Gy, gray; SRS, stereotactic radiosurgery; WBI, whole brain irradiation.

Table 16.3 Conventional fractionation dose tolerance guidelines for critical structures in the central nervous system

Site	Maximum tolerance dose
Whole brain	60 Gy
Partial brain	60–70 Gy
Brainstem	54 Gy
Spinal cord	45–55 Gy
Optic chiasm	50–54 Gy
Retina	45 Gy
Optic lens	10 Gy

Abbreviation: Gy, gray.

- A thermoplastic mask is fabricated for each patient for customized immobilization
- Imaging studies such as computed tomography and, in some cases, magnetic resonance imaging (MRI) are performed to better define tumor volume and normal surrounding critical structures
- Simulation of radiation therapy for the spinal cord is similar. However, rather than the mask used in patients receiving cranial radiation, patients receiving spinal cord radiation receive permanent marks (i.e., tattoos) on the skin to ensure consistent positioning for treatment

16.4.2 Simulation for Steriotactic Radiosurgery

- It depends on the type of SRS
  - CyberKnife simulation is similar to the simulation described earlier for EBRT. It involves a meticulous stereotactic planning process, rigorous quality assurance, and supervision of simulated radiation delivery
  - Patients undergoing Gamma Knife and CyberKnife procedures generally require collaborative treatment planning from radiation oncologists, neurosurgeons, and radiation physicists

16.4.3 Potential Side Effects

Radiation treatment is a form of local therapy, so side effects are generally confined to the treatment region.

- Acute side effects usually do not manifest until after 2 to 3 weeks of treatment
- Patients are monitored for side effects during treatment, and those side effects are managed as they occur in an effort to keep the patient comfortable, to reduce complications, and to help prevent prolonged treatment breaks

- Patients may experience emotional reactions to diagnosis and therapy, including fear, depression, and anxiety. Education, counseling, and medication should be offered as indicated to ameliorate these emotions

Early Side Effects

Acute Alopecia

- Alopecia is hair loss that occurs approximately 3 to 4 weeks into conventional therapy. It occurs as the result of radiosensitivity of the hair follicles and glands
- May occur after doses as low as 5 Gy and is usually temporary
- Doses of 45 Gy or greater may cause permanent hair loss or delayed regrowth
- Alopecia occurs regionally in the path of the radiation beam
- Hair loss over the entire scalp occurs after WBI

Acute Radiation Myelopathy

- May occur after radiation to the spinal cord; involves transient demyelination of the myelin-producing oligodendroglial cells in the targeted spinal cord segment
- May occur as transient phenomenon
- Acute myelopathy is clinically manifested by momentary electric shock–like sensations and numbness from the neck down to the extremities when the neck is flexed (i.e., Lhermitte's sign)
- Early delayed myelopathy usually occurs 1 to 6 months after cessation of radiotherapy, and often resolves within 6 to 12 months

Cerebral Edema

- Most commonly occurs when large doses of radiation are delivered to the brain
- Incidence of cerebral edema increases with higher doses per fraction (between 1.8 and 2.0 Gy is generally a well-tolerated dose)
- Potential for cerebral edema increases if patients are weaned off steroids too rapidly after surgery (Box 16.4 Clinical Alert: Treatment-Related Toxicities)
- Symptoms include headache, nausea, vomiting, and decreased neurologic function

Box 16.4 Clinical Alert: Treatment-Related Toxicities

- Clinical manifestations of certain treatment-related toxicities, such as cerebral edema, are similar to those of tumor progression

Fatigue

- An early reaction to radiotherapy that may last anywhere from several weeks to months
- Patients suffering from fatigue often report excessive sleep, low energy, and decreased appetite
- Decreased energy affects all aspects of life; therefore, the patient and family should be made aware of the potential for fatigue during treatment and advised to adjust daily activities accordingly
- Overt somnolence is a rare side effect, but acute somnolence syndrome may be indicated by extreme sleepiness and signs of increased intracranial pressure (ICP)

Mucositis, Esophagitis, Nausea, and Myelosuppression

- Not commonly seen in cranial irradiation; more common in patients who have undergone spinal irradiation, due to the large volume of bone marrow treated
- Risk of these side effects is increased in patients undergoing concurrent chemotherapy
- Mucositis, esophagitis, or nausea can occur during CSI or when the radiation beams directed at the spine exit through the oropharynx, mediastinum, or gut

Late Side Effects

Cerebral Necrosis

- Necrosis is dead tissue thought to result from radiation on replicating glial cells and on capillary endothelial cells
- Symptoms are typically observed anywhere from 6 to 36 months after therapy. These symptoms often mimic those of a recurrent tumor, with MRI revealing mass effect or enhancement
- Dose-related phenomenon, with relative threshold radiation dose of 55 Gy, if treatment was given according to a conventional fractionation schedule
- Risk of occurrence reported as 5%
- Treatment of cerebral necrosis includes corticosteroid therapy and possible surgical intervention

Endocrinopathies

- May occur from radiation alone or from a combination of radiation and chemotherapy, especially if the hypothalamic–pituitary axis is in the field of radiation
- Hypothalamic dysfunction can occur when a dose greater than 24 Gy is directed at the hypothalamic–pituitary axis

Neurocognitive Decline

- Related to cranial irradiation
- Studies report a significant decline in neurocognitive scores after WBI

Late Radiation Myelopathy

- Related to dose, amount of cord treated, and fractionation
- Induces permanent demyelination of sensory neurons, resulting in permanent and irreversible neurologic damage (i.e., weakness and loss of function) at and below the level of the radiation site
- Generally manifests between 13 and 29 months after treatment
- Doses of 45 to 54 Gy rarely impart significant damage, but unanticipated outcomes are less likely with lower dosage
- Risk of myelopathy is less than 1% with doses of 45 Gy, but risk increases to 5% with doses of greater than 57 Gy

Less Common Side Effects of Craniospinal Irradiation

- External or serous otitis
- Leukoencephalopathy
- Hearing loss
- Cataracts, visual changes, and retinopathy

Side Effects of Stereotactic Radiosurgery

Side effects of SRS differ from those of conventional fractionated radiotherapy, as SRS affects a smaller target volume and uses higher doses per fraction. Reactions to SRS are less severe, but may occur within 48 hours due to transient swelling.

- Include nausea, headache, and exacerbation of seizures or discomfort at pin sites (if rigid head frame is used)
- Acute reactions occur within 90 days of treatment
- Late reactions occur within 3 to 10 months
- Combining SRS with WBI (or any form of radiotherapy) increases the risk of side effects

16.5 Radiation Oncologic Emergencies

16.5.1 Spinal Cord Compression

- About 95% of patients with spinal cord compression have evidence of metastatic disease in the epidural or extradural space

- Manifestations of spinal cord compression vary depending on location and degree of compression but may include motor weakness, pain, autonomic dysfunction, and sensory loss
- Treatment must be initiated as soon as possible after cord compression is discovered, so early recognition and diagnosis are essential and cannot be overemphasized
- Therapy may not reverse paralysis that has been present for over 48 hours
- Tissue diagnosis or known history of metastatic disease should be obtained before initiation of radiotherapy
- High-dose steroids should be administered as indicated
- If possible, surgical decompression should be considered
- Postoperative radiotherapy is indicated to prevent recurrence
- Radiotherapy can also be used alone if surgery is not feasible
- Treatment depends on the tumor type, onset of compression and progression, and physician preference
- If the onset of symptoms occurs rapidly, large radiation doses may be administered initially

16.5.2 Cerebral Metastases

- Cerebral metastases may require rapid radiotherapeutic intervention to preserve neurologic function and to prevent further decline
- Headache and impaired cognition are the most common symptoms of cerebral metastasis
- Tissue diagnosis or known history of metastatic disease should be obtained before initiation of radiotherapy
- WBI is indicated for patients with multiple metastases
- Surgical decompression of a symptomatic lesion may be warranted
- Corticosteroids should be administered as indicated

16.6 Nursing Management for Patients Undergoing Radiotherapy

Nursing management of patients undergoing radiotherapy involves more than the radiation treatment itself, as all patients undergoing radiotherapy have an underlying disease process. Nurses caring for these patients will have many opportunities to educate and support patients and their families as they face these unfamiliar, frightening experiences (Box 16.5 Focus on Protocol-Directed Therapies). The acute effects of radiotherapy are described earlier and are presented in ▶ Table 16.4. A more detailed table, including strategies for managing the long-term effects of radiation, is included in **Appendix A14: Nursing Management of Patients Undergoing Radiation Therapy**.

Table 16.4 Radiation therapy: what to watch for

Complication	Type of radiation	Nursing action	Rationale
Cerebral edema	Large doses of radiation, usually > 1.8–2.0 Gy	Steroids may be indicated Monitor neurologic assessment closely, watching for headache, nausea, vomiting, decreased mental status, motor or sensory decline, seizures, cranial neuropathies, or speech difficulties Pain management	May occur in patients with vasogenic edema who are not on steroids, or whose steroid regimen has been tapered too rapidly May also be a sign of hemorrhage or tumor recurrence
Seizures	Any	AEDs as needed Monitor levels of AEDs, if appropriate Maintain safety precautions related to seizures	Seizures may be a symptom of cerebral edema, or they may be exacerbated by radiotherapy
Myelosuppression	Spinal irradiation (caused by treatment of large volume of bone marrow)	Monitor laboratory values closely throughout the course of treatment Patients receiving craniospinal radiation and chemotherapy are at increased risk for myelosuppression	Myelosuppression is manifested by low blood cell counts
Esophagitis, nausea, mucositis	Can occur during spinal irradiation or when the spinal fields exit through the oropharynx, mediastinum, or gut	Patient may need prophylactic antiemetic Pain management	Symptoms usually manifest 10 d after the initiation of treatment

Abbreviations: AEDs, antiepileptic drugs; d, days; Gy, gray.

This chapter is intended as a bedside reference for nurses caring for patients undergoing radiotherapy. The reader is encouraged to consult the references found at the end of this chapter to learn more about specific subjects of interest.

Box 16.5 Focus on Protocol-Directed Therapies

It is important for nurses to have knowledge of current clinical trials and where they can obtain clinical trial information at their institutions. Clinical trial information can be found on the Radiation Therapy Oncology Group website (http://www.rtog.org) or on the American College of Radiology Imaging Network's website (http://www.acrin.org). Other websites offering professional and patient information on clinical trials include the following:

• National Cancer Institute (http://www.cancer.gov)
• National Institutes of Health clinical trials website (http://www.clinicaltrials.gov)

Lack of awareness on the part of staff and physicians is a major barrier to the inclusion of patients in clinical trials. Additional barriers include misconceptions about clinical trials, quality of life issues, health insurance coverage, and practical considerations (e.g., transportation, time, etc.). Nurses play a vital role in educating patients and families about ongoing trials at their facilities and in providing patients with resources.

16.6.1 Neurologic Assessment

• Evaluate level of consciousness; see also Chapter 2: Assessment
• Assess cognition using the Karnofsky scale
• Test motor function
• Monitor sensory function
• Assess cranial nerve function
• Monitor for signs of increased ICP; see also Chapter 3: Principles of Intracranial Pressure
    ◦ Perform ICP monitoring, if appropriate
    ◦ Report decrease in neurologic function immediately

16.6.2 Integumentary Assessment

• Perform close monitoring of the skin and scalp in patients undergoing cranial radiation

16.6.3 Pain Management

• Assess the patient for immobility-related or frame-related discomfort

16.6.4 Patient and Family Teaching

- Educate the patient and the family about types of radiation, including side effects and goals of treatment
- Help manage the patient's and family's expectations of treatment
- Allow the patient and family to ask questions and to express concerns and fears
- Patient education must precede initiation of radiotherapy
- Encourage the patient and family to seek additional sources of support (e.g., clergy, local support groups), as appropriate

16.6.5 Collaborative Management

Many different specialties may be called to help support a patient undergoing radiation therapy. These specialties include the following:
- Nursing
- Radiation oncology
- Neurosurgery
- Medical or neuro-oncology
- Support groups specific to the disease process
- Therapies
  - Physical therapy
  - Occupational therapy
  - Speech therapy for cognition
- Palliative care, if appropriate
- Clergy, chaplain, or other spiritual support

Video
Video 16.1 Gamma Knife treatment.

Suggested Reading

[1] Ballonoff A. Acute complications of cranial irradiation. 2016; http://www.uptodate.com/contents/acute-complications-of-cranial-irradiation. Accessed July 12, 2017

[2] Bernstein M, Berger M, ed. Neuro-Oncology: The Essentials. 3rd ed. New York, NY: Thieme; 2014

[3] Chang EL, Wefel JS, Hess KR, et al. Neurocognition in patients with brain metastases treated with radiosurgery or radiosurgery plus whole-brain irradiation: a randomised controlled trial. Lancet Oncol. 2009; 10(11):1037–1044

[4] Chen CC, Chapman PH, Loeffler JS. Stereotactic cranial radiosurgery. 2016; http://www.uptodate.com/contents/stereotactic-cranial-radiosurgery. Accessed July 12, 2017

[5] Coia LR, Moylan DJ. Introduction to Clinical Radiation Oncology. 3rd ed. Madison, WI: Medical Physics Pub.; 1998

[6] Cox JD, Kian Ang K. Radiation Oncology: Rationale, Technique, Results. 9th ed. Philadelphia, PA: Mosby Elsevier; 2010

[7] DeAngelis LM, Posner JB. Neurologic Complications of Cancer. 2nd ed. New York, NY: Oxford University Press; 2008

[8] Hansen E, Roach M, III, eds. Handbook of Evidence-Based Radiation Oncology. 2nd ed. New York, NY: Springer; 2010

[9] Iwamoto RR, Haas ML, Gosselin T, eds. Manual for Radiation Oncology. Nursing Practice and Education. 4th ed. Pittsburgh, PA: Oncology Nursing Society; 2012

[10] Oddie K, Pinto M, Jollie S, Blasiak E, Ercolano E, McCorkle R. Identification of need for an evidence-based nurse-led assessment and management protocol for radiation dermatitis. Cancer Nurs. 2014; 37(2):E37–E42

[11] Watkins-Bruner D, Moore-Higgs GJ, Haas M. Outcomes in Radiation Therapy: Multidisciplinary Management. Burlinton, MA: Jones and Bartlett; 2001

17 Rehabilitation

Sara Stephenson and Risa Maruyama

Abstract

Rehabilitation begins as soon as the patient is admitted to the hospital. For patients with neurologic diseases or injuries, rehabilitation may include physical, occupational, and speech therapy. These services are usually provided by therapists who are specially trained in working with patients with brain and spinal cord injuries. The specific course of rehabilitation differs for each patient, but it almost always requires a multidisciplinary team that includes nurses, physicians, case managers, therapists, and family members. Given the extent of close interaction with patients with neurologic diseases or injuries, nurses are expected to play a vital role in the recovery and rehabilitation of all patients with neurologic diagnoses.

Keywords: activities of daily living (ADLs), occupational therapy, physical therapy, rehabilitation, speech therapy, therapeutic assessment

17.1 Rehabilitation

Patients who undergo neurosurgical intervention often require some form of rehabilitation. The rehabilitation team comprises many different members, and various levels of rehabilitation are available depending on each patient's needs (▶ Table 17.1). Rehabilitation and rehabilitation services are provided, in part, by therapists (e.g., speech, occupational, and physical therapists). Therapists should be involved as early as possible; in some cases, they may work with patients while they are still in the intensive care unit (ICU). Early initiation of rehabilitation services may help decrease length of stay and has been shown to reduce complications related to prolonged bed rest (e.g., pressure sores, range of motion [ROM] limitations, and loss of muscle strength).

This chapter offers a brief description of the disciplines that may be involved with a patient at each level of care, from admission through rehabilitation (Box 17.1 Diagnoses Appropriate for Therapy Referral).

Table 17.1 Collaborative management of patients with impaired physical mobility

Complication	Discipline	Therapy intervention	Rationale
Impaired ambulation	PT	Strength and sensory assessment Leg exercises Modify transfers Use of a gait belt Orthotics as indicated	Weakness or sensory loss affects gait and balance
Activity intolerance or impaired endurance	PT/OT	Progressive activity Energy conservation techniques Therapeutic exercise to increase endurance Activity with light weights and increased repetitions	Inactivity and/or prolonged bed rest leads to decreased muscle mass and diminished endurance Medical issues may be exacerbated by inactivity
Transfers	PT/OT	Thorough examination of strength and sensation prior to mobility Teach level surface transfers Use of electric lift, sliding board, and/or specialized toilet equipment Use of specific techniques, such as bracing of a paralyzed extremity Use of walkers, gait belts, and canes for stability	Limit fall risks by capitalizing on the patient's strengths and intact skills for transfer
Risk of immobility	PT/OT	Early mobility Elevate head of bed Lower extremity and upper extremity nonweight exercises Spend time sitting on edge of the bed	Strategies help prevent muscle atrophy, decreased respiratory function, DVT, pneumonia, urinary tract infections, and upper respiratory infections
Cognitive impairment Disorientation Short-term memory impairments Unable to recall daily events Agitation and emotional lability	OT/SLP	Use of simple directions and helpful external memory aids Limit environmental stimuli that may distract the patient during interactions (e.g., TV, medications)	Thorough cognitive evaluation will help identify areas of deficit and determine appropriate interventions Compensatory strategies may be initiated, and the entire medical team should be encouraged to use them

Table 17.1 (*continued*)

Complication	Discipline	Therapy intervention	Rationale
Dysphagia "Wet voice" quality Patient complains of trouble swallowing or "things not going down right" Facial weakness, coughing with oral intake	OT/SLP	Swallowing evaluation	Limit diet to food that can be swallowed safely, and teach swallowing strategies
Impairment of visual motor skills or visual field cuts Diplopia New onset deficits in eye movement Unable to reach for items (i.e., reach falls short or overshoots) Visual neglect (i.e., patient not appreciating visual stimuli on one side)	OT	Environmental control, use of bright visual markers to help identify boundaries in a visual field, use of spot patching for diplopia	Vision impairments can affect all aspects of patient care By addressing vision deficits early, strategies can be used to accommodate for deficits
Aphasia/dysarthria Abnormal voice Unclear speech Receptive or expressive speech problems, or both	SLP	Evaluation, use of techniques to strengthen speech quality and compensate for deficits	Ability to communicate is a cornerstone of rehabilitation after neurologic injury
Impairment of self-care skills (affecting one or more ADLs) Unable to manage a meal tray Unable to grip hygiene items Unable to "figure out" how to use hygiene items/tools Muscle weakness Sensory loss	OT	Instruct patient on proper use of adaptive equipment to overcome these challenges	Use of adaptive equipment and rearranging the environment can increase a patient's capacity for independence in self-care

Abbreviations: ADLs, activities of daily living; DVT, deep vein thrombosis; OT, occupational therapy; PT, physical therapy; SLP, speech and language pathology.

Box 17.1 Diagnoses Appropriate for Therapy Referral

- Aneurysm
- Brain tumor
- Hydrocephalus
- Low back pain
- Meniere's disease
- Meningitis
- Multiple sclerosis
- Myasthenia gravis
- Parkinson's disease
- Scoliosis
- Spinal cord injury
- Spinal fracture
- Spinal surgery
- Stroke
- Traumatic brain injury
- Vascular malformation

17.2 Philosophy of Rehabilitation

The primary purposes of rehabilitation are to provide preventative care, to recover function after neurologic injury, to compensate for skill loss, and to promote independence in the least restrictive environment for the patient. To achieve these goals, the main strategies of the therapy team working with neurosurgery patients include the following:
- Early mobilization
- Active and passive therapeutic exercises
- Positioning to optimize function
- Use of adaptive equipment and techniques
- Restoration of neuromuscular function

17.3 The Rehabilitation Process

The rehabilitation process begins with neurologic assessments that help therapists determine the patient's neurologic strengths and deficits.
- Clinical regulations and licensure determine which therapy discipline should perform evaluations and treatment. These regulations vary by state and institution
- Therapists from each discipline are responsible for the following needs:
  - Evaluation of the patient's strengths and deficits

- Determination of plan of care and treatment regimen (including frequency and duration of therapeutic treatment)
  - Education of patients, family members, and caregivers
  - Recommending discharge placement and ongoing treatment (if appropriate)
- Treatment plans vary by patient and should be tailored to meet individual needs
- Therapists in the neurologic setting communicate with members of the nursing and rehabilitation teams and may assist with discharge recommendations
- Therapy should be initiated as early as possible (Box 17.2 Early Therapy)
- Each discipline of therapy is governed by state and national standards of practice

---

Box 17.2 Early Therapy

- Initiation of therapy services while the patient is in the ICU can do the following:
  - Reduce complications related to extended bed rest and/or inactivity (e.g., pressure sores, ROM limitations, loss of strength)
  - Reduce length of stay
- Rehabilitation
  - Should start as early as possible, preferably at admission, given preoperative therapy may improve postoperative outcomes
  - Is geared toward preventive care
  - Increases independence

17.3.1 Therapeutic Assessments

Occupational Therapy

Despite its name, occupational therapy is not a therapy for an occupation or career. Instead, it teaches a much more essential set of abilities—skills for "the job of living." An occupational therapist may be asked to evaluate a patient or provide therapeutic assistance in the following areas:

- ADLs
- Visual perceptual training
- Visual hand–eye coordination
- Splint or brace fabrication
- Fine motor control
- Upper extremity strength and ROM
- Cognitive skills

- Upper extremity neuromuscular reeducation
- Adaptive equipment fabrication and training
- Therapeutic exercise
- Patient and family education

Physical Therapy

The goals of physical therapy may be described by the mantra, "Movement is life." Physical therapists may work with patients who aspire to achieve previous levels of activity, or they may treat patients whose mobility is severely impaired. They may provide therapeutic assistance in the following areas:
- Functional mobility, balance, and gait training
- Lower extremity strength and ROM
- Therapeutic exercise
- Neuromuscular reeducation
- Nonpharmacologic pain management
- Patient and family education

Speech and Language Pathology

Speech and language pathologists are a critical element of rehabilitation of patients, as the ability to communicate is often viewed as the most basic element of what makes us human. Speech pathologists may evaluate a patient or provide therapeutic assistance in the following areas:
- Aphasia and language deficits
- Dysarthria
- Motor skills related to speech
- Cognitive skills
- Swallowing function
- Modified barium swallowing studies
- Fiberoptic endoscopic swallowing studies
- Augmentative communication (i.e., forms of expression that do not require words)

17.3.2 Levels of Care

Patients with neurologic conditions may require rehabilitation or therapeutic assistance anywhere along the continuum of care. Below are some of the settings in which patients may receive such care.

Acute Care

- Hospital-based patient care, including the ICU, intermediate or step-down units, and regular floor units
- Physical therapy, occupational therapy, or speech therapy, as indicated

Skilled Nursing Facility and Subacute Rehabilitation

- Medical and nursing care are provided
- Therapies are less intensive, typically have 1 to 2 hours each day of one or more therapy services, as the patients in these settings usually cannot tolerate more than 3 hours of therapy every day
- Focus is on preparing the patient to return home or to transfer to another level of care

Long-Term Acute Care Hospital

- Nursing and medical care for patients who are stable but who need complex care
- Therapy is provided less frequently, at a lower level of intensity
- Patients are expected to remain in this setting for longer periods of time; they may have complex respiratory needs that inhibit opportunities for rehabilitation

Inpatient Rehabilitation Facility

- Medically stable patients may be transferred to an inpatient rehabilitation facility from acute care units, skilled nursing facilities, or from a long-term acute care hospital
- Intensive rehabilitation takes place for at least 3 hours each day
- Physical therapy, occupational therapy, or speech therapy, as indicated
- May include neuropsychological and therapeutic recreational activities
- Focus is on preparing the patient to return home

Home Health

- Home-based therapies, usually two to three times per week
- Patient must be homebound to receive home health rehabilitation

Outpatient Therapy

- Therapies take place in an outpatient clinic one to five times per week
- Physical therapy, occupational therapy, or speech therapy, as indicated

17.3.3 Therapeutic Interventions for Common Neurologic Conditions

Traumatic Brain Injury

Mobility

- Weakness or hemiparesis
- Balance impairment
- Therapeutic intervention
  - Strength and gait training
  - Neuromuscular reeducation

Tone

- Hypertonicity
- Hypotonicity
- Therapeutic intervention
  - Appropriate positioning
  - Monitoring ROM in upper extremities to prevent subluxation injury

Dysphagia

- Impaired swallowing
- Therapeutic intervention
  - Swallowing diagnostics
  - Diet modification

Vision and Perception

- Visual motor deficits
- Visual perceptual deficits
- Therapeutic intervention
  - Environmental modifications
  - Vision exercises
  - Lens adaptation

Cognition

- Traumatic brain injury may involve deficits in the following areas:
  - Short-term memory
  - Problem-solving ability
  - Attention and focus
  - Reasoning and judgment
  - Organization and sequencing
- Deficits may range from mild to severe
- Global deficits can be seen in patients with frontal, anoxic, or diffuse axonal injuries
- Therapeutic intervention strategies
  - Use of helpful external memory aids
  - A structured environment
  - Limitation of distractions; frequent redirection when patient is distracted
  - Possible 24-hour supervision after discharge from hospital

Communication

- Aphasia
- Dysarthria

- Abnormal voicing
- Apraxia
- Therapeutic intervention
  - Modified communication strategies
  - Therapeutic exercises for vocal, oral, and facial musculature

Behavior Management

- Initiation deficit or lethargy
- Impulsive behaviors
- Inability to follow commands
- Agitation (especially in individuals with frontal injuries)
- Therapeutic intervention
  - Limitation of visitors
  - Quiet, dim environment
  - One direction at a time
  - Frequent breaks from therapy to allow the patient to rest

Space-Occupying Lesions

Posterior Fossa Lesion

An individual with a lesion of the posterior fossa may experience visual deficits (e.g., diplopia), dysphagia, or cranial nerve impairment.

Mobility

- Loss of control over most movement
- Therapeutic intervention
  - Added stability to help the patient perform tasks (e.g., upper extremity support for self-feeding or oral care)

Tone

- Tone is not usually affected by posterior fossa lesions

Dysphagia

- Impaired swallowing
- Therapeutic intervention
  - Swallowing diagnostics
  - Diet modification

Vision and Perception

- Visual motor deficits
- Visual perceptual deficits
- Therapeutic intervention
  - Environmental modifications
  - Vision exercises
  - Lens adaptation

Cognition

- High-level cognitive deficits
- Therapeutic intervention
  - Thorough cognitive evaluation

Communication

- Dysarthria
- Possible cranial nerve involvement
- Therapeutic intervention
  - Therapeutic exercises for vocal, oral, and facial musculature

Behavior Management

- Behavioral issues are not usually associated with posterior fossa lesions

Frontal Lesions

Mobility

- Hemiparesis or hemiplegia
- Therapeutic intervention
  - Strength and gait training
  - Neuromuscular reeducation

Tone

- Hypertonicity
- Hypotonicity
- Therapeutic intervention
  - Appropriate positioning
  - Careful increase in ROM of upper extremities to prevent subluxation injury

Cognition

- Problem maintaining attention
- Unaware of deficits
- Poor initiation and verbal response to commands
- Memory impairments
- Difficulty with planning and organization
- Therapeutic intervention
  - Memory systems
  - Structured environment
  - Limit distractions
  - Frequent redirection

Communication

- Dysarthria
- Cadence of speech
- Therapeutic intervention
  - Structured speech and language exercises
  - Speech therapy

Behavior Management

- Poor initiation
- Impulsive behavior
- Inability to follow commands
- Difficulty taking feedback or suggestions
- Lethargy
- Agitation
- Therapeutic intervention
  - Limitation of visitors
  - Quiet, dim environment
  - One direction at a time
  - Frequent breaks from therapy to allow the patient to rest

Left or Right Hemisphere Lesions

Depending on the lesion and its location, patients may experience visual deficits (e.g., hemianopia).

Mobility

- Hemiparesis or hemiplegia
- Sensory impairments
- Therapeutic intervention
  - Strength and gait training
  - Neuromuscular reeducation

Tone

- Hypertonicity
- Hypotonicity
- Therapeutic intervention
  - Neuromuscular reeducation or bracing
  - Hypotonicity requires careful positioning and slow increases in ROM to prevent subluxation injury

Dysphagia

- Impaired swallowing
- Therapeutic intervention
  - Swallowing diagnostics
  - Diet modification

Vision and Perception

- Visual motor deficits
- Visual perceptual deficits
- Therapeutic intervention
  - Environmental modifications
  - Vision exercises
  - Lens adaptation

Cognition

- Cognitive deficits associated with lesions in the left hemisphere may include the following:
  - Lability
  - Impaired memory
- Cognitive deficits associated with lesions in the right hemisphere may include the following:
  - Stubbornness or inflexible mindset
  - Impulsive behavior
  - Poor safety awareness
- Therapeutic intervention
  - Memory aids
  - Clear, concrete questions
  - A structured and predictable environment
  - Possible 24-hour supervision after discharge from hospital

Communication

- Communicative deficits associated with lesions in the left hemisphere may include the following:
  - Aphasia
    - Receptive deficits
    - Expressive deficits
  - Apraxia
  - Dysarthria
- Communicative deficits associated with lesions in the right hemisphere may include the following:
  - Expressive deficits related to topic maintenance, completeness, organization
  - Confusion
  - Flat affect
- Therapeutic intervention
  - Structured therapy sessions to address expression
  - Memory aids that encourage or prompt repetition
  - Use of calendars, communication boards, or picture boards to assess the patient's need for alternative styles of communication

Spinal Cord Injury

Aggressive, persistent rehabilitation after spinal cord injury (SCI) is a critical component of the healing process. Chapter 12: Traumatic Spine Injury addresses SCI in detail, but this section describes what some patients may expect after surgical treatment of SCI.

Mobility

- Motor and sensation deficits at and below the level of injury
- Therapeutic intervention
  - Brace or orthosis fitting (thoracic lumbosacral orthotic, corset, cervical collar)
  - Early mobility and upright postures help avoid medical complications
  - Strength, mobility, and equipment training

Tone

- Hypotonia after injury
- Spasticity follows hypotonia
- Therapeutic intervention
  - Passive ROM exercises
  - Appropriate positioning
  - Splinting as indicated
  - Careful increases in ROM of upper extremities to avoid subluxation injury

Communication

- Respiratory compromise (tracheostomy, ventilator requirements)
- Endurance issues related to speech; patient may become easily fatigued or breathless
- Therapeutic intervention
  - Soft-touch call light within patient's reach
  - Passy-Muir speaking valve (Passy Muir Inc., Irvine, CA)
  - Alternative communication devices
  - Teach patient tongue clicks if he or she is on a mechanical ventilator

Equipment for Patients with Spinal Cord Injury

As their mobility and strength may be limited, patients with SCI may require use of special devices that help prevent complications associated with prolonged bed rest (▶ Table 17.2). These devices may include the following:

- Pressure relief cushion
- Abdominal binder
- Wheelchair or supportive seating system
- Hydraulic patient lift device
- Pressure relief boots or foot drop splints for heels and feet
- Soft-touch call lights

Table 17.2 Common therapy and adaptive equipment

Therapy equipment	Adaptive equipment
Canes	Toilet aides
• Single-point	Elevated toilet seats
• Quad-point or wide-base	Bedside commodes
Four-wheel walkers	Hand splints
Pick-up walkers	Built-up handles for utensils and ADLs tools
Wheelchairs	Spot patching for diplopia
• Electric	Adaptive self-feeding
• Manual	Shower chairs
Seating systems	
Gait belts	
Orthotics	
• Ankle–foot orthosis	
• Thoracic–lumbosacral orthotic	
• Lumbosacral orthotic	
Transfer boards	

Abbreviation: ADLs, activities of daily living.

17.3.4 Family Teaching

Therapy services should reach out to the patient's family as soon as possible, preferably at the time of the initial evaluation. This should involve written, verbal, and hands-on education for the family and/or the caregiver. The following areas should be addressed:

- Impairment information
- Speech and language techniques
- Strategies for memory compensation
- ROM training
- Neuromuscular strengthening
- Swallowing precautions
- Discharge recommendations
- Transfers
- Braces
- Adaptive equipment training
- ADLs
- Community resources

17.3.5 Discharge Planning

In most cases, discharge planning begins when the patient is admitted to the hospital. Therapists in the acute neurologic setting communicate with members of the rehabilitation team in the extended setting to coordinate discharge recommendations.

17.4 Nursing Management for Patients During Rehabilitation

The role of therapy is integral to the healing process for patients with brain or spinal cord injuries. Nurses must assume an active role in the rehabilitation of such patients. Although various subspecialties of therapy may be needed to determine whether certain activities (e.g., ambulation or swallowing) can be safely initiated, it is often the duty of the nursing staff to maintain and encourage such activities. Therapists and nurses often work together to determine when the following treatment strategies are safe and appropriate:

- Early mobilization
- Appropriate positioning
- Bracing
- Adaptive equipment for ADLs
- ROM
- Cognitive assessments, such as the Rancho Los Amigos Cognitive Scale
- Skin protection
- Patient and family teaching

17.4.1 Collaborative Management

- Nursing
- Neurosurgery
- Physiatry
- Internal medicine
- Orthotist for bracing, if indicated
- Therapies
  - Physical therapy
  - Occupational therapy
  - Speech therapy
- Social services
- Neuropsychology
- Dietician

Suggested Reading

[1] American Physical Therapy Association. http://www.apta.org. Accessed July 11, 2017

[2] American Physical Therapy Association. APTA Code of Ethics. 2011; http://www.apta.org/uploadedFiles/APTAorg/About_Us/Policies/Ethics/CodeofEthics.pdf#search=%22code of ethics%22. Accessed July 11, 2017

[3] American Speech-Language-Hearing Association. http://www.asha.org. Accessed July 11, 2107

[4] American Speech-Language-Hearing Association. Code of ethics. 2016. http://www.asha.org/Code-of-Ethics/. Accessed July 11, 2017

[5] American Stroke Association. http://www.strokeassociation.org. Accessed July 11, 2017

[6] Aydın G, Mucuk S. The evaluation of daily living activities, pressure sores and risk factors. Rehabil Nurs. 2015; 40(2):84–91

[7] Burtin C, Clerckx B, Robbeets C, et al. Early exercise in critically ill patients enhances short-term functional recovery. Crit Care Med. 2009; 37(9):2499–2505

[8] Camicia M, Black T, Farrell J, Waites K, Wirt S, Lutz B, Association of Rehabilitation Nurses Task Force. The essential role of the rehabilitation nurse in facilitating care transitions: a white paper by the association of rehabilitation nurses. Rehabil Nurs. 2014; 39(1):3–15

[9] Caraviello KA, Nemeth LS, Dumas BP. Using the beach chair position in ICU patients. Crit Care Nurse. 2010; 30(2):S9–S11

[10] Dong ZH, Yu BX, Sun YB, Fang W, Li L. Effects of early rehabilitation therapy on patients with mechanical ventilation. World J Emerg Med. 2014; 5(1):48–52

[11] Enforcement procedures for the occupational therapy code of ethics and ethics standards. Am J Occup Ther. 2014; 68 suppl 3:S3–S15

[12] Gillick BT, Marshall WJ, Rheault W, Stoecker J. Mobility criteria for upright sitting with patients in the neuro/trauma intensive care unit: an analysis of length of stay and functional outcomes. Neurohospitalist. 2011; 1(4):172–177

[13] Kim O, Kim JH. Falls and use of assistive devices in stroke patients with hemiparesis: association with balance ability and fall efficacy. Rehabil Nurs. 2015; 40(4):267–274

[14] Knier S, Stichler JF, Ferber L, Catterall K. Patients' perceptions of the quality of discharge teaching and readiness for discharge. Rehabil Nurs. 2015; 40(1):30–39

[15] Mayeda-Letourneau J. Safe patient handling and movement: a literature review. Rehabil Nurs. 2014; 39(3):123–129

[16] Miller ET. Family caregivers - a precious resource. Rehabil Nurs. 2015; 40(3):131–132

[17] Morris PE, Griffin L, Berry M, et al. Receiving early mobility during an intensive care unit admission is a predictor of improved outcomes in acute respiratory failure. Am J Med Sci. 2011; 341(5): 373–377

[18] Parker AM, Lord RK, Needham DM. Increasing the dose of acute rehabilitation: is there a benefit? BMC Med. 2013; 11:199

[19] Schweickert WD, Pohlman MC, Pohlman AS, et al. Early physical and occupational therapy in mechanically ventilated, critically ill patients: a randomised controlled trial. Lancet. 2009; 373 (9678):1874–1882

[20] Stanback R. Rebuilding lives after injury. Nurs Times. 2014; 110(15):27

Part V

Appendices

Appendix A: Nursing Management Tables

Appendix A1 Nursing management of patients with increased intracranial pressure

Problem	Nursing action	Rationale
Neurologic	Perform neurologic assessments hourly, or as directed, including LOC, motor/sensory assessment, and CN assessment Compare assessment to baseline Be aware of clinical manifestations of herniation syndromes Report any decrease in function immediately	Deterioration in neurologic assessment could indicate increase in ICP, with resulting neurologic compromise
Increased ICP		
ICP monitoring	Monitoring of ICP via EVD or other ICP device, such as parenchymal bolt or screw: • Check ICP and CPP hourly • Regular analysis of ICP waveform • Monitor CSF output and characteristics hourly Brain tissue oxygenation monitoring	Goal of ICP monitoring is to ensure adequate CPP Maintenance of normal ICP is essential to prevent further neurologic decline
Nursing duties	Limit duration of nursing activities with patient, including positioning, bathing, performing assessments, giving medications Consider the effect of external factors, such as family visitation, touch, noise (e.g., radio or television), and their effect on ICP	Any type of stimulus, including those associated with nursing care or external stimuli, may increase ICP
	Position patients with head and neck in neutral position Keep head of bed at 30 degrees, unless contraindicated	Decreases resistance to venous return
Fever management	Monitor temperature carefully, administer antipyretics as ordered Use cooling blankets, ice packs, and tepid baths as appropriate	Fever increases cerebral metabolism and is a predictor of poor neurologic outcome

Appendix A1 (*continued*)

Problem	Nursing action	Rationale
Cardiovascular		
Hemodynamic stability	Monitor cardiac rate and rhythm Monitor ECG (if available) Monitor for cardiac arrhythmias Monitor hemodynamic data via central line, arterial line	Assesses ability of the heart to oxygenate the brain adequately
Hypotension	Monitor blood pressure closely Administer vasopressors, if indicated	Hypotension is a strong indicator of poor neurologic outcome (due to cerebral hypoxia)
Anemia	Monitor CBC for hemoglobin/ hematocrit	Anemia indicates poor oxygen-carrying capacity of red blood cells and could lead to cerebral hypoxia
Respiratory		
Hypoxia	Monitor oxygen saturation levels Monitor ABGs Monitor respiratory rate and pattern Administer supplementary oxygen as indicated	Hypoxia is directly related to cerebral ischemia and poor neurologic outcome
Hypercapnia	Monitor ABGs; normal values are $Paco_2$ 35–45 mm Hg	Hyperventilation may reduce ICP; however, rapid vasoconstriction may decrease CBF with resulting cerebral ischemia
Respiratory failure	Monitor patient's ability to protect airway due to decreased LOC	Respiratory failure may result from many causes (e.g., decreased LOC, aspiration, pneumonia)
Impaired airway	Prepare for intubation and mechanical ventilation	Hypoxia is directly related to poor neurologic outcome
Electrolytes		
Hyponatremia, Hypernatremia	Monitor electrolyte levels Strict intake and output Urine specific gravity for increased urine output Administer salt supplements, including hyperosmolar intravenous solutions, as ordered	Hyponatremia usually due to SIADH, may be associated with cerebral edema Hypernatremia may be the result of dehydration, associated with hypotension and poor neurologic outcomes Could be due to the use of hyperosmolar solutions often used to reduce cerebral edema (mannitol, hyperosmolar sodium)

Appendix A1 (continued)

Problem	Nursing action	Rationale
Hyperglycemia	Monitor electrolyte levels Use Chemsticks for glucose testing Strict intake and output Implement sliding scale insulin regimen as directed Be aware that some medications may alter the absorption or metabolism of electrolytes Report all new or abnormal findings	Hyperglycemia is a known contributor to poor neurologic outcome; therefore, strict glucose control is important
Pain		
Sedation and analgesia	Administer sedation as directed Monitor changes in neurologic assessment carefully	Agitation due to pain or confusion increases ICP Use caution when administering analgesics or sedating drugs to neurologically compromised patients to balance the risk of secondary injury and to maintain normal ICP See also Table 3.2. Pharmacology for management of patients with increased intracranial pressure

Abbreviations: ABGs, arterial blood gases; CBC, complete blood cell count; CBF, cerebral blood flow; CN, cranial nerve; CPP, cerebral perfusion pressure; CSF, cerebrospinal fluid; ECG, electrocardiogram; EVD, external ventricular drain; ICP, intracranial pressure; LOC, level of consciousness; SIADH, syndrome of inappropriate antidiuretic hormone.

Appendix A2 Nursing management of patients with hydrocephalus and shunt failure

Problem	Nursing action	Rationale
Headache	Neurologic assessment, vitals	Assesses for possible increased ICP, possibly caused by shunt failure
	Headache diary	Diary helps determine whether there is a pattern to headaches (e.g., time of day, or causative/alleviating issues)
	Consider shunt tap	Measure ICP

Appendix A2 (*continued*)

Problem	Nursing action	Rationale
Vomiting	Neurologic assessment	Assesses for possible increased ICP, possibly caused by shunt failure
Fever	If shunt was placed > 6 mo ago, look for other causes of fever	Likelihood of shunt infection decreases with time; more common within 3 mo of placement surgery
	Obtain CBC, CRP. Consider shunt tap if no other source is found	Obtain CSF to test for infection (Gram stain, culture, glucose, protein, cell count)
	If patient has a VA shunt, obtain blood cultures and 24-h urine to test for total protein	Complications of VA shunt infection include endocarditis and shunt nephritis
Redness or swelling along shunt tract or wound	Vital signs, CBC, possible shunt tap	Looking for possible infection
Other signs of increased ICP	Changes in vision or personality (e.g., irritability) decline in work or school performance	Shunt failure can result in personality changes
Exposed hardware	Cover with sterile dressing, call for neurosurgical consult and intervention	Exposed hardware is a nidus for infection and must be surgically repaired
Seizures	Take measures to ensure patient safety	Rarely occur as a result of shunt failure, but patients with seizure disorders may have an increase in seizures associated with shunt failure

Abbreviations: CBC, complete blood cell count; CRP, C-reactive protein; CSF, cerebrospinal fluid; ICP, intracranial pressure; VA, ventriculoatrial.

Appendix A3 Nursing management of patients with electrolyte imbalances

Problem	Nursing action	Rationale
Hyponatremia		
SIADH	Fluid restriction Strict intake and output Administer salt supplements and hyperosmolar saline solutions as ordered	SIADH is characterized by volume overload
	Monitor serum sodium and serum osmolality every 6 h, or as ordered	Subtle changes in serum sodium can result in neurologic compromise Overcorrection of hyponatremia may result in CPM, with devastating neurologic consequences
	Monitor neurologic status	Hyponatremia is associated with cerebral edema
	Record patient's weight daily	Weight gain is a possible sign of fluid overload
CSW	Strict intake and output Volume replacement, as directed Administer salt supplements and hyperosmolar saline solutions as ordered	CSW is characterized by sodium deficiency with volume depletion
	Monitor serum sodium and serum osmolality every 6 h, or as ordered	Subtle changes in serum sodium can result in neurologic compromise Overcorrection of hyponatremia may result in CPM, with devastating neurologic consequences
	Monitor neurologic status	Hyponatremia is associated with cerebral edema
Hypernatremia		
DI	Strict intake and output Urine specific gravity test Replace fluids as directed Record patient's weight daily	Avoid fluid depletion and dehydration
	Monitor serum sodium and urine osmolality every 6 h, or as ordered Administer desmopressin acetate, if indicated Monitor neurologic status	Overcorrection of hypernatremia may result in CPM, with devastating neurologic consequences
Hypoglycemia		
	Monitor glucose at bedside via Accucheck every 6 h, or before meals or at bedtime, as ordered Administer glucose as ordered Monitor for signs of hypoglycemia Monitor neurologic status	Hypoglycemia is associated with increased risk of cerebral hypoxia, which can result in cerebral edema and increased ICP

Appendix A3 *(continued)*

Problem	Nursing action	Rationale
Hyperglycemia		
	Monitor glucose at bedside via Accucheck every 6 h, or before meals or at bedtime, as ordered Administer insulin as ordered, per sliding scale Monitor for signs of hyperglycemia Monitor neurologic status	Avoid hyperglycemia due to risk of cerebral edema and resulting increased ICP
	Be aware of potential interactions of medications with nutrition that the patient is receiving	Some steroids (e.g., dexamethasone) are associated with increased glucose levels

Abbreviations: CPM, central pontine myelinolysis; CSW, cerebral salt wasting; ICP, intracranial pressure; SIADH, syndrome of inappropriate antidiuretic hormone.

Appendix A4 Nursing management of patients with seizures or epilepsy

Problem	Nursing action	Rationale
Safety during seizure event	Assess the patient to ensure he or she has an adequate airway and that the event does not have a cardiac cause (e.g., asystole)	Always begin emergency intervention and assessment with the ABCs (i.e., airway, breathing, and circulation)
	Place a cushion under the patient's head and loosen restrictive clothing or linens Do not restrain the patient Do not place anything between the patient's teeth	Protect the patient from harm or danger present in the surrounding environment
	Turn the patient on his or her side to allow drainage of secretions	Prevent aspiration
Assessment after seizure event	Perform assessment and documentation of the seizure event; see Box 6.7. Nursing Assessment of Seizure Event Check and record vital signs and neurologic status	Nursing observations during the seizure event are critical for appropriate treatment of the patient after seizure
AEDs	Knowledge of patient's AEDs, dosage, and potential interactions with other drugs or food	Many AEDs have significant interactions with other drugs or food

Appendix A4 (*continued*)

Problem	Nursing action	Rationale
	Be knowledgeable about the appropriate dosage for AEDs	AEDs may be ineffective if the prescribed level is subtherapeutic Drug toxicity may also be seen, and can result in serious medical complications
	Be aware of common side effects associated with AEDs (including allergic reactions)	Side effects of AEDs may be problematic to the patient, possibly requiring a change of medication Allergic reactions can be so severe that they lead to serious—even fatal—medical complications
Patient and family education	Teach patients and families about the measures they can take during a seizure to ensure patient safety Educate patients and their families about their AEDs, including information about potential side effects and drug or food interactions Give patient and family necessary information regarding legality of driving in their state	Patients who are well educated on their condition are better equipped for effective self-care Educating the family improves the support system for the patient, especially after hospital discharge
Prevention	Provide patients and family with information needed to reduce possibility of seizures	Many seizures can be prevented by compliance with prescribed AEDs

Abbreviation: AEDs, antiepileptic drugs.

Appendix A5 Nursing management of patients with brain tumors

Problem	Nursing action	Rationale
Decreased LOC or neurologic function (neurologic deficits vary based on location of tumor and surgical approach)	Perform complete neurologic assessment and monitor for any changes in assessment Always know the location of the tumor and the possible associated deficits	Increased vasogenic edema is possible depending on tumor histology Hemorrhage from tumor bed is also possible
Cerebral edema (vasogenic edema)	Administer dexamethasone (Decadron) Do not skip doses or discontinue abruptly	Patient could experience increased edema if dexamethasone is abruptly decreased or discontinued
Decreased visual acuity	Visual acuity testing should be part of the neurologic assessment for all patients, especially those with pituitary tumors	Decreased visual acuity may result from compression of the optic nerve. It is more common with tumors in the vicinity of the optic nerve or in the occipital lobe
CSF leak	Monitor patient for rhinorrhea; ask patient if he or she notices fluid leaking from the nose or dripping down the back of the throat	CSF leak is a possible complication of many surgical approaches for pituitary tumor resection
	Report presence of CSF immediately	CSF leak increases the risk of meningitis
Seizures	Monitor blood levels of AEDs, if warranted Watch for side effects, allergic reactions, or interactions with food or other drugs Take measures to ensure patient safety	Patient is at increased risk for seizure activity if levels of AEDs are subtherapeutic
Hyponatremia	Monitor serum sodium levels Restrict fluids, if ordered Maintain strict intake and output Administer salt supplements or hyperosmolar solutions if ordered	Hyponatremia, usually SIADH, may result in cerebral edema
Hypercoaguable states, DVT, PE	Encourage early ambulation, unless contraindicated SCDs at all times while in bed Administer enoxaparin or heparin, unless contraindicated Assess for DVT every shift; if DVT is suspected, report immediately	Patients with brain tumors, especially those with GBM, are at increased risk for DVT and PE

Abbreviations: AEDs, antiepileptic drugs; CSF, cerebrospinal fluid; DVT, deep vein thrombosis; GBM, glioblastoma multiforme; LOC, level of consciousness; PE, pulmonary embolism; SCD, sequential compression device; SIADH, syndrome of inappropriate antidiuretic hormone.

Appendix A6 Nursing management of patients with stroke

Problem	Nursing action	Rationale
Neurologic decline	Monitor neurologic status closely, report any decrease in function immediately Monitor patient for signs of increased ICP	It is possible for the area affected by an ischemic stroke to enlarge or for a hemorrhagic stroke to re-bleed "Time is brain"—acting quickly in response to any change in patient status can save brain tissue from irreversible damage
	Nursing measures to protect normal ICP; see also Chapter 3: Principles of Intracranial Pressure	Take appropriate measures to protect patient from increased ICP and neurologic decline
Respiratory	Assess patient for adequate airway Use oxygen saturation monitor, if warranted	Hypoxia potentiates cerebral edema, increased ICP, and neurologic decline
Cardiovascular	Monitor blood pressure frequently Medicate with antihypertensive medications as ordered	Hypertension after hemorrhagic stroke may increase the likelihood of rehemorrhage
	Notify physician of any change in blood pressure, based on noted parameters	Blood pressure parameters in ischemic stroke may be somewhat flexible to facilitate cerebral perfusion
	Critical to know the desired blood pressure range	Treatment may differ depending on stroke type—know the difference!
Electrolytes	Monitor serum sodium Strict intake and output Know desired range for serum sodium; report abnormal values	Hyponatremia may cause neurologic decline, including cerebral edema. See also Chapter 5: Electrolyte Disturbances
	Monitor serum glucose Use Chemsticks as ordered; administer insulin accordingly	Both hypoglycemia and hyperglycemia can cause cerebral edema
Pain	Check with patient frequently for presence of pain or discomfort; medicate as ordered	An increase in pain or discomfort may increase ICP or blood pressure, presenting an unnecessary risk to the patient
Postoperative implications of CEA	Measure neck circumference hourly or as directed	Potential for postoperative bleeding
	Watch incision for signs of bleeding or hematoma	Hematoma or swelling can obstruct the patient's airway

Appendix A6 (*continued*)

Problem	Nursing action	Rationale
Patient and family education	Teach patient and family about risk factors for stroke Provide patients and family with educational materials, including appropriate websites and support groups	Identifying risk factors and making lifestyle modifications may decrease risk of further stroke

Abbreviations: CEA, carotid endarterectomy; ICP, intracranial pressure.

Appendix A7 Nursing management of patients with subarachnoid hemorrhage

Problem	Nursing action	Rationale
Neurologic decline		
	Monitor neurologic status hourly or as ordered	The mortality and morbidity associated with SAH are high, with potential for further neurologic decline due to cerebral edema, vasospasm, rehemorrhage, hydrocephalus, or any number of other medical complications
	Take appropriate measures to maintain normal ICP; see also Chapter 3: Principles of Intracranial Pressure. Perform ICP monitoring per institutional protocol	Ensure adequate CBF to prevent cerebral edema, increased ICP, and further neurologic damage
Respiratory		
	Ensure adequacy of airway Be prepared for intubation and mechanical ventilation if GCS score is < 8, or if the airway is unprotected	Patients with decreased LOC may have unprotected airways, resulting in insufficient oxygenation for cerebral oxygenation
Vasospasm (triple H therapy)		
Hypertension (i.e., MAP 20–30 mm Hg above baseline systolic blood pressure)	Maintain blood pressure at ordered parameters Administer vasopressors as indicated	Increases CBF

Problem	Nursing action	Rationale
Hypervolemia (increase in cerebral blood volume)	Administer intravenous fluids as ordered (about 125–150 mL/h) Monitor laboratory values (e.g., serum sodium, osmolality) Strict intake and output	Increases CBF
Hemodilution (hematocrit <35%)	Monitor laboratory values (e.g., hemoglobin and hematocrit)	Increases CBF
Hyponatremia		
	Monitor laboratory values (e.g., serum sodium, osmolality) Be aware of desired range for serum sodium; it is common for target to be ≥140 mEq/L Strict intake and output Administer medications, including oral salt tablets or hypertonic saline solutions, if indicated	Hyponatremia can increase the risk of cerebral edema In patients with SAH, hyponatremia is usually caused by CSW
	Fluid restriction is absolutely contraindicated	Fluid restriction in this population may exacerbate vasospasm and result in further neurologic compromise
Hydrocephalus		
	Monitor neurologic status Report any changes in status, including LOC, gait, vision, or urinary incontinence	Hydrocephalus is common in patients with SAH, as the subarachnoid blood clogs the arachnoid granulations, impairing CSF absorption
Seizures		
	Ensure patient safety in the event of a seizure Administer AEDs as ordered Monitor drug levels, if indicated Be aware of interactions between AEDs and food or other drugs	Seizures are relatively common in the presence of SAH Seizure may exacerbate cerebral edema Many common medications and foods may interact with AEDs, causing increased risk of seizures

Appendix A7 (continued)

Problem	Nursing action	Rationale
Pain		
	Monitor pain and discomfort, and medicate as ordered	Pain can increase ICP
Patient and family education		
	Provide patient and family with educational material, including websites and support groups	Patients who are well educated on their condition are better equipped for effective self-care Educating the family improves the support system for the patient, especially after hospital discharge

Abbreviations: AEDs, antiepileptic drugs; CBF, cerebral blood flow; CSF, cerebrospinal fluid; CSW, cerebral salt wasting; GCS, Glasgow Coma Scale; ICP, intracranial pressure; LOC, level of consciousness; MAP, mean arterial pressure; SAH, subarachnoid hemorrhage.

Appendix A8 Nursing management of patients with traumatic brain injury

Problem	Nursing action	Rationale
CSF leaks		
Maintenance of normal ICP	Take appropriate measures to maintain normal ICP; see also Table 3.4. Increased intracranial pressure	Normal ICP is essential to prevent secondary injury and further neurologic decline
Prevention of secondary injury	Perform neurologic assessment hourly, or as directed. Should include LOC, motor, sensory, and CN assessments	Depending on the type of hematoma (e.g., epidural hematomas), patients may present with a period of lucidity, followed by rapid neurologic decline Patients with an expanding space-occupying lesion (e.g., hematoma, blossoming contusion, or edema) are at risk for brain herniation. See also Chapter 2: Assessment

Problem	Nursing action	Rationale
Prevent complications due to CSF leak	Observe patient for signs of otorrhea and rhinorrhea CSF may be seen directly or may be visible on linens CSF leakage is usually more evident when the patient is sitting upright and slightly forward (i.e., reservoir sign) CSF is distinguishable by appearance of fluid with a yellow ring surrounding it (i.e., "halo sign" on linens) Report any sign of CSF leak	Patients with skull fractures may have CSF leak through the nose or ear (this may indicate basal skull fracture) Patients with CSF leak are at risk for meningitis
Prevent blood loss due to scalp lacerations	Observe patient for presence of scalp or facial lacerations	Patients with scalp lacerations are at risk for excessive blood loss
Prevent blood loss due to other trauma	Monitor hemoglobin and hematocrit Observe for bleeding in other parts of the body (e.g., retroperitoneum, bladder, chest) Observe urine for presence of blood Report new findings of bleeding, tenderness, difficulty breathing, or possible expanding hematomas Transfuse as necessary	Prevent anemia and resulting hypoxemia associated with excessive blood loss from trauma Hypoxemia may lead to cerebral hypoxia and, ultimately, cerebral edema Patients with trauma-related head injuries may have injuries to other parts of the body
Respiratory		
Airway protection	Monitor patient's ability to protect the airway (may not be possible, depending on LOC) Prepare for intubation, mechanical ventilation	Respiratory failure may result from many causes (e.g., aspiration, pneumonia, or decreased LOC)
Prevention of respiratory failure	Perform regular respiratory assessments, including visual inspection of respiratory rate and pattern and auscultation of lungs	Hypoxia is directly related to poor neurologic outcome Patients with TBI often have other injuries, especially to the chest (e.g., flail chest, pneumothorax, hemothorax, rib fractures)

Appendix A8 (*continued*)

Problem	Nursing action	Rationale
Seizure		
Seizure management	Administer AEDs as directed Monitor laboratory values, especially drug levels, if patient is on AED regimen Be aware of how other medications and/or foods may interact with absorption or metabolism of AEDs Ensure patient safety in the event of a seizure	Certain medications, including antibiotics, may affect absorption of certain AEDs, placing the patient at risk for seizures Seizures may increase cerebral edema, a known predictor of poor neurologic outcome
Patient and family		
Education	Support and educate the family and patient about possible outcomes, immediate and long-term implications of injury	Because TBIs occur suddenly, family is often ill-prepared to cope with injury and is not informed on injury, possible plans, and prognosis
Support	Involve clergy or chaplain services as appropriate Educate the patient and family about risks associated with TBI, especially postconcussion syndrome	The patient and family must be made aware of the importance of continued observation and commit to following up in the event of lingering complaints (e.g., headache, difficulty concentrating, visual problems)

Abbreviations: AED, antiepileptic drug; CN, cranial nerve; CSF, cerebrospinal fluid; ICP, intracranial pressure; LOC, level of consciousness; TBI, traumatic brain injury.

Appendix A9 Nursing management of patients with infection of the central nervous system

Problem	Nursing action	Rationale
Decline in neurologic assessment	Nursing measures to protect normal ICP; see also Chapter 3: Principles of Intracranial Pressure Monitor neurologic status closely, report any decrease in function immediately	Deterioration of neurologic status could indicate increase in ICP, with resulting neurologic compromise
Meningism and fever	Perform complete neurologic assessment, including assessment for the presence of meningism Monitor vital signs, including temperature Document and report all pertinent information, including assessment outcomes, vital signs, current medications, recent surgeries and procedures, and current laboratory test results (e.g., CBC) Prepare patient for lumbar puncture	Fever may be an indication of meningitis, which must be diagnosed by laboratory examination of CSF Early diagnosis of meningitis is a positive indicator of good neurologic outcome
Inflamed, swollen, or draining incision	Monitor vital signs, including temperature	Inflammation or redness of an incision may indicate infection. Wound infections from some surgeries (e.g., craniotomies, shunts, or spinal surgeries) may be the first sign of systemic infection, including infection of CSF (i.e., meningitis or ventriculitis)

Abbreviations: CBC, complete blood cell count; CSF, cerebrospinal fluid; ICP, intracranial pressure.

Appendix A10 Nursing management of patients with spine disorders

Problem	Nursing action	Rationale
Decrease in motor or sensory function	Perform regular neurologic assessments, including motor and sensory assessment	Worsening assessment may indicate edema or hemorrhage
Urinary retention	Accurate intake and output Check PVR	Urinary retention is a common complication of lumbar surgery or lumbar myelopathy Urinary retention can also be a side effect of opioid use
Constipation	Administer stool softeners or laxatives as directed Keep track of patient's bowel movements Patient may need to adhere to a high-fiber diet	Constipation can result from opioid use, decreased physical mobility, or myelopathy
Pain	Administer analgesics and muscle relaxants as ordered and as necessary based on patient's pain level Record the patient's response to the medications Use alternative methods of pain management (e.g., ice or heat, massage, repositioning) when feasible	Presence of pain may cause the patient to refrain from activity or mobility, which may exacerbate some spinal disorders
Immobility	Use SCDs when the patient is in bed Administer enoxaparin as ordered Encourage early ambulation and activity as appropriate Involve rehabilitation services as appropriate	Immobility places patients at risk for DVT and PE Early mobilization is usually recommended
Patient and family education	Assess risk factors for complications associated with spinal disorders (e.g., smoking, excess weight, lack of exercise) Educate patient on proper body mechanics to help avoid injury Recommend appropriate exercise program	Many spinal disorders (e.g., degenerative disk disease) are aggravated by repeated movements or stressors caused by poor body mechanics
	Encourage smoking cessation, provide materials to help patients learn effective ways to quit	Smoking contributes to a less healthy lifestyle and overall wellness and is detrimental to bone health and healing

Abbreviations: DVT, deep vein thrombosis; PE, pulmonary embolism; PVR, postvoid residual; SCD, sequential compression device.

Appendix A11 Nursing management of patients with spinal cord injury

Problem	Nursing action	Rationale
Neurologic		
Neurologic deterioration	Perform a thorough neurologic examination, especially motor and sensory assessment, with continued assessments as indicated	Neurologic deterioration and secondary injury are possible outcomes of increased swelling of the spinal cord
Autonomic dysreflexia	See Table 12.5 Autonomic dysreflexia	Autonomic dysreflexia is a potentially life-threatening condition that must be recognized immediately
Cardiovascular		
Hypovolemic shock	Monitor blood pressure, heart rate, and heart rhythm regularly	Shock may be the result of underhydration or blood loss from trauma or surgery
Orthostatic hypotension and neurogenic shock (neurogenic shock is more common in SCI at C6 or higher)	Monitor patient for signs of hypotension, including taking orthostatic blood pressure bilaterally A central line and a pulmonary artery catheter may be needed to monitor central venous pressure and cardiac output Administer volume replacement, vasopressors, if indicated Monitor peripheral pulses and temperature of the extremities Strict intake and output An abdominal binder may be indicated for blood pressure support	Orthostatic hypotension may be caused by loss of sympathetic vascular tone and arteriole vasomotor control
DVT	Encourage early mobility, if possible Use SCDs when the patient is in bed Administer enoxaparin, if not contraindicated	DVT is a common complication of SCI that could lead to PE
Respiratory		
Respiratory insufficiency or respiratory failure	Closely monitor respiratory rate, volume, oxygen saturation Prepare for intubation if the patient's airway is not protected	SCI, especially at the cervical level, may result in compromised respiratory functions if the diaphragm is innervated (results from disruption of the phrenic nerve above C5)

Appendix A11 (*continued*)

Problem	Nursing action	Rationale
Atelectasis and pneumonia	If the patient is not intubated, encourage the use of an incentive spirometer Encourage the patient to cough and to practice deep breathing exercises Suction may be needed if the patient is intubated or unable to manage secretions independently	Atelectasis and pneumonia are common complications of SCI Ventilated patients are at increased risk for ventilator-acquired pneumonia
PE	Encourage early mobility, if possible Use SCDs when the patient is in bed Enoxaparin, if not contraindicated Watch for signs of DVT	PE is a potentially life-threatening complication that is more likely to occur in immobile patients
Gastrointestinal		
Gastroparesis and ileus	Assess bowel sounds frequently and monitor abdomen for distention and tenderness Monitor patient for nausea and vomiting Nasogastric tube may be needed to decompress the abdomen in case of ileus Encourage appropriate diet and fluids based on the patient's GI status	Gastroparesis, loss of intestinal peristalsis, and ileus are common complications of spinal shock Aspiration due to emesis is a life-threatening complication that can lead to respiratory failure
Gastric stress ulcer	Monitor hematocrit Check nasogastric tube for vomit that resembles coffee grounds Administer peptic ulcer prophylaxis if ordered (e.g., H2-receptor antagonist or proton pump inhibitor)	Gastric stress ulcers can result in superficial hemorrhages and GI blood loss
Constipation	Establish a bowel care program early in the acute phase of SCI. This program should institute consistent schedule for defecation, based on the patient's patterns of elimination before injury, and	SCI will likely cause abnormalities in both sensory and motor function of the bowel. This results from disruption of the spinal tracts responsible for

Appendix A11 *(continued)*

Problem	Nursing action	Rationale
	anticipated future demands (based on level and extent of injury) Bowel care program should include stool softeners, chemical stimulants (e.g., suppositories), mechanical stimulation (i.e., digital stimulation), and a high-fiber diet	bowel control (based on level and extent of injury) Constipation is a potential cause of autonomic dysreflexia
Integumentary		
Decubitus ulcer	Perform a thorough baseline skin assessment, followed by frequent skin checks Reposition the patient frequently, if warranted Clothing and linens under the patient should be kept clean and dry	Decubitus ulcers are a common source of infection in patients with SCI
Other		
Pain	Administer pain medications as directed Watch for urinary retention and/or constipation	SCI may be painful, especially if it is associated with vertebral fracture Narcotics may cause urinary retention and/or constipation (see above)
Urinary retention	Monitor strict intake and output Check PVR Use a straight catheter if the PVR exceeds 250 mL Monitor patient closely for signs of UTIs	Urinary retention is a common source of infection and/or discomfort in patients with SCI Urinary retention is a potential cause of autonomic dysreflexia

Abbreviations: DVT, deep vein thrombosis; GI, gastrointestinal; PE, pulmonary embolism; PVR, postvoid residual; SCD, sequential compression device; SCI, spinal cord injury; UTI, urinary tract infection.

Appendix A12 Nursing management of patients undergoing craniotomy

Problem	Nursing action	Rationale
Cerebral edema with increased ICP	Close monitoring of neurologic status, including LOC, motor/sensory assessment, and CN assessment Close monitoring of vital signs Avoid activities known to increase ICP as much as possible Nursing measures to protect normal ICP; see also Chapter 3: Principles of intracranial pressure; use of ICP monitoring, if appropriate	Changes in mental status, neurologic examination, and vital signs may be indications of cerebral edema and increased ICP
Hydrocephalus	Watch for signs of hydrocephalus (e.g., change in LOC, gait disturbance, incontinence)	Hydrocephalus may require temporary treatment with ventriculostomy or lumbar drain. If it persists, VPS may be indicated
Seizures	Manage AEDs, being conscientious about possible interactions of AEDs with other drugs or food Patient safety; see also Chapter 6: Seizures	Seizures may occur after craniotomy; they must be recognized and treated rapidly Status epilepticus is a serious complication associated with increased morbidity and mortality
Pneumocephalus	Keep head of bed elevated higher than 30 degrees 100% O_2 if ordered Pain management	May occur after surgery, especially with certain operative approaches. May cause pain and neurologic changes
CSF leak	Keep head of bed elevated higher than 30 degrees or as ordered. The patient should not blow his or her nose if rhinorrhea is present Serial lumbar punctures may help decrease pressure, lumbar drain may be used to divert CSF pathway, and persistent leaks may require surgical repair	CSF leak may be observed at operative site or draining from ears or nose. Any time the dura is opened for an extended period, the risk of infection or meningitis increases

Abbreviations: AED, antiepileptic drug; CN, cranial nerve; CSF, cerebrospinal fluid; ICP, intracranial pressure; LOC, level of consciousness; VPS, ventriculoperitoneal shunt.

Appendix A13 Nursing management of patients undergoing neurosurgery

Problem	Nursing action	Rationale
Cardiovascular		
Arrhythmias, hypo- or hypertension	Hemodynamic monitoring, if appropriate	Monitor for hypovolemia or cardiac arrhythmias (standard for any postoperative patient)
Stunned myocardium	Hemodynamic monitoring, if appropriate	Occasionally seen in patients with SAH
Respiratory		
Airway compromise, respiratory failure, pneumonia, and PE	Perform regular airway assessments Monitor respiratory rate and rhythm Assess ABGs, oxygen saturation	Patients who have undergone craniotomy are at increased risk for aspiration (especially patients who have undergone posterior fossa craniotomy, in which nausea and vomiting are more common), airway compromise, and respiratory depression due to neurologic deficit. Effects of anesthesia may compound respiratory depression, so patients must be monitored closely
Electrolyte disturbances		
Hypo- or hypernatremia, DI, SIADH, or CSW	Monitor serum sodium level Watch for signs of hypo or hypernatremia Report any new findings	DI, SIADH, and CSW are common after craniotomy. Electrolytes must be monitored closely, and abnormalities must be addressed promptly to prevent further neurologic decline
Hyperglycemia	Monitor glucose levels, especially if the patient is on steroids Administer insulin as directed	
Immobility		
DVT	Watch for signs and symptoms of DVT Administer enoxaparin (Lovenox) as ordered Use antiembolism stockings	DVT can increase morbidity, mortality, and length of stay in the hospital. In serious cases, DVT can lead to greater permanent disability
Balance difficulties	Encourage mobility and early ambulation	

Appendix A13 (*continued*)

Problem	Nursing action	Rationale
Nutrition		
Nausea and vomiting	Evaluate and treat nausea and/or vomiting	Vomiting can lead to aspiration pneumonia and increases in ICP
Other		
Pain	Evaluate and treat pain, administering pain medication as ordered Be mindful of the effect of environmental changes. Keeping the room dark and quiet may help diminish pain Distraction, if appropriate Ice or teabags may increase patient's comfort, especially in cases of periorbital or other facial edema	Pain issues need to be addressed promptly in all patients to enhance comfort and keep ICP at a safe level
Fever management	Monitor the patient's temperature, administering antipyretics as necessary Obtain cultures for fever as ordered Administer antibiotics as ordered	Increases in temperature can increase cerebral metabolic demands, sometimes resulting in secondary brain injury Treatment goal is normothermia
Wound infection	Craniotomy incision must be kept clean and dry If the dressing is saturated, replace it with a dry dressing The surgeon may prefer to remove the first dressing after surgery Monitor incision for erythema, edema, and drainage Monitor WBCs postoperatively Treatment for infection may include wound care, topical antimicrobials, and intravenous or oral antibiotics	Infection of a surgical site prolongs recovery and hospital stay, as well as increases morbidity and mortality. Infections should therefore be addressed promptly
Specialty therapies	Various therapy specialties may be involved in patient care after neurosurgery, including physical and occupational therapy Speech therapy, including swallowing evaluation, if appropriate	An early focus on mobility and rehabilitation lessens the negative effects of inactivity and immobility

Appendix A13 (*continued*)

Problem	Nursing action	Rationale
	Rehabilitation consult, if appropriate	
Patient and family education	The patient and family should be informed about neurosurgical interventions, precipitating illness, expected recovery, pre- and postoperative medications, and what to expect upon hospital discharge	Patients who are well educated on their condition are better equipped for effective self-care Educating the family improves the support system for the patient, especially after hospital discharge

Abbreviations: ABGs, arterial blood gases; CSW, cerebral salt wasting; DI, diabetes insipidus; DVT, deep vein thrombosis; ICP, intracranial pressure; PE, pulmonary embolism; SAH, subarachnoid hemorrhage; SIADH, syndrome of inappropriate antidiuretic hormone; WBC, white blood cells.

Appendix A14 Nursing management of patients undergoing radiation therapy

Problem	Associated radiation characteristics	Nursing action	Rationale
Cerebral edema	Large doses of radiation (usually > 1.8–2.0 Gy)	Administer steroids as ordered Monitor neurologic status closely, watching for headache, nausea, vomiting, decreased mental status, motor/ sensory decline, seizures, cranial neuropathies, or speech difficulties Ensure the patient's pain is being managed effectively	Cerebral edema may occur in patients with vasogenic edema who are not on steroids, or in patients whose steroid dosage is tapered too rapidly
Seizures	Any	Administer AEDs as ordered, monitoring levels of AEDs carefully Maintain seizure-related safety precautions	Seizures may be a symptom of cerebral edema, or they may be exacerbated by radiation therapy

Appendix A14 (*continued*)

Problem	Associated radiation characteristics	Nursing action	Rationale
Alopecia	May occur after radiation doses as low as 5 Gy Occurs only regionally, in the path of the ionizing beam Complete scalp hair loss may occur after WBRT	Encourage use of hat and sunscreen Use water-soluble lubricant to ease discomfort associated with dermatitis Educate patient and family to prepare them for potential hair loss	Hair loss causes scalp sensitivity Care must be taken to protect the sensitive scalp and avoid further injury
Acute radiation myelopathy	Radiation to the spinal cord causes transient demyelination May occur 1–6 mo after radiation therapy is complete Usually resolves within 6–12 mo	Educate patient and family in order to reduce anxiety about acute myelopathy, reminding them that it is a temporary side effect of radiation therapy	Patients who are well educated on their condition are better equipped for effective self-care Educating the family improves the support system for the patient, especially after hospital discharge
Late radiation myelopathy	Permanent demyelination of sensory fibers causing severe irreversible weakness and functional loss from the radiation portal inferiorly. Usually present 13 y after treatment	Educate patient and family in order to reduce anxiety about late myelopathy, informing them that it may be a permanent side effect of radiation therapy	Patients who are well educated on their condition are better equipped for effective self-care Educating the family improves the support system for the patient, especially after hospital discharge
Fatigue	A side effect for most patients who receive cranial irradiation	Educate patient and family to prepare them for increased fatigue and resulting limitation of ADLs	Families need to be prepared to help patients with ADLs

Problem	Associated radiation characteristics	Nursing action	Rationale
Myelosuppression	Occurs with spinal irradiation due to the large volume of bone marrow that may be irradiated	Monitor laboratory values closely throughout the course of treatment Patients receiving craniospinal radiation and chemotherapy are at high risk for myelosuppression	The clinical manifestation of myelosuppression is low blood cell counts
Esophagitis, nausea, mucositis	Can occur during spinal irradiation or when the spinal fields exit through the oropharynx, mediastinum, or gut	May need to pre-medicate the patient with an antiemetic Ensure the patient's pain is being managed effectively	Symptoms usually manifest 10 d after the initiation of treatment
Cerebral necrosis	Noted approximately 6–36 mo after RT Signs of cerebral necrosis mimic those of recurrent tumor; MRI often shows mass or enhancement Dose-related phenomenon, with threshold dose of 55 Gy fractionated.	Administer steroids as indicated Possible surgical decompression with resection of necrosis Monitor neurologic status closely, report changes Monitor laboratory values, especially glucose, if steroids are initiated	Cerebral necrosis may cause cerebral edema, which is associated with neurologic deficits
Endocrinopathies	May occur if the hypothalamic–pituitary axis is in the field of radiation May occur with doses > 24 Gy	May require close monitoring of laboratory values, specific to the area of the pituitary gland that is affected Strict intake and output May require endocrine consultation	Children are especially at risk Hypothalamic dysfunction seen in doses > 24 Gy

Appendix A14 (*continued*)

Problem	Associated radiation characteristics	Nursing action	Rationale
Neurocognitive decline	Any cranial irradiation, especially WBRT	Perform cognitive testing Monitor cognitive status compared to baseline assessment. Suggest screening or testing, if appropriate Administer modafinil (Provigil) or armodafinil (Nuvigil) to promote wakefulness, if ordered	Cognitive decline is a common effect of the underlying disease process and of treatment
Patient and family education	All forms of radiation therapy	Be aware of the type of radiation the patient is to receive, the treatment schedule, patient expectations, and possible side effects Discuss goals of treatment, type of treatment, schedule, simulation, and possible side effects of treatment with patient and family	Knowledgeable patients are less apprehensive about their procedures, and are better equipped for independence and self-care after radiation therapy
Emotional needs	All forms of radiation therapy	Give emotional support Be aware of patients' mental status, ask about eating and sleeping habits, and be available to talk or listen, if needed	Patients may experience fear, depression, and anxiety related to their treatment and underlying disease process

Abbreviations: ADLs, activities of daily living; AEDs, antiepileptic drugs; Gy, gray; MRI, magnetic resonance imaging; RT, radiotherapy; WBRT, whole brain radiation therapy.

531

Appendix B: Sample Discharge Instructions

You recently underwent a surgical procedure called *placement of a ventriculoperitoneal shunt*. This shunt has a valve or pump that looks and feels like a small lump under your skin just above the ear. Attached to either end of the pump is a tube. One end of the tube penetrates the fluid-filled space in the brain (i.e., the ventricle) and drains cerebrospinal fluid (CSF) to the other end of the tube, which drains into the abdomen. The instructions below provide important information regarding your care at home.

- Incision care
  - You may shower with mild soap and shampoo daily. Gently wash your incision and pat dry. **This is the only time you may touch your incisions**
  - Do not apply ointments, lotions, or creams to your incisions
  - Do **not** swim, use a hot tub, or take a bath until your incisions are completely healed (this usually takes about 3 weeks)
  - Stop smoking tobacco; smoking delays healing and may result in infection at the incision sites
- Activity
  - Start with light activity around the house for the first 3 days you are home
  - Gradually increase your activity, beginning with a short walk 1–2 times every day
  - Avoid contact sports, skating, riding a bicycle, or other physically demanding activities for 6 weeks
  - You may **not** drive until your neurosurgeon clears you to do so
- Nutrition
  - Eat plenty of fruits and vegetables to prevent constipation
- Medication
  - Take your pain medications with food, and use these medications sparingly to avoid nausea, vomiting, and constipation
  - Take your pain medications as prescribed and gradually taper them as your pain decreases
- Follow-up
  - Call your neurosurgeon when you get home from the hospital to schedule your follow-up appointment
  - Follow up with your primary care physician for all medical issues

- Call your doctor or return to the emergency department if you experience any of the following:
  - A fever of more than 100 °F
  - Redness, swelling, odor, or drainage at your incision site
  - Sleepiness or difficulty waking up
  - Nausea or vomiting that will not stop
  - Headaches while you are in an upright position that resolve when you lie down
  - Confusion or changes in personality
  - Difficulty walking
  - Neck stiffness
  - Loss of bladder control

Appendix B2. Sample Discharge Instructions After Observation or Treatment in the Epilepsy Monitoring Unit

You recently underwent seizure monitoring in an epilepsy monitoring unit. During your hospital stay, you were likely asked to stop taking your antiepileptic medications, which were then restarted before discharge. You may have the same side effects that you experienced when you first started taking these medications (e.g., fatigue, unsteadiness, and memory problems). The instructions below provide important information regarding your care at home.

- Medication
  - Take your medications as they were prescribed at the time of discharge, bearing in mind that the dosages may differ from what they were before you came to the hospital
  - If you suddenly stop taking your medications, you are at risk for having life-threatening seizures
  - If you have trouble remembering to take your medications, establish a reminder system to help you. Take your medication with a routine you do every day, such as brushing your teeth or eating meals. You can also set alarms or post reminders where you will see them every day. A pill dispenser, which you can purchase from any pharmacy or drugstore, is an easy way to organize your medications and keep track of missed doses
  - Report any side effects to your doctor. Most are temporary, but your doctor needs to be made aware so he or she can determine whether your doses need to be adjusted
  - Avoid drinking alcohol while you are taking seizure medications
  - Let your doctor know if you are taking medication for any other conditions, given there may be a risk for interactions
- Keep all appointments with your doctors

- Safety
  - Most seizure-related injuries result from falls, altered consciousness, or abrupt, powerful body movements
  - Knowing your seizure pattern can help you plan for your safety
  - Avoid driving until cleared by your doctor. Check with your state motor vehicle department for information on laws regarding seizures and driving
  - Do not operate heavy equipment
  - **Do not bathe, swim, or use a hot tub alone**
  - Avoid working or playing above ground level to diminish the impact of falls
  - Stress and lack of sleep can increase the frequency of seizures. Be sure to get plenty of sleep each night, and plan time every day to relax
  - See Appendix B4 for more information on seizure safety
- Nutrition
  - It is important for you to eat a balanced diet and to have your meals at regular times
- **Call your doctor or return to the emergency department if you experience any of the following**
  - Intolerable or severe side effects
  - Increase in seizure frequency, or different types of seizures
  - Questions about the dosages of your medications
  - Follow up with your primary care physician for all medical issues

Appendix B3. Sample Discharge Instructions After Craniotomy for Treatment of Epilepsy

You recently underwent a surgical procedure called *craniotomy for treatment of epilepsy*. During this procedure, your skull was opened so your surgeon could remove or treat an abnormality in your brain. The goal of this surgery is to help reduce the frequency of your seizures. The instructions below provide important information regarding your care at home.

- Incision care
  - You may shower with mild soap and shampoo daily. Gently wash your incision and pat dry. **This is the only time you may touch your incision**
  - Do not apply ointments, lotions, or creams to your incision
  - Apply an ice pack or a clean bag of frozen peas to your incision to help reduce the swelling and discomfort every 30 minutes or as needed
  - You may have some itching at your incision site, some jaw tightness, or trouble opening your mouth wide for a few days after surgery. These side effects will resolve as your incision begins to heal
  - Wear a hat outdoors to protect your incision until your doctor has removed the staples or sutures (usually 7–14 days after surgery)
  - Do not put anything in your ears and do not submerge your head in water

- Activity
  - Start with light activity around the house for the first 3 days you are home
  - Gradually increase your activity, beginning with a short walk 1 or 2 times every day
  - You may **not** drive
  - **Do not bathe, swim, or use a hot tub alone**
  - Avoid contact sports, skating, riding a bicycle, or other physically demanding activities for 6 weeks
  - Avoid straining to have a bowel movement
- Nutrition
  - Eat plenty of fruits and vegetables to prevent constipation
- Medication
  - Take your pain medications with food, and use these medications sparingly to avoid nausea, vomiting, and constipation
  - Take your pain medications as prescribed and gradually taper them as your pain decreases
  - Your seizure medications should have been restarted before you were discharged from the hospital. As your body gets used to them again, you may have the same side effects that you experienced when you first started taking these medications (e.g., fatigue, unsteadiness, and memory problems). **Continue to take your seizure medications**
  - Stool softeners such as Colace or laxatives such as Dulcolax are available at pharmacies; these medications may be helpful until your bowel movements return to normal
  - You may need to use a suppository (e.g., Dulcolax or glycerin) or an enema if you have not had a bowel movement in 3 days
- Follow-up
  - Call your neurosurgeon when you get home from the hospital to schedule your follow-up appointment
  - Follow up with your neurologist as directed
  - Follow up with your primary care physician for all medical issues
- **Call your doctor or return to the emergency department if you experience any of the following**
  - Increased seizure activity or jerking or twitching of the face, arms, or legs
  - Difficulty or discomfort moving your neck
  - Difficulty moving or weakness in your face, arms, or legs
  - **A fever of more than 100 °F**
  - Redness, swelling, odor, or drainage at your incision site
  - Clear or bloody drainage from your nose or ears
  - Worsening headache
  - Dizziness or ringing in your ears

Appendix B4. Sample Handout with Seizure Information and Safety Instructions

A *seizure* is a sudden surge of electrical activity in the brain that usually affects how a person feels or acts for a short time. A seizure may cause facial twitching, difficulty speaking, arm or leg shaking, weakness, and loss of consciousness. Epilepsy is a condition that affects the nervous system and is characterized by recurring seizures. It is usually diagnosed after a person has had at least 2 seizures that were not attributable to a known cause (e.g., alcohol withdrawal or low blood sugar). Many conditions may cause seizures, including head injury, brain tumor, brain surgery, stroke, infection, or fever; however, the cause of a seizure may not always be determined. **If you have had a seizure, you are at an increased risk of having more seizures**. The instructions below provide important information to help you manage seizures and maintain safety at home.

- Seizure medication
  - Take your medications as they were prescribed at the time of discharge from the hospital
  - If you suddenly stop taking your medications, you are at risk for having life-threatening seizures
  - If you have trouble remembering to take your medications, establish a reminder system to help you. Take your medication with a routine you do every day, such as brushing your teeth or eating meals. You can also set alarms or post reminders where you will see them every day. A pill dispenser, which you can purchase from any pharmacy or drugstore, is an easy way to organize your medications and keep track of missed doses
  - Report any side effects to your doctor. Most are temporary, but your doctor needs to be made aware so he or she can determine whether your doses need to be adjusted
  - **Keep all appointments with your doctor**
  - Avoid drinking alcohol while you are taking seizure medications
  - Let your doctor know if you are taking medication for any other conditions because there may be a risk of interactions
- Safety
  - Most seizure-related injuries result from falls, altered consciousness, or abrupt, powerful body movements
  - Knowing your seizure pattern can help you plan for your safety
  - Be extra careful when handling hot objects or cooking
  - **Do not bathe, swim, or use a hot tub alone**
  - Do not operate heavy equipment
  - Avoid working or playing above ground level to diminish the impact of falls
  - Stress and lack of sleep can increase the frequency of seizures. Be sure to get plenty of sleep each night, and plan time every day to relax

- **Nutrition**
  - It is important for you to eat a balanced diet and to have your meals at regular times
- **When can you drive again?**
  - Talk with your doctor about driving. All 50 states have laws restricting access to driver's licenses for individuals with seizures not controlled by medication
  - It is your responsibility to report your seizures to the motor vehicle department; check with your local motor vehicle department for information on laws regarding seizures and driving
- **First aid during a seizure: information for your family and friends**
  - Try to cushion the person's head
  - Remove eyeglasses
  - Time the seizure with a watch
  - Loosen tight clothing
  - Turn the person on his or her side
  - Do not put anything in the person's mouth
  - Do not hold the person down
- **When to call 911**
  - If the seizure lasts longer than 5 min
  - If the person is having trouble breathing or is not waking up
  - For any signs of serious injury or sickness
- **Call your doctor if you have the following**
  - Intolerable or severe side effects
  - Increase in seizure frequency, length of seizures, and/or different types of seizures
  - Questions about the dosages of your medications
  - Any medical issues
  - More seizures than usual (return to the emergency department if necessary)
- **Resources**
  - Centers for Disease Control and Prevention Epilepsy Program: http://www.cdc.gov/epilepsy/index.html
  - National Institute of Neurological Disorders and Stroke (NINDS): http://www.ninds.nih.gov/disorders/epilepsy/epilepsy.htm
  - Epilepsy Foundation: http://www.epilepsy.com/

Appendix B5. Sample Discharge Instructions After Resection of a Pituitary Tumor

You recently underwent a surgical procedure called a *transnasal transsphenoidal craniotomy for removal of a pituitary tumor*. Your neurosurgeon accessed the space behind the bridge of your nose via your nasal passages, then made an incision in this space (called the *sphenoid* sinus) to access and remove as much of your tumor as possible. If you also have an incision in your abdomen, your surgeon probably took fat from this area to patch the opening where he or she entered your skull. The instructions below provide important information regarding your care at home.

- Incision care
  - You may shower with mild soap and shampoo daily. Gently wash your incision and pat dry. **This is the only time you may touch your incision**
  - You will not be able to see the incision in your nose. After surgery, it is normal to have some nasal and facial swelling, bruising, pain, and a small amount of bloody nasal drainage
  - You may also have a headache due to sinus congestion; this may last several days but should resolve after the swelling improves
  - You may irrigate your nose using saline nasal spray 5 times per day, or as needed for dryness or comfort. **Do not** put anything else in your nose
  - Do **not** swim, use a hot tub, or take a bath until your incision is completely healed (this usually takes about 4 weeks)
  - Stop smoking tobacco; smoking delays healing and may result in infection at the incision site
- Activity
  - If your surgeon tells you that there was a leak of cerebrospinal fluid (CSF) during surgery, sleep with your head elevated at least 30 degrees for 10 days after surgery
  - Do not blow your nose or drink from a straw for 12 weeks
  - It is important to cough when necessary to avoid getting pneumonia, but avoid **hard** coughing, sneezing, or holding your breath for 12 weeks
  - Do not bend over or lower your head more than 20–30 degrees for 12 weeks
  - Avoid lifting more than 10 lb for 12 weeks
  - Avoid any activity that involves holding your breath and bearing down with your abdomen for 12 weeks
  - Use a humidifier as needed to keep your nasal membranes moist
  - Start with light activity around the house for the first 3 days you are home
  - Gradually increase your activity, beginning with a short walk 1 or 2 times every day

- Avoid contact sports, skating, riding a bicycle, golfing, jogging, or other physically demanding activities for 12 weeks
- Avoid straining to urinate or to have a bowel movement
- **Nutrition**
  - A decrease in your ability to taste or smell is normal. It usually improves after a few weeks, but can take up to several months
  - Eat plenty of fruits and vegetables to prevent constipation
  - Take your pain medications with food, and use these medications sparingly to avoid nausea, vomiting, and constipation
- **Medication**
  - You may take seasonal allergy medications as directed; however, use oral decongestants sparingly, as they tend to dry out the nose and cause crusting and discomfort
  - Patients with allergies may use a steroid nasal spray (e.g., Nasonex). Consult with your doctor about the acceptable dose (usually 2 sprays per nostril, once a day, beginning 10–14 days after surgery)
  - Take your pain medications as prescribed and gradually taper them as your pain decreases
  - Stool softeners such as Colace or laxatives such as Dulcolax are available at pharmacies; these medications may be helpful until your bowel movements return to normal
  - You may need to use a suppository (e.g., Dulcolax or glycerin) or an enema if you have not had a bowel movement in 3 days
- **Follow-up**
  - Call your neurosurgeon when you get home from the hospital to schedule your follow-up appointment (this appointment is usually scheduled for 2–3 weeks after surgery)
  - If directed to do so, follow up with an endocrinologist after discharge from the hospital (this appointment is usually scheduled for 2–6 weeks after surgery)
  - Follow up with your primary care physician for all medical issues
- **Call your doctor or return to the emergency department if you experience any of the following**
  - A salty taste in your mouth or liquid running down the back of your throat
  - Double vision, blurred vision, or impaired peripheral vision
  - An intense feeling of thirst accompanied by frequent urination
  - Headache that is not relieved by your pain medication, or a headache that worsens when you stand up
  - Clear or bloody drainage from your ears or nose
  - Neck stiffness or discomfort moving your neck
  - **A fever of more than 100 °F**
  - Redness, swelling, or odor at your incision site

Appendix B6. Sample Discharge Instructions After Craniotomy for Acoustic Neuroma

You recently underwent a surgical procedure called a *craniotomy for removal of an acoustic neuroma*. An acoustic neuroma, also called a *vestibular schwannoma*, is usually a benign tumor on the cells that cover the nerve that runs from your brain to your inner ear. During this procedure, your surgeons made an incision on your head and opened your skull to remove as much of your tumor as could be removed safely. After this surgery, some people experience mild hearing loss, facial weakness, nausea, or dizziness. The instructions below provide important information regarding your care at home.

- Incision care
  - You may shower with mild soap and shampoo daily. Gently wash your incision and pat dry. **This is the only time you may touch your incision**
  - Do not apply ointments, lotions, or creams to your incision
  - Apply an ice pack or a clean bag of frozen peas to your incision to help reduce the swelling and discomfort every 30 minutes or as needed
  - Wear a hat outdoors to protect your incision until your doctor has removed the staples or sutures (usually 7–14 days after surgery)
  - Do not put anything in your ears and do not submerge your head in water
- Activity
  - When getting out of bed, slowly sit up and then stand up. Keeping your eyes open when you stand up will help reduce motion sickness
  - Start with light activity around the house for the first 3 days you are home
  - Gradually increase your activity, beginning with a short walk 1 or 2 times every day for 6 weeks
  - Avoid contact sports, skating, riding a bicycle, or other physically demanding activities
  - You may **not** drive until your neurosurgeon clears you to do so
  - Avoid straining to have a bowel movement
- Nutrition
  - Eat plenty of fruits and vegetables to prevent constipation
- Medication
  - Take your pain medications with food, and use these medications sparingly to avoid nausea, vomiting, and constipation
  - Take your pain medications as prescribed and gradually taper them as your pain decreases
  - Stool softeners such as Colace or laxatives such as Dulcolax are available at pharmacies; these medications may be helpful until your bowel movements return to normal

- You may need to use a suppository (e.g., Dulcolax or glycerin) or an enema if you have not had a bowel movement in 3 days
- **Follow-up**
  - Call your neurosurgeon when you get home from the hospital to schedule your follow-up appointment
  - Follow up with your primary care physician for all medical issues
- **Call your doctor or return to the emergency department if you experience any of the following**
  - Clear or bloody drainage from your nose or ears
  - Worsening headache
  - Seizure activity or jerking or twitching of the face, arms, or legs
  - Dizziness or ringing in your ears
  - Difficulty or discomfort moving your neck
  - Difficulty moving or weakness in your face, arms, or legs
  - Worsening dizziness or nausea
  - **A fever of more than 100 °F**
  - Redness, swelling, odor, or drainage at your incision site

Appendix B7. Sample Discharge Instructions After Craniotomy for Resection of a Brain Tumor

You recently underwent a surgical procedure called a *craniotomy for removal of a brain tumor*. During this procedure, your skull was opened so your surgeon could remove all or part of your tumor. The instructions below provide important information regarding your care at home.

- **Incision care**
  - You may shower with mild soap and shampoo daily. Gently wash your incision and pat dry. **This is the only time you may touch your incision**
  - Do not apply ointments, lotions, or creams to your incision
  - Apply an ice pack or a clean bag of frozen peas to your incision to help reduce the swelling and discomfort every 30 minutes or as needed
  - You may have some itching at your incision site, some jaw tightness, or trouble opening your mouth wide for a few days after surgery. These side effects will resolve as your incision begins to heal
  - Wear a hat outdoors to protect your incision until your doctor has removed the staples or sutures (usually 7–14 days after surgery)
  - Do not put anything in your ears and do not submerge your head in water

- **Activity**
  - Start with light activity around the house for the first 3 days you are home
  - Gradually increase your activity, beginning with a short walk 1 or 2 times every day
  - Avoid contact sports, skating, riding a bicycle, or other physically demanding activities for 6 weeks
  - You may **not** drive until your neurosurgeon clears you to do so
  - Avoid straining to have a bowel movement
- **Nutrition**
  - Eat plenty of fruits and vegetables to prevent constipation
- **Medication**
  - Take your pain medications with food, and use these medications sparingly to avoid nausea, vomiting, and constipation
  - Take your pain medications as prescribed and gradually taper them as your pain decreases
  - Stool softeners such as Colace or laxatives such as Dulcolax are available at pharmacies; these medications may be helpful until your bowel movements return to normal
  - You may need to use a suppository (e.g., Dulcolax or glycerin) or an enema if you have not had a bowel movement in 3 days
- **Follow-up**
  - Call your neurosurgeon when you get home from the hospital to schedule your follow-up appointment
  - Follow up with your primary care physician for all medical issues
  - Call your neuro-oncologist and radiation oncologist to schedule your follow-up appointment when you are discharged from the hospital (if instructed to do so)
- **Call your doctor or return to the emergency department if you experience any of the following**
  - Clear or bloody drainage from your nose or ears
  - Worsening headache
  - Seizure activity or jerking or twitching of the face, arms, or legs
  - Dizziness or ringing in your ears
  - Difficulty or discomfort moving your neck
  - Difficulty moving or weakness in your face, arms, or legs
  - **A fever of more than 100 °F**
  - Redness, swelling, odor, or drainage at your incision site

Appendix B8. Sample Discharge Instructions After Craniotomy for Aneurysm Clipping

You recently underwent a surgical procedure called a *craniotomy for aneurysm clipping*. During this procedure, your skull was opened so your surgeon could apply a small, titanium clip to your brain aneurysm. When clipped, blood will stop flowing to the aneurysm, which decreases the chance of the aneurysm bursting or bleeding. The instructions below provide important information regarding your care at home.

- Incision care
  - You may shower with mild soap and shampoo daily. Gently wash your incision and pat dry. **This is the only time you may touch your incision**
  - Do not apply ointments, lotions, or creams to your incision
  - Apply an ice pack or a clean bag of frozen peas to your incision to help reduce the swelling and discomfort every 30 minutes or as needed
  - You may have some itching at your incision site, some jaw tightness, or trouble opening your mouth wide for a few days after surgery. These side effects will resolve as your incision begins to heal
  - Wear a hat outdoors to protect your incision until your doctor has removed the staples or sutures (usually 7–14 days after surgery)
  - Do not put anything in your ears and do not submerge your head in water
- Activity
  - Start with light activity around the house for the first 3 days you are home
  - Gradually increase your activity, beginning with a short walk 1 or 2 times every day
  - Avoid contact sports, skating, riding a bicycle, or other physically demanding activities for 6 weeks
  - You may **not** drive until your neurosurgeon clears you to do so
  - Avoid straining to have a bowel movement
- Nutrition
  - Eat plenty of fruits and vegetables to prevent constipation
- Medication
  - Take your pain medications with food, and use these medications sparingly to avoid nausea, vomiting, and constipation
  - Take your pain medications as prescribed and gradually taper them as your pain decreases
  - Stool softeners such as Colace or laxatives such as Dulcolax are available at pharmacies; these medications may be helpful until your bowel movements return to normal
  - You may need to use a suppository (e.g., Dulcolax or glycerin) or an enema if you have not had a bowel movement in 3 days

- **Follow-up**
  - Call your neurosurgeon when you get home from the hospital to schedule your follow-up appointment
  - Follow up with your primary care physician for all medical issues
- **Call your doctor or return to the emergency department if you experience any of the following**
  - Clear or bloody drainage from your nose or ears
  - Sudden severe headache not relieved by pain medications
  - Seizure activity or jerking or twitching of the face, arms, or legs
  - Dizziness or ringing in your ears
  - Difficulty or discomfort moving your neck
  - Difficulty moving or weakness in your face, arms, or legs
  - **A fever of more than 100 °F**
  - Redness, swelling, odor, or drainage at your incision site

Appendix B9. Sample Discharge Instructions After Carotid Endarterectomy

You recently underwent a surgical procedure called a *carotid endarterectomy*. This surgery is commonly performed to prevent stroke. During this procedure, your neurosurgeon made an incision in your neck and opened the carotid artery to remove the plaque (the plaque results from a buildup of fat and cholesterol). The instructions below provide important information regarding your care at home.

- **Incision care**
  - You may shower with mild soap and shampoo daily. Gently wash your incision and pat dry. **This is the only time you may touch your incision**
  - Do not apply ointments, lotions, or creams to your incision
  - Apply an ice pack or a clean bag of frozen peas to your incision to help reduce the swelling and discomfort every 30 minutes or as needed
  - Stop smoking tobacco; smoking delays healing and may result in infection at the incision site
- **Activity**
  - Start with light activity around the house for the first 3 days you are home
  - Gradually increase your activity, beginning with a short walk 1 or 2 times every day
  - Allow your body time to heal by resting for short periods during the day
  - Avoid contact sports, skating, riding a bicycle, or other physically demanding activities for 6 weeks
  - You may **not** drive until your neurosurgeon clears you to do so

- ○ Avoid lifting, pushing, or pulling heavy objects (more than 10 lb) for 6–12 weeks
- ○ Avoid bending over to pick things up
- **Nutrition**
  - ○ Eat plenty of fruits and vegetables to prevent constipation
  - ○ Warm liquids and soft foods are usually easiest to swallow after this surgery
  - ○ A soft diet usually includes shakes, soup, pasta, soft vegetables, tender meat, and breads
- **Medication**
  - ○ Take your pain medications with food, and use these medications sparingly to avoid nausea, vomiting, and constipation
  - ○ Take your pain medications as prescribed and gradually taper them as your pain decreases
  - ○ Stool softeners such as Colace or laxatives such as Dulcolax are available at pharmacies; these medications may be helpful until your bowel movements return to normal
  - ○ You may need to use a suppository (e.g., Dulcolax or glycerin) or an enema if you have not had a bowel movement in 3 days
- **Follow-up**
  - ○ Call your neurosurgeon when you get home from the hospital to schedule your follow-up appointment
  - ○ Follow up with your primary care physician for all medical issues
- **Call your doctor or return to the emergency department if you experience any of the following**
  - ○ Difficulty breathing or swallowing
  - ○ Constipation (i.e., no bowel movement for more than 3 days)
  - ○ Nausea or vomiting that won't stop
  - ○ Your pain is not well controlled by your pain medications
  - ○ **A fever of more than 100 °F**
  - ○ Redness, swelling, odor, or drainage at your incision site
  - ○ Headache
  - ○ Slurred speech
  - ○ Weakness on one side of your body or face
  - ○ Confusion

Appendix B10. Sample Discharge Instructions After Concussion (or Other Closed Head Injury)

You hit your head and sustained an injury to your brain called a *concussion*. Concussions, which result in *temporary* loss of normal brain function, are commonly caused by motor vehicle or bicycle accidents, or by falls around the home. The instructions below provide important information regarding your care at home.

- Activity
  - Someone should stay with you for the next several days to watch for worsening of symptoms (see bottom section of discharge instructions) and to allow you to rest
  - Limit yourself to light activity around the house for the first 72 hours after injury
  - Allow your body time to heal by resting for short periods during the day
  - Gradually increase your activity, beginning with a short walk 1 or 2 times every day
  - Avoid contact sports, skating, riding a bicycle, or other physically demanding activities for 6 weeks
  - You may drive and return to work when your doctor says it is safe to do so
- Nutrition
  - Avoid alcoholic beverages for 6 weeks after injury
  - Eat plenty of fruits and vegetables to prevent constipation
- Medication
  - Take your pain medications as prescribed and gradually taper them as your pain decreases
  - Take your pain medications with food, and use these medications sparingly to avoid nausea, vomiting, and constipation
- Follow-up
  - Call your doctor when you get home from the hospital to schedule your follow-up appointment
  - Follow up with your primary care physician for all medical issues
- **Call your doctor or return to the emergency department if you experience any of the following**
  - Your pain is not well controlled by your pain medications
  - Clear or bloody drainage from your nose or ears
  - Worsening headache
  - Changes in vision or difference in pupil size
  - Sleepiness or difficulty waking up
  - Memory loss
  - Irritability
  - Nausea or vomiting that won't stop

- Confusion or difficulty talking
- Seizures
- **A fever of more than 100 °F**
- Weakness in the face, arms, or legs
- Difficulty walking, loss of balance, or dizziness
- Stiff neck

Appendix B11. Sample Discharge Instructions After Subdural Hematoma

You have recently been diagnosed with a subdural hematoma, which is an accumulation of blood between the protective membranes that cover the surface of your brain. A subdural hematoma may be the result of a bump on the head or a fall, or it may occur due to use of blood-thinning medications. The instructions below provide important information regarding your care at home.

- **Activity**
  - Someone should stay with you for the next several days to watch for worsening of symptoms (see bottom section of discharge instructions) and to allow you to rest
  - Limit yourself to light activity around the house for the first 72 hours after injury
  - Allow your body time to heal by resting for short periods during the day
  - Gradually increase your activity, beginning with a short walk 1 or 2 times every day
  - Avoid contact sports, skating, riding a bicycle, or other physically demanding activities for 6 weeks
  - You may drive and return to work when your doctor says it is safe to do so
- **Nutrition**
  - Avoid alcoholic beverages and nonsteroidal anti-inflammatory drugs (NSAIDs) (e.g., Motrin, Advil) and aspirin for 12 weeks
  - Eat plenty of fruits and vegetables to prevent constipation
- **Medication**
  - Take your pain medications as prescribed and gradually taper them as your pain decreases
  - Take your pain medications with food, and use these medications sparingly to avoid nausea, vomiting, and constipation
- **Follow-up**
  - Call your doctor when you get home from the hospital to schedule your follow-up appointment
  - Follow up with your primary care physician for all medical issues

- **Call your doctor or return to the emergency department if you experience any of the following**
  - Severe or worsening headache
  - Changes in vision or difference in pupil size
  - Sleepiness or difficulty waking up
  - Memory loss
  - Irritability
  - Nausea or vomiting that won't stop
  - Confusion or difficulty talking
  - Seizures
  - **A fever of more than 100 °F**
  - Weakness in your face, arm, or leg
  - Difficulty walking, loss of balance, or dizziness
  - Neck stiffness

Appendix B12. Sample Discharge Instructions After Anterior Cervical Discectomy with Fusion and Plating

You recently underwent a surgical procedure called an *anterior cervical diskectomy with fusion and plating*. During this procedure, your neurosurgeon made an incision in the front of your neck and removed your damaged disks, replaced them with bone material, and applied a plate and screws to hold the bone material in place. As your neck heals over the next 6–12 weeks, the bones at the level of surgery will fuse together. The instructions below provide important information regarding your care at home

- **Incision Care**
  - You may shower with mild soap and shampoo daily. Gently wash your incision and pat dry. **This is the only time you may touch your incision**
  - Do not apply ointments, lotions, or creams to your incision
  - Apply an ice pack or a clean bag of frozen peas to your incision to help reduce the swelling and discomfort every 30 minutes or as needed
  - Occasional episodes of neck pain and arm pain are not unusual immediately after surgery
  - Discomfort between your shoulder blades is a common part of healing
  - Wear a neck collar if your neurosurgeon has instructed you to do so
- **Activity**
  - Start with light activity around the house for the first 3 days you are home
  - Gradually increase your activity, beginning with a short walk 1 or 2 times every day
  - Allow your body time to heal by resting for short periods during the day

- Avoid contact sports, skating, riding a bicycle, or other physically demanding activities for 6 weeks
- You may **not** drive until your neurosurgeon clears you to do so
- Avoid lifting, pushing, or pulling heavy objects (more than 10 lb) for 6–12 weeks
- Avoid bending over to pick things up, turning your head from side to side, and nodding
- Avoid sitting in soft chairs or slumping while seated
- Stretch while seated or get up and move around every 30 minutes

- **Nutrition**
  - Eat plenty of fruits and vegetables to prevent constipation
  - Warm liquids and soft foods are usually easiest to swallow after this surgery
  - A soft diet usually includes shakes, soup, pasta, soft vegetables, tender meat, and breads
  - A sore throat and soft voice is common for about 2–3 weeks after surgery. You should still be able to swallow food and beverages without choking or coughing

- **Medication**
  - Take your pain medications with food, and use these medications sparingly to avoid nausea, vomiting, and constipation
  - Take your pain medications as prescribed and gradually taper them as your pain decreases
  - Stool softeners such as Colace or laxatives such as Dulcolax are available at pharmacies; these medications may be helpful until your bowel movements return to normal
  - You may need to use a suppository (e.g., Dulcolax or glycerin) or an enema if you have not had a bowel movement in 3 days

- **Follow-up**
  - Call your neurosurgeon when you get home from the hospital to schedule your follow-up appointment
  - Follow up with your primary care physician for all medical issues

- **Call your doctor or return to the emergency department if you experience any of the following**
  - Difficulty breathing or swallowing
  - Constipation (i.e., no bowel movement for more than 3 days)
  - Difficulty moving or weakness in your face, arms, or legs
  - Nausea or vomiting that won't stop
  - Your pain is not well controlled by your pain medications
  - **A fever of more than 100 °F**
  - Redness, swelling, odor, or drainage at your incision site

You recently underwent a surgical procedure called a *laminectomy*. During this procedure, your neurosurgeon made an incision in your back or neck to remove a piece (i.e., the lamina) of one or more of your vertebrae. Surgeons may perform a laminectomy to remove tumors, herniated disks, or other spinal abnormalities. The instructions below provide important information regarding your care at home.

- Incision care
  - You may shower with mild soap and shampoo daily. Gently wash your incision and pat dry. **This is the only time you may touch your incision**
  - Do not apply ointments, lotions, or creams to your incision
  - Apply an ice pack or a clean bag of frozen peas to your incision to help reduce the swelling and discomfort every 30 min or as needed
  - Do **not** swim, use a hot tub, or take a bath until your incision is completely healed (this usually takes about 4 weeks)
  - Stop smoking tobacco; smoking delays healing and may result in infection at the incision site
- Activity
  - Start with light activity around the house for the first 3 days you are home
  - Gradually increase your activity, beginning with a short walk 1 or 2 times every day
  - Allow your body time to heal by resting for short periods during the day
  - Avoid contact sports, skating, riding a bicycle, or other physically demanding activities for 6 weeks
  - You may **not** drive while you are taking pain medications. Do not drive until your neurosurgeon clears you to do so
  - Avoid lifting, pushing, or pulling heavy objects (more than 10 lb) for 6–12 weeks
  - Avoid bending over or twisting to pick things up
  - Avoid sitting in soft chairs or slumping while seated
  - Stretch while seated or get up and move around every 30 min
- Nutrition
  - Eat plenty of fruits and vegetables to prevent constipation
- Medication
  - Take your pain medications as prescribed and gradually taper them as your pain decreases
  - Stool softeners such as Colace or laxatives such as Dulcolax are available at pharmacies; these medications may be helpful until your bowel movements return to normal
  - You may need to use a suppository (e.g., Dulcolax or glycerin) or an enema if you have not had a bowel movement in 3 days

- **Follow-up**
  - Call your neurosurgeon when you get home from the hospital to schedule your follow-up appointment
  - Follow up with your primary care physician for all medical issues
- **Call your doctor or return to the emergency department if you experience any of the following**
  - Constipation (i.e., no bowel movement for more than 3 days)
  - Difficulty moving or weakness in your legs
  - You are experiencing back pain that is not well controlled by your pain medications
  - **A fever of more than 100 °F**
  - Redness, swelling, odor, or drainage at your incision site
  - Loss of bowel or bladder control
  - Headaches while you are in an upright position that resolve when you lie down
  - Difficulty feeling your legs
  - Difficulty walking

Appendix B14. Sample Discharge Instructions After Lumbar Diskectomy

You recently underwent a surgical procedure called a *lumbar diskectomy*. During this procedure, your neurosurgeon made an incision in your lower back to remove a piece (i.e., the lamina) of one or more of your vertebrae. Your neurosurgeon then removed the portion of the disk that compressed your spinal nerve(s), which likely caused pain or leg weakness. The rest of the disk was left in place. The instructions below provide important information regarding your care at home

- **Incision care**
  - You may shower with mild soap and shampoo daily. Gently wash your incision and pat dry. **This is the only time you may touch your incision**
  - Do not apply ointments, lotions, or creams to your incision
  - Apply an ice pack or a clean bag of frozen peas to your incision to help reduce the swelling and discomfort every 30 minutes or as needed
  - Do **not** swim, use a hot tub, or take a bath until your incision is completely healed (this usually takes about 4 weeks)
  - Stop smoking tobacco; smoking delays healing and may result in infection at the incision site
- **Activity**
  - Start with light activity around the house for the first 3 days you are home

- Gradually increase your activity, beginning with a short walk 1 or 2 times every day
- Allow your body time to heal by resting for short periods during the day
- Avoid contact sports, skating, riding a bicycle, or other physically demanding activities for 6 weeks
- You may **not** drive while you are taking pain medications. Do not drive until your neurosurgeon clears you to do so
- Avoid lifting, pushing, or pulling heavy objects (more than 10 lb) for 12 weeks
- Avoid bending over or twisting to pick things up
- Avoid sitting in soft chairs or slumping while seated
- Stretch while seated or get up and move around every 30 minutes
- **Nutrition**
  - Eat plenty of fruits and vegetables to prevent constipation
- **Medication**
  - Take your pain medications as prescribed and gradually taper them as your pain decreases
  - Stool softeners such as Colace or laxatives such as Dulcolax are available at pharmacies; these medications may be helpful until your bowel movements return to normal
  - You may need to use a suppository (e.g., Dulcolax or glycerin) or an enema if you have not had a bowel movement in 3 days
- **Follow-up**
  - Call your neurosurgeon when you get home from the hospital to schedule your follow-up appointment
  - Follow up with your primary care physician for all medical issues
- **Call your doctor or return to the emergency department if you experience any of the following**
  - Constipation (i.e., no bowel movement for more than 3 days)
  - Difficulty moving or weakness in your legs
  - You are experiencing back pain that is not well controlled by your pain medications
  - **A fever of more than 100 °F**
  - Redness, swelling, odor, or drainage at your incision site
  - Loss of bowel or bladder control
  - Headaches while you are in an upright position that resolve when you lie down
  - Difficulty feeling your legs
  - Difficulty walking
  - Worsened or new leg pain

Appendix B15. Sample Discharge Instructions After Anterior Lumbar Spinal Fusion

You recently underwent a surgical procedure called an *anterior lumbar spinal fusion*. During this procedure, your neurosurgeon made an incision in your abdomen to expose your spinal bones and nerves. Disks were removed from your lower spine, and hardware (such as rods, screws, and spacers) and bone material were used to properly align and stabilize your spine. Your spinal bones will fuse together to form a solid bone mass in about 12 weeks. The instructions below provide important information regarding your care at home.

- Incision care
  - You may shower with mild soap and shampoo daily. Gently wash your incision and pat dry. **This is the only time you may touch your incision**
  - Do not apply ointments, lotions, or creams to your incision
  - Apply an ice pack or a clean bag of frozen peas to your incision to help reduce the swelling and discomfort every 30 minutes or as needed
  - Do **not** swim, use a hot tub, or take a bath until your incision is completely healed (this usually takes about 4 weeks)
  - Stop smoking tobacco; smoking delays healing and may result in infection at the incision site
- Activity
  - Wear your lumbar brace or corset when you are out of bed for up to 12 weeks, as directed by your neurosurgeon
  - Hold a pillow against your incision to support or splint your sore muscles when you cough or when you reposition yourself in bed
  - Start with light activity around the house for the first 3 days you are home
  - Gradually increase your activity, beginning with a short walk 1 or 2 times every day
  - Allow your body time to heal by resting for short periods during the day
  - Avoid contact sports, skating, riding a bicycle, or other physically demanding activities for 12 weeks
  - You may **not** drive while you are taking pain medications. Do not drive until your neurosurgeon clears you to do so
  - Avoid lifting, pushing, or pulling heavy objects (more than 10 lb) for 12 weeks
  - Avoid bending over or twisting to pick things up
  - Avoid sitting in soft chairs or slumping while seated
  - Stretch while seated or get up and move around every 30 minutes
- Nutrition
  - Eat plenty of fruits and vegetables to prevent constipation
- Medication
  - Take your pain medications as prescribed and gradually taper them as your pain decreases

- Stool softeners such as Colace or laxatives such as Dulcolax are available at pharmacies; these medications may be helpful until your bowel movements return to normal
- You may need to use a suppository (e.g., Dulcolax or glycerin) or an enema if you have not had a bowel movement in 3 days

- **Follow-up**
  - Call your neurosurgeon when you get home from the hospital to schedule your follow-up appointment
  - Follow up with your primary care physician for all medical issues
- **Call your doctor or return to the emergency department if you experience any of the following**
  - Constipation (i.e., no bowel movement for more than 3 days)
  - Difficulty moving or weakness in your legs
  - You are experiencing back pain that is not well controlled by your pain medications
  - **A fever of more than 100 °F**
  - Redness, swelling, odor, or drainage at your incision site
  - Loss of bowel or bladder control
  - Headaches while you are in an upright position that resolve when you lie down
  - Difficulty feeling your legs
  - Difficulty walking

Appendix B16. Sample Discharge Instructions After Baclofen Pump Placement

You recently underwent a surgical procedure to place a *baclofen pump*. During this procedure, your neurosurgeon made incisions in your abdomen and lower back and inserted a catheter through a needle, which was guided into the spinal canal. The other end of the catheter was tunneled under the skin to the abdomen, and the pump was placed there under your skin. The incisions were then closed, and the pump reservoir was filled with a dose of baclofen. The instructions below provide important information regarding your care at home.

- **Incision care**
  - You may shower with mild soap and shampoo daily. Gently wash your incisions and pat dry. **This is the only time you may touch your incisions**
  - Do not apply ointments, lotions, or creams to your incisions
  - Apply an ice pack or a clean bag of frozen peas to your incisions to help reduce the swelling and discomfort every 30 minutes or as needed
  - Do **not** swim, use a hot tub, or take a bath until your incisions are completely healed (this usually takes about 4 weeks)

○ Stop smoking tobacco; smoking delays healing and may result in infection at the incision sites

- **Activity**
  - ○ Start with light activity around the house for the first 3 days you are home
  - ○ Gradually increase your activity, beginning with a short walk 1 or 2 times every day
  - ○ Avoid contact sports, skating, riding a bicycle, or other physically demanding activities for 6 weeks
  - ○ You may **not** drive until your neurosurgeon clears you to do so
  - ○ Avoid straining to have a bowel movement. Stool softeners such as Colace or laxatives such as Dulcolax are available at pharmacies; these medications may be helpful until your bowel movements return to normal
- **Nutrition**
  - ○ Eat plenty of fruits and vegetables to prevent constipation
- **Medication**
  - ○ Take your pain medications with food, and use these medications sparingly to avoid nausea, vomiting, and constipation
  - ○ Take your pain medications as prescribed and gradually taper them as your pain decreases
  - ○ Your doctor can adjust your baclofen pump using an external programmer
  - ○ Side effects of baclofen may include dizziness, drowsiness, headache, nausea, and weakness
- **Follow-up**
  - ○ Call your neurosurgeon when you get home from the hospital to schedule your follow-up appointment
  - ○ Your doctor will refill or adjust your baclofen pump as needed (typically every 2–3 months)
  - ○ Follow up with your primary care physician for all medical issues
- **Call your doctor or return to the emergency department if you experience any of the following**
  - ○ Signs of baclofen overdose, such as muscle weakness, drowsiness, vomiting, dilated or pinpoint pupils, weak or shallow breathing, fainting, or coma
  - ○ Signs of baclofen withdrawal, such as anxiety, fever, altered mental status, increased spasticity, muscle stiffness, or muscle rigidity
  - ○ Pain at your pump site
  - ○ Difficulty or discomfort moving your neck or back
  - ○ Difficulty moving or weakness in your face, arms, or legs
  - ○ **A fever of more than 100 °F**
  - ○ Redness, swelling, odor, or drainage at your incision site

Appendix B17. Sample Discharge Instructions After Spinal Fracture

You have recently been diagnosed with one or more spinal fractures. Spinal fractures can result from falls, vehicle or bicycle accidents, osteoporosis, or other causes. The instructions below provide important information regarding your care at home.

- **Activity**
  - Start with light activity around the house for the first 2 days you are home
  - Gradually increase your activity, beginning with a short walk 1 or 2 times every day
  - Allow your body time to heal by resting for short periods during the day
  - Avoid contact sports, skating, riding a bicycle, or other physically demanding activities for 12 weeks
  - You may **not** drive until your neurosurgeon clears you to do so
  - Avoid lifting, pushing, or pulling heavy objects (more than 10 lb) for 6–12 weeks
  - Avoid bending over or twisting to pick things up
  - Avoid sitting in soft chairs or slumping while seated
  - Stretch while seated or get up and move around every 30 minutes
  - Wear your brace or corset when you are out of bed for up to 12 weeks, as directed by your neurosurgeon
- **Nutrition**
  - Eat plenty of fruits and vegetables to prevent constipation
- **Medication**
  - Take your pain medications as prescribed and gradually taper them as your pain decreases
  - Stool softeners such as Colace or laxatives such as Dulcolax are available at pharmacies; these medications may be helpful until your bowel movements return to normal
  - You may need to use a suppository (e.g., Dulcolax or glycerin) or an enema if you have not had a bowel movement in 3 days
- **Follow-up**
  - Call your neurosurgeon when you get home from the hospital to schedule your follow-up appointment
  - Follow up with your primary care physician for all medical issues
- **Call your doctor or return to the emergency department if you experience any of the following**
  - Constipation (i.e., no bowel movement for more than 3 days)
  - Difficulty moving or weakness in your legs
  - You are experiencing back pain that is not well controlled by your pain medications

- A fever of more than 100 °F
- Loss of bowel or bladder control
- Difficulty feeling your legs
- Difficulty walking
- Increased back or leg pain

Appendix B18. Sample Discharge Instructions After Repair of Chiari Malformation

You recently underwent a surgical procedure called *repair of a Chiari malformation*. During this procedure your neurosurgeon made an incision in the back of your head or neck and removed a small piece of bone from the first level of your neck and the base of your skull. This was done to decompress and surgically remove or repair the malformation. The instructions below provide important information regarding your care at home.

- **Incision care**
  - You may shower with mild soap and shampoo daily. Gently wash your incision and pat dry. **This is the only time you may touch your incision**
  - Do not apply ointments, lotions, or creams to your incision
  - Apply an ice pack or a clean bag of frozen peas to your incision to help reduce the swelling and discomfort every 30 minutes or as needed
  - Do **not** swim, use a hot tub, or take a bath until your incision is completely healed (this usually takes about 4 weeks)
  - Stop smoking tobacco; smoking delays healing and may result in infection at the incision site
- **Activity**
  - Start with light activity around the house for the first 3 days you are home
  - Gradually increase your activity, beginning with a short walk 1 or 2 times every day
  - Allow your body time to heal by resting for short periods during the day
  - Avoid contact sports, skating, riding a bicycle, or other physically demanding activities for 6 weeks
  - You may **not** drive while you are taking pain medications. Do not drive until your neurosurgeon clears you to do so
  - Avoid lifting, pushing, or pulling heavy objects (more than 10 lb) for 6–12 weeks
  - Gentle shoulder shrugs may help relieve some of the tension you feel in your neck or shoulders
  - You may wear a soft neck collar for comfort as needed
- **Nutrition**
  - Eat plenty of fruits and vegetables to prevent constipation

- Medication
  - Take your pain medications as prescribed and gradually taper them as your pain decreases
  - Stool softeners such as Colace or laxatives such as Dulcolax are available at pharmacies; these medications may be helpful until your bowel movements return to normal
  - You may need to use a suppository (e.g., Dulcolax or glycerin) or an enema if you have not had a bowel movement in 3 days
- Follow-up
  - Call your neurosurgeon when you get home from the hospital to schedule your follow-up appointment
  - Follow up with your primary care physician for all medical issues
- **Call your doctor or return to the emergency department if you experience any of the following**
  - Constipation (i.e., no bowel movement for more than 3 days)
  - Difficulty moving or weakness in your face, arms, or legs
  - Your pain is not well controlled by your pain medications
  - **A fever of more than 100 °F**
  - Redness, swelling, odor, or drainage at your incision site
  - Loss of bowel or bladder control
  - Headaches while you are in an upright position that resolve when you lie down
  - Difficulty feeling your arms or legs
  - Difficulty walking

Appendix B19. Sample Discharge Instructions After Cerebral Angiogram for Cerebral Aneurysm Embolization or Coiling

You recently underwent a surgical procedure called a *cerebral angiogram* for aneurysm embolization or coiling. During this procedure, a sheath (plastic tube) was inserted into your femoral artery (near your upper leg/groin). Various wires and medical devices were inserted through this sheath and passed through your body to embolize (i.e., close off) or coil your cerebral aneurysm. The instructions below provide important information regarding your care at home.

- Incision care
  - Apply pressure to puncture site for small amounts of bleeding or oozing. If bleeding is persistent or uncontrolled even when you apply pressure, call 911—This is a medical emergency

- You may shower with mild soap. Gently wash your leg puncture site and pat dry. This is the only time you may touch your puncture site
- Keep your puncture site clean and dry (except when showering) and change the dressing within 24 hours or if it becomes wet or saturated. Never leave a wet dressing in place
- Do **not** submerge your puncture site in water (e.g., by swimming, bathing, or using a hot tub) for 1 week or until your wound is completely healed
- Do not apply ointments, lotions, creams, or powders to your puncture site
- Mild bruising and soreness at the puncture site is normal and should resolve within 1 or 2 weeks

- **Activity**
  - Avoid strenuous activity for 2 weeks (e.g., weight training, work-related lifting, sexual activity, or lifting anything weighing more than 10 lb)
  - Allow your body time to heal by resting for short periods during the day
  - You may **not** drive until your neurosurgeon clears you to do so
  - Avoid contact sports, skating, riding a bicycle, or other physically demanding activities for 6 weeks
  - Avoid straining to have a bowel movement. Stool softeners such as Colace or laxatives such as Dulcolax are available at pharmacies; these medications may be helpful until your bowel movements return to normal

- **Nutrition**
  - Eat plenty of fruits and vegetables to prevent constipation

- **Medication**
  - Continue all normal medications, unless directed otherwise by your primary care physician

- **Follow-up**
  - Call your neurosurgeon when you get home from the hospital to schedule your follow-up appointment
  - Follow up with your primary care physician for all medical issues

- **Call 911 or return to the emergency department if you experience any of the following**
  - Pain, numbness, cold feeling, or bluish color to your leg below the puncture site
  - Redness, swelling, odor, drainage, or bleeding at your puncture site
  - Headache or neck stiffness
  - Confusion or deteriorating mental capabilities
  - Chills
  - A fever of more than 100 °F
  - Weakness in the face, arm, or leg
  - Difficulty with balance or walking
  - Any change in vision or speech

Appendix B20. Sample Discharge Instructions After Kyphoplasty

You recently underwent a surgical procedure called a *kyphoplasty* to treat your spinal compression fracture(s). During this procedure, your neurosurgeon used X-rays of your spine to locate your fractured vertebrae and made 2 small incisions in your back. A tube was inserted into the center of the fractured vertebral body, and a balloon was used to push the bone back to its normal height and shape. The cavity created by the balloon was completely filled with bone cement. By elevating the fractured vertebrae, the spinal nerves that were compressed were freed from pressure. This should significantly decrease the pain caused by your fracture and increase the stability of your spine. The instructions below provide important information regarding your care at home.

- Incision care
  - You may shower with mild soap and shampoo daily. Gently wash your incision and pat dry. **This is the only time you may touch your incisions**
  - Do not apply ointments, lotions, or creams to your incisions
  - Apply an ice pack or a clean bag of frozen peas to your incisions to help reduce the swelling and discomfort every 30 minutes or as needed
  - Do **not** swim, use a hot tub, or take a bath until your incisions are completely healed (this usually takes about 2 weeks)
  - Stop smoking tobacco; smoking delays healing and may result in infection at the incision sites
- Activity
  - Start with light activity around the house for the first 3 days you are home
  - Gradually increase your activity, beginning with a short walk 1 or 2 times every day
  - Allow your body time to heal by resting for short periods during the day
  - Avoid contact sports, skating, riding a bicycle, or other physically demanding activities for 6 weeks
  - You may **not** drive until your neurosurgeon clears you to do so
  - Avoid lifting, pushing, or pulling heavy objects (more than 10 lb) for 6–12 weeks
  - Avoid bending over or twisting to pick things up
  - Avoid sitting in soft chairs or slumping while seated
  - Stretch while seated or get up and move around every 30 minutes
  - Wear your brace as instructed by your doctor at all times when you are out of bed
- Nutrition
  - Eat plenty of fruits and vegetables to prevent constipation
- Medication

- Take your pain medications as prescribed and gradually taper them as your pain decreases
- Stool softeners such as Colace or laxatives such as Dulcolax are available at pharmacies; these medications may be helpful until your bowel movements return to normal
- You may need to use a suppository (e.g., Dulcolax or glycerin) or an enema if you have not had a bowel movement in 3 days
- **Follow-up**
  - Call your neurosurgeon when you get home from the hospital to schedule your follow-up appointment
  - Follow up with your primary care physician for all medical issues
- **Call your doctor or return to the emergency department if you experience any of the following**
  - Constipation (i.e., no bowel movement for more than 3 days)
  - Difficulty moving or weakness in your legs
  - Back pain that is not well controlled by your pain medications
  - **A fever of more than 100 °F**
  - Redness, swelling, odor, or drainage at your incision sites
  - Loss of bowel or bladder control
  - Difficulty feeling your legs
  - Difficulty walking
  - Increased pain in your back or legs

Appendix B21. Sample Discharge Instructions After Vertebroplasty

You recently underwent a surgical procedure called a *vertebroplasty*. During this procedure, your neurosurgeon used X-rays of your spine to locate your fractured vertebra. Bone cement was injected into the fractured vertebra to repair the fracture. This procedure should have relieved the pressure on your spinal nerves, thereby significantly decreasing your back pain and stabilizing your spine. The instructions below provide important information regarding your care at home.

- **Incision care**
  - You may shower with mild soap and shampoo daily. Gently wash your incision and pat dry. **This is the only time you may touch your incision**
  - Do not apply ointments, lotions, or creams to your incision
  - Apply an ice pack or a clean bag of frozen peas to your incision to help reduce the swelling and discomfort every 30 minutes or as needed
  - Do **not** swim, use a hot tub, or take a bath until your incision is completely healed (this usually takes about 2 weeks)

- Stop smoking tobacco; smoking delays healing and may result in infection at the incision site
- **Activity**
  - Start with light activity around the house for the first 3 days you are home
  - Gradually increase your activity, beginning with a short walk 1 or 2 times every day
  - Allow your body time to heal by resting for short periods during the day
  - Avoid contact sports, skating, riding a bicycle, or other physically demanding activities for 6 weeks
  - You may **not** drive until your neurosurgeon clears you to do so
  - Avoid lifting, pushing, or pulling heavy objects (more than 10 lb) for 6–12 weeks
  - Avoid bending over or twisting to pick things up
  - Avoid sitting in soft chairs or slumping while seated
  - Stretch while seated or get up and move around every 30 minutes
  - Wear your brace as instructed by your doctor at all times when you are out of bed
- **Nutrition**
  - Eat plenty of fruits and vegetables to prevent constipation
- **Medication**
  - Take your pain medications as prescribed and gradually taper them as your pain decreases
  - Stool softeners such as Colace or laxatives such as Dulcolax are available at pharmacies; these medications may be helpful until your bowel movements return to normal
- **Follow-up**
  - Call your neurosurgeon when you get home from the hospital to schedule your follow-up appointment
  - Follow up with your primary care physician for all medical issues
- **Call your doctor or return to the emergency department if you experience any of the following**
  - Constipation (i.e., no bowel movement for more than 3 days)
  - Difficulty moving or weakness in your legs
  - Back pain that is not well controlled by your pain medications
  - **A fever of more than 100 °F**
  - Redness, swelling, odor, or drainage at your incision sites
  - Loss of bowel or bladder control
  - Difficulty feeling your legs
  - Difficulty walking
  - Increased pain in your back or legs

Appendix B22. Sample Discharge Instructions After Placement of a Deep Brain Stimulator

You recently underwent a surgical procedure called a *craniotomy for placement of a deep brain stimulator* to treat Parkinson's disease or other neurologic symptoms. During this procedure, your skull was opened so that your neurosurgeon could place the deep brain stimulators. The pulse generator was then placed through an incision in your chest. The instructions below provide important information regarding your care at home.

- Incision care
  - You may shower with mild soap and shampoo daily. Gently wash your incision and pat dry. **This is the only time you may touch your incision**
  - Do not apply ointments, lotions, or creams to your incision
  - Apply an ice pack or a clean bag of frozen peas to your incision to help reduce the swelling and discomfort every 30 minutes or as needed
  - You may have some itching at your incision site, some jaw tightness, or trouble opening your mouth wide for a few days after surgery. These side effects will resolve as your incision begins to heal
  - Wear a hat outdoors to protect your incision until your doctor has removed the staples or sutures (usually 7–14 days after surgery)
  - Do not put anything in your ears and do not submerge your head in water
- Activity
  - Start with light activity around the house for the first 3 days you are home
  - Gradually increase your activity, beginning with a short walk 1 or 2 times every day
  - Avoid contact sports, skating, riding a bicycle, or other physically demanding activities for 6 weeks
  - You may **not** drive until your neurosurgeon clears you to do so
  - Avoid straining to have a bowel movement. Stool softeners such as Colace or laxatives such as Dulcolax are available at pharmacies; these medications may be helpful until your bowel movements return to normal
- Nutrition
  - Eat plenty of fruits and vegetables to prevent constipation
- Medication
  - Take your pain medications with food, and use these medications sparingly to avoid nausea, vomiting, and constipation
  - Take your pain medications as prescribed and gradually taper them as your pain decreases
- Follow-up
  - Call your neurosurgeon when you get home from the hospital to schedule your follow-up appointment

- Follow up with your primary care physician for all medical issues
- Follow up with your neurologist as directed
- **Call your doctor or return to the emergency department if you experience any of the following**
  - Clear or bloody drainage from your nose or ears
  - Worsening headache
  - Seizure activity or jerking or twitching of the face, arms, or legs
  - Dizziness or ringing in your ears
  - Difficulty or discomfort moving your neck
  - Difficulty moving or weakness in your face, arms, or legs
  - Signs of mania (e.g., hypersexuality, overshopping, or not sleeping)
  - Worsening of symptoms associated with Parkinson's disease
  - **A fever of more than 100 °F**
  - Redness, swelling, odor, or drainage at your incision site

Appendix B23. Sample Discharge Instructions After Craniotomy for Microvascular Decompression

You recently underwent a surgical procedure called *microvascular decompression*, which relieves compression of a cranial nerve. It may be performed to treat trigeminal neuralgia, vagoglossopharyngeal neuralgia, or hemifacial spasm. These conditions often result from an artery or vein compressing a nerve root. During this procedure, your surgeons made an incision on your head and opened your skull to decompress the nerve. The instructions below provide important information regarding your care at home.

- **Incision care**
  - You may shower with mild soap and shampoo daily. Gently wash your incision and pat dry. **This is the only time you may touch your incision**
  - Do not apply ointments, lotions, or creams to your incision
  - Apply an ice pack or a clean bag of frozen peas to your incision to help reduce the swelling and discomfort every 30 minutes or as needed
  - Wear a hat outdoors to protect your incision until your doctor has removed the staples or sutures (usually 7–14 days after surgery)
  - Do **not** put anything in your ears and do not submerge your head in water
- **Activity**
  - Start with light activity around the house for the first 3 days you are home
  - Gradually increase your activity, beginning with a short walk 1 or 2 times every day
  - Avoid contact sports, skating, riding a bicycle, or other physically demanding activities for 6 weeks
  - You may **not** drive until your neurosurgeon clears you to do so

- **Nutrition**
  - Eat plenty of fruits and vegetables to prevent constipation
- **Medication**
  - Take your pain medications with food, and use these medications sparingly to avoid nausea, vomiting, and constipation
  - Take your pain medications as prescribed and gradually taper them as your pain decreases
  - Stool softeners such as Colace or laxatives such as Dulcolax are available at pharmacies; these medications may be helpful until your bowel movements return to normal
  - You may need to use a suppository (e.g., Dulcolax or glycerin) or an enema if you have not had a bowel movement in 3 days
- **Follow-up**
  - Call your neurosurgeon when you get home from the hospital to schedule your follow-up appointment
  - Follow up with your primary care physician for all medical issues
- **Call your doctor or return to the emergency department if you experience any of the following**
  - Clear or bloody drainage from your nose or ears
  - Worsening headache
  - Seizure activity or jerking or twitching of the face, arms, or legs
  - Dizziness or ringing in your ears
  - Difficulty or discomfort moving your neck
  - Difficulty moving or weakness in your face, arms, or legs
  - Worsening dizziness or nausea
  - **A fever of more than 100 °F**
  - Redness, swelling, odor, or drainage at your incision site

Appendix C: Preoperative Nursing Checklist

- Informed consents
  - Surgical consent
  - Blood consent or refusal of blood or blood products
  - Anesthesia consent
- Preoperative teaching
  - Patient and family education about procedure, expected timeline, and outcomes
  - History and physical examination
  - Allergies, including reactions
- Laboratory tests as ordered. These may include the following
  - CBC
  - Coagulation profile
  - Urinalysis
  - Blood tests
    - Type and screen
    - Crossmatch
    - Number of units ordered and availability
    - Pregnancy test, if appropriate
  - Comprehensive metabolic profile or basic metabolic profile
  - Electrocardiogram
  - Chest radiograph
  - Old chart, if available
- Special preparatory measures, if ordered
  - Identification bracelet
  - Compliance with orders for nil per os (NPO), or nothing by mouth, and ordered duration
  - Removal of undergarments
  - Removal of bobby pins, combs, wig, hair piece, and false eyelashes
  - Removal of jewelry, watches, and/or religious medals. Document placement (e.g., with a specific family member or with hospital security staff)
  - Rings taped

- Removal of dentures (bridge, plates, partials), container labeled
- Removal of prostheses, with documentation of placement. Prostheses may include the following
  - Artificial eye (if removal is necessary for surgical access)
  - Contact lenses
  - Glasses
  - Hearing aids
  - Prosthetic limbs
  - Other
- Identification labels with chart
- Face sheet, or a one-page sheet that summarizes important patient information, attached to chart
- Measures to prevent deep vein thrombosis (DVT)
  - Sequential compression devices or antiembolism stockings, unless contraindicated
  - Documentation of the time of last void or catheter placement
  - Compliance with necessary isolation precautions
  - Medication reconciliation on chart
  - List of medications administered preoperatively, with documented drug/dose/time
- Time of last dose of β-blockers, if applicable
  - For patients on β-blocker therapy at home, the β-blocker must be administered 24 hours before surgery or within the perioperative period (within 6 hours of the end of surgery for patients going directly to intensive care unit (ICU) postoperatively)
    - Document whether a β-blocker was given within 24 h of surgery
    - Document whether a β-blocker was not administered before surgery
- Safety
  - Side rails up
  - Call light within reach
- Vital signs
  - Blood pressure
  - Temperature
  - Pulse
  - Respiration rate
  - Oxygen saturation
  - Special comments and considerations for operating room and recovery room nurses
- Communication of patient limitations
  - Sight
  - Motion
  - Hearing

- ○ Speech
- ○ Other
- Measure patient's height and weight
- Test bedside blood glucose level (for patients with diabetes mellitus or on steroids)
- Document last dose of insulin or oral hypoglycemic agent (include type and amount)
- The night before or day of surgery
  - ○ Preoperative shower and shampoo (preferably with chlorhexidine)

Index

Note: Page numbers set **bold** or *italic* indicate headings or figures, respectively.

C

Index